Cysts of the Oral Regions

Cysts of the Oral Regions

Third edition

Mervyn Shear DSc(Dent), MDS, FRCPath, HDipDent, FRSSAf, FOS(SA)
Deputy Vice-Chancellor and Honorary Professor of Oral Pathology, University of the Witwatersrand; Past Professor and Head of the Department of Oral Pathology in the School of Pathology of the University of the Witwatersrand and South African Institute for Medical Research, Johannesburg, South Africa

With a contribution by

Gordon R. Seward MDS, FDS, RCS, FRCS(Eng), FRCS(Edin)
Emeritus Professor of Oral and Maxillofacial Surgery, University of London

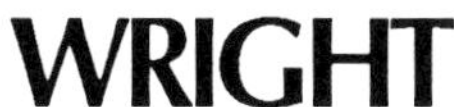

Wright
An imprint of Butterworth-Heinemann Ltd
Linacre House, Jordan Hill, Oxford OX2 8DP

 PART OF REED INTERNATIONAL BOOKS

OXFORD LONDON BOSTON
MUNICH NEW DELHI SINGAPORE SYDNEY
TOKYO TORONTO WELLINGTON

First published 1976
Second edition 1983
Third edition 1992

British Library Cataloguing in Publication Data
Shear Mervyn
Cysts of the Oral Regions. – 3Rev. ed
I. Title
616.99231

ISBN 0 7236 0987 X

Library of Congress Cataloguing in Publication Data
Shear, Mervyn.
Cysts of the oral regions/Mervyn Shear; with a contribution by Gordon R. Seward. – 3rd ed.
p. cm.
Includes bibliographical references and index.
ISBN 0 7236 0987 X
1. Mouth – Cysts. 2. Jaw – Cysts. 3. Odontogenic cysts.
I. Title.
[DNLM: 1. Cysts – diagnosis. 2. Cysts – therapy. 3. Mouth Diseases – diagnosis. 4. Mouth Diseases – Therapy. WU 280 S539c]
RC8 15.S46 1992
617.5′22–dc20
DNLM/DLC
for Library of Congress 92 – 69
CIP

Composition by Genesis Typesetting, Laser Quay, Rochester, Kent
Printed in Great Britain at the University Press, Cambridge

Contents

Preface to the third edition vii
Preface to the second edition viii
Preface to the first edition ix

Introduction xi

1 History 1
2 Odontogenic keratocyst (primordial cyst) 4
3 Gingival cyst and midpalatal raphe cyst of infants 46
4 Gingival cyst of adults, lateral periodontal cyst, botryoid odontogenic cyst and glandular (sialo-)odontogenic cyst 51
5 Dentigerous (follicular) cyst 75
6 Eruption cyst 99
7 Calcifying odontogenic cyst 102
8 Nasopalatine duct (incisive canal) cyst 111
9 The so-called median palatine, median alveolar, median mandibular and globulomaxillary cysts 124
10 Nasolabial (nasoalveolar) cyst 130
11 Radicular cyst, residual cyst, paradental cyst and mandibular infected buccal cyst 136
12 Solitary bone cyst (traumatic, simple, haemorrhagic bone cyst) 171
13 Aneurysmal bone cyst 179
14 Cysts associated with the maxillary antrum 187
15 Developmental cysts of the soft tissues of the mouth, face and neck 196
16 Cysts of the salivary glands 212
17 Parasitic cysts 223
18 Treatment of cysts 227
Gordon R. Seward

References 257
Index 283

Preface to the third edition

Over the past 8 years since publication of the second edition of this book, the subject of jaw cysts and cysts of the soft tissues in and around the mouth has continued to evoke considerable interest among clinicians, pathologists and basic scientists, and numerous papers have been published on these topics. Advances in immunocytochemistry have provided the opportunity for studies on the epithelium of cyst linings in an attempt to clarify the pathogenesis of the many varieties and to improve the accuracy of microscopic diagnosis; while further immunological investigations have been undertaken to identify the changes which initiate the formation of radicular cysts in periapical granulomas, and into other aspects of cyst pathology. Basic research has also led to progress in the understanding of the mechanisms involved in the enlargement of cysts. A few new entities have been identified such as the mandibular infected buccal cyst, the glandular odontogenic cyst and AIDS-related bilateral lympho-epithelial cysts of the parotid glands; while our understanding of lesions such as the unicystic ameloblastoma, the botryoid odontogenic cyst and the postoperative maxillary cyst has been enhanced by careful clinicopathological research.

In order to do justice to all this recent work and to bring it to the attention of others in the field, I have added references to about 250 new papers. In preparing the book I have tried to make the work useful to undergraduate and postgraduate students, dentists, oral and general surgeons, radiologists, oral and general pathologists, and anyone doing research in the field. I trust that readers will not find it difficult to gain access to the information they seek.

In consultation with the publishers, Butterworth-Heinemann, it was decided to take the book out of the *Dental Practitioner Handbook* series, and to produce it in a new format. We have also invited the collaboration of Professor Gordon Seward, who kindly agreed to write a chapter on the treatment of cysts. His expert input will undoubtedly enhance the value of the book to those who treat these lesions.

As with past editions, I have received invaluable assistance from a number of people. I am greatly indebted to Professor Mario Altini, Head of the Department of Oral Pathology of the University of the Witwatersrand, for allowing me access to the material in the department, and to him and other members of his staff who were generous in assisting me with the preparation of material. Likewise, Dr Jos Hille, Head of the Department of Oral Pathology of the University of the Western Cape, was most helpful. Many other colleagues were also extremely kind in lending me good sections and good illustrations, and these have been acknowledged in the text.

M.S.
Johannesburg

Preface to the second edition

In the period since the first edition of this book, there have been many publications in the field. This has given me the opportunity of doing an extensive revision of the text by introducing the newer concepts and reassessing the older. Some 160 references have been added, not all of them published since the first edition. The numbers of jaw cysts from my own department which have been used in this edition, particularly for the clinical analyses, have been increased from 750 to 1345. Most of the diagrams have therefore been redrawn and the tables revised to include the new data. These additional cases were extracted from the departmental archives by Dr A. Rudick in preparation for his research dissertation leading to the degree of MSc(Dent), and it is a pleasure to acknowledge his contribution in this regard.

The classification used in the first edition has been modified slightly as a result of my experience using it in teaching undergraduate and postgraduate students.

The number of figures used has been increased by 24 and many of the original illustrations have been replaced. Colleagues have been most generous in allowing me to use their clinical photographs and radiographs and this is greatly appreciated.

Members of staff and students in my Department have been extremely helpful in many ways and I should like to record my indebtedness to Mario Altini, Simon Bender, Mark Cohen, David Fleming, Chris Rachanis, Stevan Thompson, Archibald Scott, Christine Stewart and Lenah Free. Miss Ann Line typed the manuscript and checked the reference list with great skill and I am very grateful to her. Mrs Marlies Jansen of the Photographic Division of our School was of considerable assistance in reproducing illustrations.

M.S.
Johannesburg

Preface to the first edition

Cysts of the jaws and mouth have been recognized as clinical problems for a long time. During the past few years, however, there have been a large number of publications on the subject, reflecting a great increase in interest in the causes, pathogenesis, behaviour, diagnosis and treatment of the various types of cyst.

This book was written in an attempt to record, in one volume, current views on these cysts. Clinical data, primarily from my own records, radiological features, discussion on pathogenesis, descriptions of the pathology and brief comments on treatment have been included for each variety. It is hoped that the work will be helpful to undergraduate and postgraduate students, general dental practitioners, surgeons, radiologists and pathologists.

A considerable proportion of this book was written during a sabbatical leave spent in the Department of Oral Pathology, Royal Dental College, Copenhagen, Denmark, and I am extremely grateful to Professor Jens Pindborg, Head of this Department, for so kindly allowing me access to his material and for letting me use some of it for this book. I should also like to record my gratitude to Denmark's National Bank for generously inviting my family and me to live in one of their flats in Nyhavn 18 during our stay in Copenhagen.

In the preparation of this book, I have been very greatly helped by colleagues who have kindly lent me clinical photographs and radiographs of their cases. I am particularly indebted to Professor John Lemmer for allowing me access to the records of the Division of Radiology in his Department of our School of Dentistry. It is a pleasure to acknowledge the very considerable assistance which I have received from members of my Department, especially Mario Altini, Archibald Scott, Janice Croft, Renee Goldstein, Lenah Free, Miriam Nadel and Barbara Marcus, as well as from Marlies Jansen in the Photographic Division of our School.

M.S.
Johannesburg

Introduction

A cyst is a pathological cavity having fluid, semifluid or gaseous contents and which is not created by the accumulation of pus (Kramer, 1974). It is frequently, but not always, lined by epithelium.

Numerous classifications have been published of cysts of the jaws. Most of these are perfectly satisfactory and the reader is advised to use any classification which he finds valuable as an aid to memory and understanding. The classification of the epithelial lined cysts used in this book, is based on that recommended in the World Health Organization's publication *Histological Typing of Odontogenic Tumours* (Kramer, Pindborg and Shear, 1992). An exception is that I include the calcifying odontogenic cyst here, whereas this entity is classified as an odontogenic tumour in the WHO work. There is also merit in Main's proposal (1985) that the midpalatal cyst (midpalatal raphe cyst) of infants be given a place in a classification of jaw cysts. The remainder of the classification shown below is the one which I use in my own teaching.

The order in which the various entities are dealt with in the book does not strictly follow their order in the classification.

Classification

I. Cysts of the jaws

A. Epithelial

1. DEVELOPMENTAL

(A) Odontogenic

i. Gingival cyst of infants
ii. Odontogenic keratocyst (primordial cyst)
iii. Dentigerous (follicular) cyst
iv. Eruption cyst
v. Lateral periodontal cyst
vi. Gingival cyst of adults
vii. Botryoid odontogenic cyst
viii. Glandular odontogenic (sialo-odontogenic; mucoepidermoid odontogenic) cyst
ix. Calcifying odontogenic cyst

(B) Non-odontogenic

i. Nasopalatine duct (incisive canal) cyst
ii. Nasolabial (nasoalveolar) cyst
iii. Midpalatal raphe cyst of infants
iv. Median palatine, median alveolar and median mandibular cysts*
v. Globulomaxillary cyst*

2. INFLAMMATORY

i. Radicular cyst, apical and lateral
ii. Residual cyst
iii. Paradental cyst and mandibular infected buccal cyst
iv. Inflammatory collateral cyst

B. Non-epithelial

1. Solitary bone cyst (traumatic, simple, haemorrhagic bone cyst)
2. Aneurysmal bone cyst

II. Cysts associated with the maxillary antrum

1. Benign mucosal cyst of the maxillary antrum
2. Postoperative maxillary cyst (surgical ciliated cyst of the maxilla)

III. Cysts of the soft tissues of the mouth, face and neck

1. Dermoid and epidermoid cysts
2. Lympho-epithelial (branchial cleft) cyst
3. Thyroglossal duct cyst
4. Anterior median lingual cyst (intralingual cyst of foregut origin)
5. Oral cysts with gastric or intestinal epithelium (oral alimentary tract cyst)
6. Cystic hygroma
7. Nasopharyngeal cysts
8. Thymic cyst
9. Cysts of the salivary glands: mucous extravasation cyst; mucous retention cyst; ranula; polycystic (dysgenetic) disease of the parotid
10. Parasitic cysts: hydatid cyst; *Cysticercus cellulosae*; trichinosis

* These cysts, previously regarded as developmental non-odontogenic cysts, are of debatable origin.

Chapter 1

History

Jaw cysts are not lesions confined to modern man. Ruffer (1921) in his studies on the palaeopathology of Egypt has described lesions in the jaws of three mummified specimens which appear to be radicular cysts. The first, from a predynastic era, Naga el Deir (*circa* 4500 BC), shows a root remnant in the right second premolar region of the maxilla. A cavity is present in the bone at its apex.

In the second specimen, which is thought to be from the same period, the mandibular teeth show marked attrition and there is a cystic area in the bone involving the first permanent molar. The third specimen is from Cleopatra's period, Ras el Tin. An oval opening with smooth borders measuring 12 × 8 mm is present in the outer wall of the alveolar bone in the premolar region. An aperture artificially made through the external wall of the mandible leads into a smooth-walled cavity, 36 × 20 mm, in which the roots of the canine, lateral incisor and anterior root of the second molar are exposed.

Salama and Hilmy (1951) reported on two specimens from a collection of skulls excavated at Sakara. All belonged to the period of King Unas of the fifth dynasty (*circa* 2800 BC). One is an adult skull showing a large radicular cyst in relation to $\underline{|234}$. The teeth in relation to the cyst are missing but sockets are present, suggesting that the teeth were lost post mortem. The remaining teeth show marked attrition. The cyst has expanded almost to the midline of the palate. The second specimen shows a large multilocular cyst in the left body of an edentulous mandible. There is expansion of both the inner and outer plates of bone. A skull thought to be from the Hellenistic period has been examined by Dascoulis (1960), who found that it contained a radicular cyst.

Celcus, writing in the early part of the first century AD, is quoted by Lufkin (1938):

> It also happens, that from an ulcer of the gums . . . one may have for a long period a discharge of pus, on account of a broken or rotten tooth, or else on account of a disease of the bone; in this case there often exists a fistula.
>
> Then the latter must be opened, the tooth extracted and if any bony fragment exist, this should be removed; and if there be anything else diseased, this should be scraped away.

Lufkin also pointed out that alveolar and perialveolar abscesses are commonly seen in palaeopathological studies, particularly in Egyptian mummies.

Neiburger (1977) has described a cystic lesion in the angle of a mandible excavated from a burial mound (Dodge County, Wisconsin) of the middle

Woodland cultural period, AD 700–1100. The lesion is described as being composed of three depressed areas grouped around an elevation of bone. The radiograph shows a 'multicystic' defect. The subject was thought to be a 24- to 38-year-old female. Neiburger suggested a diagnosis of 'multilocular cyst or ameloblastoma'. It might also, however, be an odontogenic keratocyst (primordial cyst) of the variety which presents radiologically with scalloped margins.

A photograph of a skull housed in the Abelholt monastery museum in Denmark of a subject buried in the Middle Ages, shows a cystic cavity involving the apices of the left maxillary central and lateral incisors. The incisal edge of the central has been notched, possibly for ritual purposes (*FDI Newsletter*, 1983).

Fauchard (1746), having described the dentoalveolar abscess and its treatment, wrote:

> I have seen many very considerable tumours which could only have been caused by carious teeth. . . . Nothing is more frequent than to see these sort of large tumours, of which the results are insignificant or troublesome according to the exciting causes or the treatment applied to dissipate them and to cure radically when they have formed. I have treated a great number with success.
>
> When incisions in the gums have to be made, for the tumours or to keep them open, sufficient dilation is made with sharp instruments and the incision held open so as not to allow it to close too soon. Not to frighten the patient by the introduction of a fresh cutting instrument, recourse must be had to the use of dossils and tampons of charpie or cotton or to properly made tents covered with wax of some ceriate or convenient plaster which should not be disgusting by its taste or smell. . . . A prepared sponge will do as well. But the tents must be gradually reduced in size as the wound heals for if used too long it may be very dangerous as I know from experience, and this happens too often.
>
> Sometimes it is necessary to take away, to file and remove some portion not only of the gum but even of the alveolus carious or otherwise to procure sufficient aperture for the discharge of matter and for the introduction of medicaments.

Fauchard's 'Sixth Observation' in Chapter 35 of the same work appears to be a case report of a radicular cyst, although he does not give any specific name to the condition he describes.

> *On the effect of caries of two roots of a tooth which gave rise to a tumour and abscess on the left side of the lower jaw.*
>
> On the 6th December 1723 the wife of M. Brizard Concierge and keeper of furniture of the Hotel de Conti having two roots of a second large molar of the left side of the lower jaw carious for some years, this caused a considerable tumour on the same side. I was called to examine this tumour and to extirpate the two roots which I did in the presence of M. Finot (a) and M. Darmagnac (b). The gap which was left by this enabled me to insert my stiletto into the tumour. By this means I ascertained the depth which extended to the base of the maxillary bone. I knew then that the bone was exposed. I made a sufficient incision in the upper part of the gum to give vent to the matter, and, to prevent the opening of the wound being closed too soon, I dressed this lady with a tent of lint covered over with a little white wax. I renewed this tent night and morning and syringed out the wound every time that I dressed it with a lotion made of two ounces of water of ound wort, barley water with cinnamon, balsam of Fioravanti and honey

> of roses of each one ounce, the whole mixed together. The fourth day I ceased to use the tents and continued to syringe the wound as formerly until the twenty-fifth day when the patient was perfectly cured.

Reflexion

> If one deferred at first to draw the carious roots and to open up the abscess sufficiently the lodgement of the matter would have formed a new sinus and made greater progress: when it would not have been perhaps possible to end thus happily the cure of this patient.

John Hunter, writing in about 1780 of diseases of the jaw bones, described a type of lesion which appears to be a cyst.

> The second of these diseases in the bone . . . is an accumulation of curdly substance; probably it is coagulable lymph, and may be reckoned among the encysted tumours. The ossific inflammation often goes on here, till the bone acquires great size, but in these the outer ossific accumulation is not in proportion to the absorption, and therefore, being only a thin shell, it gives way.

The lingual mandibular bone defect, or Stafne cavity, which is sometimes mistaken for a solitary bone cyst on radiographs, has been identified in archaeological studies and the literature on the subject has been reviewed by Keene (1990).

Early work on the nature and treatment of jaw cysts appears in the English literature in papers by Spence (1853–54), Harvey (1855), Moon (1877–78), Heath (1880, 1887), Pedley (1886), Baker (1891), and Turner (1898).

Chapter 2

Odontogenic keratocyst (primordial cyst)

There has been a great deal of interest in the odontogenic keratocyst (primordial cyst) since it became apparent that it may grow to a large size before it manifests clinically and that, unlike other jaw cysts, it has a particular tendency to recur following surgical treatment.

In the earlier literature, the keratocyst was described as a cholesteatoma (Hauer, 1926; Kostečka, 1929). In his detailed study of the cyst, Forssell (1980) concluded that the first account of this lesion was that of Mikulicz who, in 1876, described it as a dermoid cyst.

The term 'odontogenic keratocyst' was introduced by Philipsen (1956) and is now very widely used. In this and in a subsequent paper (Pindborg, Philipsen and Henriksen, 1962), and in a paper by Pindborg and Hansen (1963), the designation 'keratocyst' was used to describe any jaw cyst in which keratin was formed to a large extent. Some dentigerous, radicular and residual cysts were therefore included in the category of odontogenic keratocyst. Moreover, keratocysts may give an erroneous radiographic impression that they are dentigerous, lateral periodontal, residual, or even so-called fissural cysts, thus giving rise to the view that these latter entities are lined by keratinized epithelium (Forssell, 1980).

Although a few radicular and residual cyst linings may become keratinized by metaplasia (**Figure 2.1**), these linings are distinctly different from the characteristic lining epithelium of the odontogenic keratocyst (Browne, 1971a; Forssell and Sainio, 1979). There are however other histological features that distinguish them and it is these which are responsible for their biological behaviour, rather than the presence of keratin. Lucas (1972) has made the point that the emphasis that has been placed on keratinization is to some extent misleading, in that there is the implication that cysts of widely differing types may all keratinize and that if they do they are then liable to recur. There is now a great deal of evidence that the cyst under discussion here is a distinct entity of developmental origin, arising from primordial odontogenic epithelium, and it is for this reason that I have tended to prefer the term 'primordial cyst' to the non-specific histological term 'keratocyst', a preference which I have emphasized in previous editions of this book. However, the designations 'odontogenic keratocyst' or 'keratocyst' are now so firmly established in the literature that they will be used in the present edition.

Browne (1969, 1972) has shown that keratinizing cysts have a significantly ($P < 0.01$) different age distribution (mean age 32.1 years; peak in second and third decades) from dentigerous (mean age 36.6 years; peak in fifth decade) and radicular cysts (mean age 40.2 years; peak from third to sixth decades). He

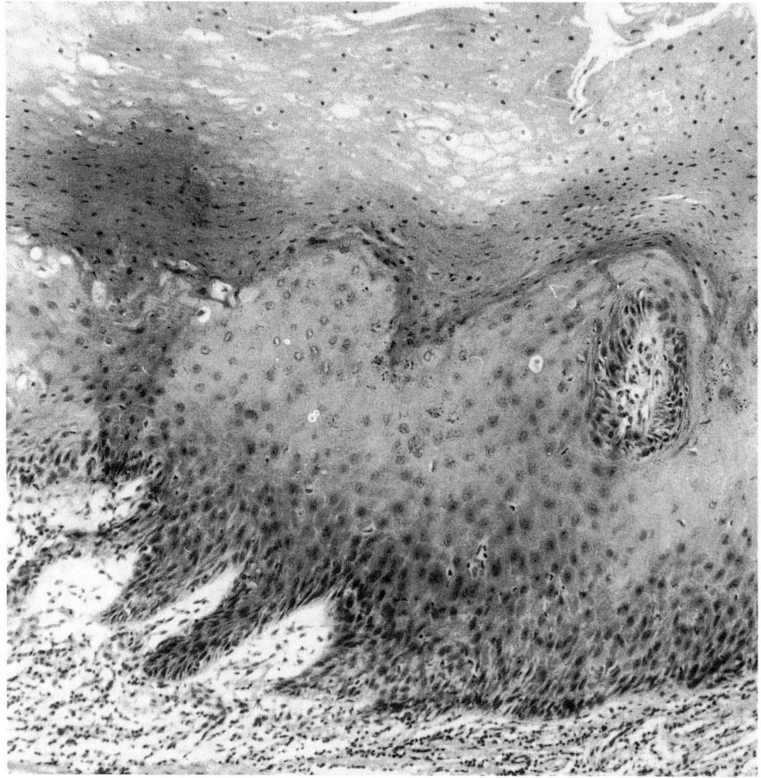

Figure 2.1. Parakeratinized stratified squamous epithelium lining a radicular cyst. (H & E; × 115.)

concluded from this that the three types of cyst arise from different populations and that the keratocyst is therefore a distinct lesion in its own right. The fact that it occurs at a younger age than the others makes it unlikely that it has arisen in long-standing dentigerous or radicular cysts.

Browne (1969) and Hjørting-Hansen, Andreasen and Robinson (1969) have demonstrated, moreover, that the site distribution of keratinizing cysts differs significantly ($P < 0.01$) from that of non-keratinized cysts; a fact which has been confirmed by Rud and Pindborg (1969) who believed that this supported the assumption that keratocysts are actually primordial cysts. Forssell and Sainio (1979), who also had a preference for the term 'primordial cyst', have shown that in these lesions ('genuine keratocysts') the epithelium was distinctly parakeratotic with cuboidal or columnar palisaded basal cells, and occasionally orthokeratotic. Cysts which show local orthokeratinization in otherwise non-keratinized epithelium; cysts with epithelium similar to that seen in parakeratotic oral mucosa; and cysts with scanty areas of thin parakeratinization, should not be regarded as primordial cysts. None of these varieties, moreover, has accentuated basal cells.

Despite agreeing that these cysts are distinct entities, Browne (1969) argued that they cannot be primordial cysts because he defines a primordial cyst, according to the original description of Robinson (1945), as one which arises by breakdown of the stellate reticulum of the enamel organ before any mineralized tissue is formed and hence develops in place of a tooth which may be one of the normal series or a supernumerary. Despite an extensive literature on the subject of primordial cysts and odontogenic keratocysts over the 47 years since Robinson published his paper, there has been no convincing evidence to support the theory which he postulated. Later in this chapter, we shall however present the evidence supporting origin of the keratocyst from primordial odontogenic epithelium, i.e. dental lamina or its remnants (Soskolne and Shear, 1967; Toller, 1967), or odontogenic basal cell hamartias (Stoelinga, 1971a, 1973; Voorsmit, 1984).

Clinical features

Frequency

Over the past 32 years, 292 keratocysts (11.2 per cent) have been diagnosed in our department of a total of 2616 cysts of the jaws (**Table 2.1**). The 292 cysts occurred in 255 patients.

Table 2.1 Distribution of 2616 jaw cysts according to diagnosis

Cysts	*Number*	*Percentage*
Radicular/residual	1368	52.3
Dentigerous	433	16.6
Keratocyst	292	11.2
Nasopalatine	287	11.0
Paradental	65	2.5
Solitary	26	1.0
Calcifying odontogenic	25	1.0
Eruption	21	0.8
Lateral periodontal	18	0.7
Nasolabial	18	0.7
Globulomaxillary	18	0.7
Gingival cyst of adults	14	0.5
Inflammatory collateral	13	0.5
Aneurysmal bone cyst	12	0.5
Postoperative maxillary	4	0.2
Mucosal cyst of maxillary antrum	2	0.1
Total	2616	100.3

The frequency in other studies is shown in **Table 2.2**. The varying frequencies in different reported series probably reflect, to a large extent, the range of material seen in these departments. The age-standardized incidence rates for keratocysts (primordial cysts), standardized against a World Standard population, per million per year, were shown to be 0.61, 0, 4.86 and 3.50 for black males and females and white males and females, respectively, on the Witwatersrand (Rachanis and Shear, 1978) (**Table 2.3**).

Age

Keratocysts occur over a wide age range and cases have been recorded as early as the first decade and as late as the ninth. In most series there has been a pronounced

Table 2.2 Frequency of keratocysts in different series

Author(s)	*Material*	*%*
Pindborg *et al.*, 1962	26 of 791 odontogenic	3.3
Toller, 1967	33 of 300 cysts, all types	11.0
Hjørting-Hansen *et al.*, 1969	56 of 502 odontogenic	11.2
Browne, 1970	41 of 537 odontogenic	7.6
Main, 1970a	12 of 289 epithelial jaw cysts	4.2
Stoelinga, 1971	54 of 486 jaw cysts	11.1
Killey *et al.*, 1977	25 of 746 jaw cysts	3.3
Payne, 1972	103 of 1313 odontogenic	7.8
Radden and Reade, 1973	64 of 368 odontogenic	17.4
Brannon, 1976	312 of 2972 oral cysts	10.5
Craig, 1976	85 of 1051 odontogenic	8.1
Djamshidi, 1976	91 of 417 odontogenic	21.8
Hodgkinson *et al.*, 1978	79 of 1100 jaw cysts	7.2
Magnusson, 1978	52 of 1420 odontogenic	3.2
Ahlfors *et al.*, 1984	319 of 5914 jaw cysts	5.4
Reff-Eberwein *et al.*, 1985	82 of 3328 odontogenic	2.5
Hoffmeister and Härle, 1985	51 of 3353 jaw cysts	1.5
Höndell and Wiberg, 1988	29 of 531 jaw cysts	5.4
Shear, present study	292 of 2616 jaw cysts	11.2

Table 2.3 Age-standardized incidence rates of keratocysts on the Witwatersrand, 1965–74, standardized against standard European, World and African populations (from Rachanis and Shear, 1978)

	Per million per year		
	European	*World*	*African*
Black male	0.67	0.61	0.63
Black female	0	0	0
White male	5.37	4.86	4.78
White female	3.64	3.50	3.54

peak frequency in the second and third decades, with figures ranging from 40 per cent to 60 per cent of patients being in this age group. The ages at diagnosis of 106 keratocysts from our own material are shown in **Figure 2.2.**

Some workers have demonstrated a bimodal age distribution with a second peak in the fifth decade or later (Toller, 1967; Magnusson, 1978; Vedtofte and Praetorius, 1979; Forssell, 1980; Ahlfors, Larsson and Sjögren, 1984; Donath, 1985; Partridge and Towers, 1987; Voorsmit, 1984; Woolgar, Rippin and Browne, 1987b). The study on age-specific morbidity rates done in our department confirmed this bimodal trend (Rachanis and Shear, 1978). It showed, moreover, that the incidence was highest in the older age groups (**Table 2.4**, **Figure 2.3**). This finding indicates that although the number of cases diagnosed is greatest in the second and third decades, the older age groups are in fact at greater risk for the diagnosis of keratocysts.

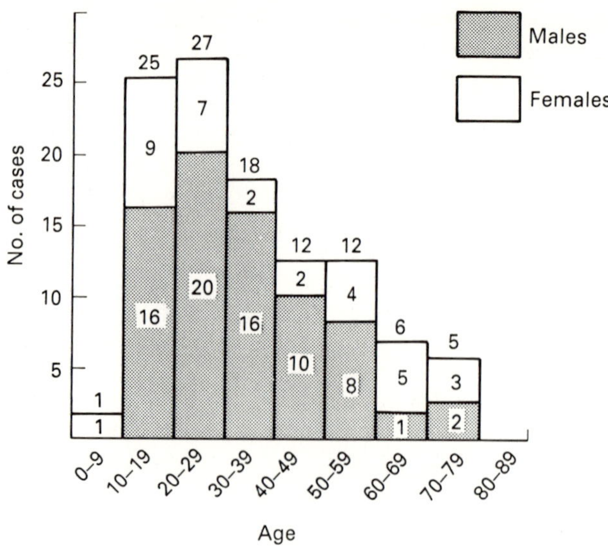

Figure 2.2. Ages of patients at diagnosis of 106 keratocysts.

Table 2.4 Average annual incidence rates for keratocysts on the Witwatersrand, South Africa, 1965–74

	Average annual incidence per million by age group (years)							
	0–9	*10–19*	*20–29*	*30–39*	*40–49*	*50–64*	*65–74*	*75+*
Black male	0	0.65	0.44	1.24	0.85	1.28	0	0
Black female	0	0	0	0	0	0	0	0
White male	0.94	4.56	5.73	7.00	1.81	11.58	6.84	0
White female	0	6.02	5.88	1.49	5.47	1.62	4.97	8.90

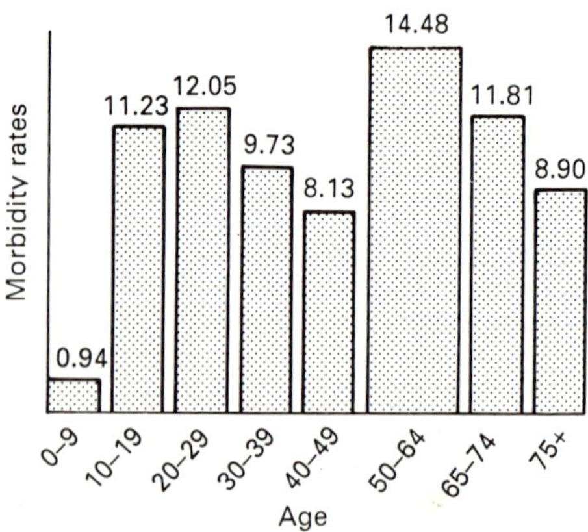

Figure 2.3. Age-specific morbidity rates for keratocysts (primordial cysts) on the Witwatersrand, 1965–74, shown as cases per million population per year.

We then addressed ourselves to the question of whether two different types of keratocyst might exist, one in younger and one in older age groups (Rachanis, Altini and Shear, 1979). All cases of keratocyst from patients in the age groups 10–29 and 50–64 years which had been accessioned in our department, were reviewed clinically and histologically. The data were analysed statistically. No significant differences were observed between the two groups. We concluded, therefore, that it is unlikely that these are different varieties of keratocyst and subscribe to the view of Browne (1975) that the cysts in older age groups have probably been present but undiagnosed for many years. This is in keeping with the observation made elsewhere in this chapter, that keratocysts may involve the body and ascending ramus of the mandible extensively, with little or no bony expansion.

Woolgar, Rippen and Browne (1987c) have pointed out that the mean age of patients with multiple keratocysts, with or without the naevoid basal cell carcinoma syndrome, is considerably lower than the mean age of patients with single non-recurrent keratocysts and that pooling patients from the three groups will account for differences in age distribution reported in different studies.

Sex

Keratocysts are generally found more frequently in males than in females ($P < 0.05$) and this sex predilection is more pronounced in black than in white patients. In a series of 119 of our patients, there were approximately twice as many males as females. Of these, 53 were white males and 36 white females (1.5:1); 25 were black males and 5 black females (5.0:1) (**Table 2.5**).

Table 2.5 Sex distribution of black and white patients with keratocysts

	Male	*Female*	*Total*	*M:F ratio*
Black	25	5	30 (25%)	5.0:1
White	53	36	89 (75%)	1.5:1
Total	78 (66%)	41 (34%)	119	1.9:1
W:B ratio	2.1:1	7.2:1	3.0:1	

A more accurate assessment of the sex and race distribution of patients with keratocysts may be obtained from standardized incidence studies. The age-standardized incidence rates for black and white males and females on the Witwatersrand are shown in **Table 2.3** and the age-specific morbidity rates for these four groups in **Table 2.4**. These figures confirm the observation that the incidence of keratocysts is higher in males than in females, that they are considerably more common in whites than in blacks and that they are particularly rare in black women. In some studies, however, an equal sex distribution has been observed (Vedtofte and Praetorius, 1979). In a sample of 20 patients with multiple keratocysts, of whom 10 had the naevoid basal cell carcinoma syndrome, Brannon (1976) observed a female preponderance of 17:1.

Site

The mandible is involved far more frequently than the maxilla. In our own material, 94 of 125 cysts (75 per cent) have occurred in the mandible. The frequency of mandibular involvement in other series is 77 per cent (Hansen, 1967); 83 per cent (Browne, 1970); 65 per cent (Brannon, 1976); 72 per cent (Hodgkinson *et al.*, 1978); 71 per cent (Vedtofte and Praetorius, 1979); 78 per cent (Forssell, 1980); 75 per cent (Ahlfors, Larsson and Sjögren, 1984) and 69 per cent (Voorsmit, 1984). About one-half of all keratocysts occur at the angle of the mandible extending for varying distances into the ascending ramus and forward into the body. As to the site distribution of the other cases, reports of a number of studies indicate that they can occur anywhere in the jaws, including the midline of the mandible and maxilla and the 'globulomaxillary area' in the maxilla (Soskolne and Shear, 1967; Browne, 1971a; Brannon, 1976; Vedtofte and Praetorius, 1979; Forssell, 1980). Woolgar, Rippen and Browne (1987c) have shown that keratocysts occur with much greater frequency in the maxilla after the age of 50.

Clinical Presentation

Patients with keratocysts complain of pain, swelling or discharge. Occasionally they experience paraesthesia of the lower lip or teeth. Some of our patients have been unaware of the lesions until they developed pathological fractures. Some of these cysts have been discovered fortuitously during dental examination when radiographs were taken. In many instances, patients are remarkably free of symptoms until the cysts have reached a large size, involving the maxillary sinus and the entire ascending ramus, including the condylar and coronoid processes. This is because the keratocyst tends to extend in the medullary cavity and clinically observable expansion of the bone occurs late. Although the cysts vary considerably in size, Forssell (1980) has shown that about one-half of his cases were 40 mm or more in diameter and that this was particularly the case with cysts of the ascending ramus and angle of the mandible compared with cysts of the maxilla or body of the mandible. Forssell suggested that the maxillary cysts are more likely to become infected even when small, than the mandibular cysts and will probably, therefore, be diagnosed at an earlier stage in their development. As with many other intraosseous jaw lesions, the enlarging cyst may lead to displacement of the teeth and Voorsmit (1984) and Lund (1985) have described the occurrence of large keratocysts which involved the maxillary sinus and led to displacement and destruction of the floor of the orbit and proptosis of the eyeballs. Neurological symptoms are occasionally seen (Browne, 1970; Brannon, 1976).

Dayan *et al.* (1988) have described the occurrence of a lesion entirely within the gingiva, which had the clinical features of a gingival cyst of adults but the histological characteristics of a typical keratocyst. They have suggested the term peripheral odontogenic keratocyst for this rare presentation of the lesion; a useful proposal in view of its apparently unaggressive nature.

An analysis of the location and frequency of bony expansion has been made by Browne (1970). In his study, expansion of bone occurred in about 60 per cent of cases. One-third of maxillary cysts caused buccal expansion, but palatal expansion was very rarely seen. About one-half of the mandibular lesions produced buccal expansion and one-third produced lingual expansion. The great majority of the latter group were in the third molar or ascending ramus regions. Forssell (1980) observed expansion of bone in 53 per cent of his material and this occurred significantly more frequently in the angle or ascending ramus of the mandible than in the maxilla or in the body of the mandible. Perforation of bone, as observed in orthopantomograms, occurred in 39 per cent of his cases. Brannon (1976), however, reported only a 25 per cent frequency of bony expansion or perforation.

Multiple keratocysts are found in some patients. Of 122 patients in our series, 113 had single cysts and nine (7 per cent) had more than 1. In three of the latter, the cysts were part of the naevoid basal cell carcinoma syndrome. Of these patients, one has had six cysts, another five and one has had two.

The naevoid basal cell carcinoma syndrome

Binkley and Johnson (1951) reported the case of a 30-year-old woman with multiple 'dental follicular cysts' involving both sides of the mandible. She also had numerous hard papules situated over various parts of the body which histological examination showed were 'basal cell nevi'. A radiograph of the chest revealed an anteriorly bifid sixth rib. Gorlin and Goltz (1960) established the association of multiple basal cell epitheliomas, jaw cysts (which they described as 'true cysts, having a typical stratified squamous epithelium') and bifid ribs, a combination which is now frequently referred to as the 'Gorlin–Goltz syndrome', as well as the naevoid basal cell carcinoma syndrome. Gorlin, Yunis and Tuna (1963) and Meerkotter and Shear (1964) identified the jaw cysts as keratocysts, and several studies have been undertaken on the keratocysts occurring in patients with the syndrome. The syndrome is inherited as a set of autosomal dominant characteristics with strong penetrance. It has variable expressivity, producing skin, jaw, other skeletal, central nervous system and eye lesions, as well as fairly typical facial features with frontal bossing and ocular hypertelorism. Keratocysts are one of the most consistent features of the syndrome, occurring in 65 to 75 per cent of cases and skeletal anomalies are also common.

Recurrences

Brief reference has already been made to the fact that the keratocyst has a particular tendency to recur after surgical treatment. The recurrences in various reported series is shown in **Table 2.6**. Pindborg and Hansen (1963) were the first to point out this peculiarly aggressive behaviour. They reported a recurrence rate of 62 per cent in a series of 16 cysts and observed that there was no correlation between the size or location of the cyst and its tendency to recur; nor was there any difference in recurrence rate between cases which were treated by 'extirpation' and those treated by 'fenestration'. Hansen (1967) found a recurrence rate of 52 per cent in a series of 52 cases followed for a period of at least 6 months. Browne (1970) reported a 25 per cent recurrence rate in 85 cysts followed for 6 months or longer. He found that most recurrences were in the first 5 years after surgery but one of his cases recurred 20 years after operation. Bramley (1971) reported a case with a recurrence 40 years after surgical treatment. Browne (1970) could find no statistically significant correlation between the frequency of recurrence and the age of the patient, location of the cyst, the method of treatment (enucleation or marsupialization), the nature of the cyst lining, and the presence of cortical perforation. In a later paper Browne (1971a) showed that there was a very similar rate of recurrence following removal of cysts with satellite cysts (23.7 per cent) and

Table 2.6 Recurrences of keratocysts in various series

Authors	*Number of cases followed*	*Recurrence rate (%)*
Pindborg and Hansen, 1963	16	62
Hansen, 1967	52	52
Toller, 1967	55	51
Cernéa *et al.*, 1969	28	18
Rud and Pindborg, 1969	21	33
Panders and Hadders, 1969	22	14
Browne, 1970	85	25
Ebling *et al.*, 1971	24	38
Stoelinga, 1971a	54	10
Klammt, 1972	32	22
Machtens *et al.*, 1972	44	59
McIvor, 1972	43	5
Payne, 1972	20	45
Borg *et al.*, 1974	25	24
Butz, 1975	38	11
Eversole *et al.*, 1975	35	20
Brannon, 1976	283	12
Hodgkinson *et al.*, 1978	74	39
Vedtofte and Praetorius, 1979	57	51
Forssell, 1980	121	40
Voorsmit *et al.*, 1981 (Group 1)	52	14
Voorsmit *et al.*, 1981 (Group 2)	40	3
Anniko *et al.*, 1981	21	50
Ahlfors *et al.*, 1984	255	27
Reff-Eberwein *et al.*, 1985	82	56
Niemeyer *et al.*, 1985	64	36
Zachariades *et al.*, 1985	16	25
Partridge and Towers, 1987	45	27
Forssell *et al.*, 1988	75	43
Köndell and Wiberg, 1988	29	24
Stoelinga and Bronkhorst, 1988	27	10

those without satellite cysts (24.4 per cent). There was a higher frequency of recurrence of cysts without epithelial residues (28.1 per cent) than with (8.3 per cent) but the difference was not statistically significant. These observations were confirmed by Vedtofte and Praetorius (1979).

Toller (1971) summarized the findings of a number of different groups of workers. In a total of 195 patients there were 85 first recurrences (44 per cent). In our own sample, 38 patients were followed-up from between 8 months and 17 years. There were two definite recurrences, proved at operation and histologically, and a further two probable cases on the basis of radiological evidence (Butz, 1975). This constitutes a recurrence rate of 11 per cent. Of the definite recurrences, one was discovered 2½ years and the other 1 year after the original operation. Lower recurrence rates than in most other studies have also been reported by Panders and Hadders in 1969 (14 per cent), by Stoelinga (1971a), (10 per cent), by Stoelinga and Bronkhorst (1988), (10 per cent) and by Brannon in 1976 (12 per cent). Forssell (1980) found a higher recurrence rate when cysts were located in the angle or ascending ramus of the mandible. The size of the cyst did not, however, appear to influence the recurrence rate.

Niemeyer *et al.* (1985) reported that their experience of recurrences in a series of 62 patients with keratocysts related to the operative procedure employed. Thirty-three of their patients were followed for at least 6 years. The highest frequency of recurrences occurred in their patients treated by cystostomy.

Wright (1981) followed 24 patients with orthokeratinized keratocysts for periods of 6 months to 8 years and found only one recurrence which occurred 6½ years postoperatively. He suggested that orthokeratinized keratocysts may be less aggressive than the parakeratinized type.

The considerable variation in recurrence rate reported by different workers may be ascribed partly to the variability in the follow-up period. Vedtofte and Praetorius (1979), Forssell (1980) and Forssell, Forssell and Kahnberg (1988) have shown quite clearly that in their own material the recurrence rate increased with extension of the follow-up period to 5 years or more. The latter authors (Forssell, Forssell and Kahnberg, 1988) found that of 75 cases in 63 patients followed for periods ranging from 5 to 17 years (mean 8.3), 32 (43 per cent) recurred. The cumulative recurrence rate of 67 of these cysts in patients examined annually, increased from 3 per cent after the first year to 37 per cent after the third year. Thereafter no new recurrences were noted. They observed that recurrences were more frequent (63 per cent) with cysts in patients with the naevoid basal cell carcinoma syndrome than with cysts in patients without the syndrome (37 per cent). Keratocysts enucleated in one piece recurred significantly less often ($P < 0.01$) than cysts enucleated in several pieces, and the recurrence rate in cases with a clinically observable infection, a fistula or with a perforated bony wall was higher than when these features were not present. The size of the cyst did not seem to influence its prognosis after surgery, but those whose radiographic appearance was multilocular had a higher recurrence rate than those with a unilocular appearance.

There are a number of possible reasons why keratocysts recur so frequently. The first of these is related to their tendency to multiplicity in some patients, including the occurrence of satellite cysts which are retained during an enucleation procedure. Some instances of recurrence are likely therefore to be new cysts rather than true recurrences. Secondly, keratocyst linings are very thin and fragile, particularly when the cysts are large, and are therefore more difficult to enucleate than cysts with thick walls. Portions of the lining may be left behind (Kramer, 1963; Fickling, 1965) and constitute the origin of a recurrence. The studies of Forssell, Sorvari and Oksala (1974); Forssell (1980) and Forssell, Forssell and Kahnberg (1988) showed that recurrences were extremely infrequent if the cyst was enucleated in one piece but occurred in more than one-half of the cases when the cyst was removed in several pieces. An attempt to save vital adjacent teeth or nerves during the operation may lead to incomplete eradication and hence to recurrence. Likewise, enucleation in one piece may be more difficult with cysts which have scalloped margins and this may explain the higher recurrence rates than with those with a smoother contour. A relationship between perforation of the lingual plate of the mandible and recurrence after treatment has been observed (Borg, Persson and Thilander, 1974).

Toller (1967) suggested that the epithelial linings of keratocysts have intrinsic growth potential and believed that there was some basis for regarding them as benign neoplasms. Ahlfors, Larsson and Sjögren (1984) also proposed that the keratocyst should be regarded as a benign cystic neoplasm.

A further possible reason for an apparently unsuccessful treatment is provided by evidence derived from patients with the naevoid basal cell carcinoma syndrome.

These patients have a particular predisposition to form keratocysts from the dental lamina (Soskolne and Shear, 1967). This suggests that keratocysts in patients without the syndrome are also likely to arise from the dental lamina. If these individuals also have an innate tendency to develop such cysts, then any remnants of dental lamina may form the target for new keratocyst formation.

Yet another potential source of the recurrences has been proposed by Stoelinga (1971a) and Stoelinga and Peters (1973) who have demonstrated that the cysts may arise from proliferations of the basal cells of the oral mucosa particularly in the third molar region and ascending ramus of the mandible. They referred to the fact that there is often firm adhesion of the cysts to the overlying mucosa and recommended that when they are surgically removed, the overlying mucosa should be excised with them in an attempt to prevent possible recurrence (or the formation of new cysts) from residual basal cell proliferations. Voorsmit, Stoelinga and van Haelst (1981) believed that a recurrent keratocyst may develop in three different ways: by incomplete removal of the original cyst lining; by the retention of daughter cysts, microcysts or epithelial islands in the wall of the original cyst; or by the development of new keratocysts from epithelial off-shoots of the basal layer of the oral epithelium. In the latter respect, the authors supported the hypothesis of Shear and Altini (1976) that there may be residual ectomesenchymal inductive influence on the overlying epithelium to initiate this process. Emerson, Whitlock and Jones (1972) reported two examples of keratocysts which involved related soft tissues. DeGould and Goldberg (1991) described the recurrence of a keratocyst in a bone graft after partial mandibulectomy, and the source of this may well have been the mucosa.

Numbers of studies have been done on patients with multiple keratocysts and in patients with the naevoid basal cell carcinoma syndrome in an attempt to find explanations for the recurrences. Payne (1972) compared the histological features of recurrent keratocysts with non-recurrent specimens and those from patients with the syndrome. The presence of inflammation and the type of keratin produced did not seem to be significant. He found bud-like proliferations of the basal cell layer in five of 11 recurrent cysts (45 per cent) and four of nine cysts from patients with the syndrome (44 per cent). By comparison, only six of 72 non-recurrent keratocysts (8 per cent) showed this feature. Satellite microcysts were observed in the cyst walls of 78 per cent of cysts from patients with the syndrome, 18 per cent of the recurrent cysts and 4 per cent of the non-recurrent cysts. Donatsky *et al.* (1976) found only five of 55 cysts (9 per cent) in patients with the syndrome to have bud-like proliferations of the basal layer of epithelium. There was, however, a significantly higher ($P < 0.01$) occurrence of epithelial islands and/or microcysts in the walls of the syndrome cysts (51 per cent) and solitary recurring cysts (53 per cent) than in the solitary non-recurring cysts (17 per cent).

Woolgar, Rippin and Browne (1987a and b) compared the clinical presentation and histological features of single keratocysts and those occurring in the naevoid basal cell carcinoma syndrome. The sex distribution of their sample without the syndrome (62 per cent male and 38 per cent female; $n = 377$) was significantly different ($P < 0.025$) from the sample with the syndrome (45 per cent male and 55 per cent female; $n = 60$). The mean ages were significantly different between the groups ($P < 0.001$). In the group without the syndrome, the mean age at removal of the cyst was 40.4 years (SD ±19.2) with a bimodal distribution, the first peak from 15 to 45 years and the second smaller peak from 55 to 65 years. In patients with the syndrome, there is a single peak at 10 to 30 years and a mean of 26.2 years

(SD ±17.3). Log linear modelling of the variables showed that in their sample there were significantly more syndrome than non-syndrome patients before the age of 36 years and that in both groups of patients females are more likely to be seen in the younger age group. Their findings indicated that female patients with keratocysts who are younger than 36 years, are the group most likely to have the syndrome. With regard to site, there was a higher frequency in the mandibular molar-ramus area (60 per cent) of cysts unassociated with the syndrome than those with (44 per cent); whereas more syndrome cysts (21 per cent) than non-syndrome cysts (11 per cent) occurred in the maxillary molar region. Eighteen patients with the syndrome initially had only one cyst. In all except three, further cysts have since developed. Of 24 syndrome patients with cysts in two quadrants, 13 had bilateral mandibular cysts related to third molar teeth. Five patients had cysts in three quadrants and 13 patients had cysts in all four quadrants. The time interval at which subsequent cysts were diagnosed, varied from 1 to 23 years.

The authors emphasized that the term multiple when applied to cysts occurring in patients with the syndrome refers to the lifetime history of the patient and not that more than one cyst is present at any one time. They also made the important point that any patient with more than one keratocyst other than a recurrence will show some other features of the syndrome, albeit only minor anomalies which may be revealed only on full examination.

In a third paper, Woolgar, Rippen and Browne (1987c) were able to identify no significant differences in age, sex or site between a sample of patients with single, non-recurrent keratocysts followed for 5 years or more and another sample of patients with keratocysts which had recurred in the same sites as their original lesions. In a histological comparison of material from both samples, the only significant difference was that the recurrences were less inflamed than the primary cysts or the controls.

In their histological study, Woolgar, Rippen and Browne (1987a) compared 164 keratocysts from 60 patients having the naevoid basal cell carcinoma syndrome with a similar number of keratocysts from patients without the syndrome, matched for age and size. Significantly higher numbers of satellite cysts ($P < 0.001$), solid islands of epithelial proliferation ($P < 0.001$), odontogenic rests within the capsule ($P < 0.01$), and in the numbers of mitotic figures in the epithelium lining the parent cyst cavity ($P < 0.001$), were found in the syndrome group. The authors derived an index of activity by grading the solid proliferations, satellite cysts, ameloblastomatoid proliferations and the mitotic rate, and found that this was significantly higher in the syndrome group ($P < 0.001$). Epithelial rests were strikingly more prevalent in the capsules of cysts from the younger age group and in the mandibular molar region. They found no association to support the theory that satellite cysts arise by basal budding of epithelium lining the parent cyst. Their results did, however, support the view that satellite cysts are formed when islands of proliferating epithelial cells derived from small epithelial rests reach a size where cystic breakdown occurs. They found no evidence that the ameloblastomatoid proliferations develop into true ameloblastomas. They suggested that there is some inherent genetic potential for proliferation of odontogenic epithelium in the syndrome patients.

Dominguez and Keszler (1988) compared solitary and syndrome-associated keratocysts histologically and histometrically. Satellite cysts and/or epithelial islands were present in 36 per cent of the syndrome-associated cysts and in only 6 per cent of the solitary group ($P < 0.005$). Histometric analysis showed that total nuclear numbers and numbers of basal nuclei were significantly higher ($P < 0.001$) in solitary keratocysts. Solitary cysts also had a significantly greater epithelial height ($P < 0.01$). They suggested that the solitary and the syndrome-associated keratocysts could be two distinct populations.

A number of authors have referred to the occurrence of multiple keratocysts in patients without obvious signs of other features of the syndrome, or of a familial trend. Brannon (1976) reported a frequency of 3 per cent with multiple cysts in his sample, Vedtofte and Praetorius (1979) 4 per cent, Ahlfors, Larsson and Sjögren (1984) 6 per cent, Voorsmit (1984) 2 per cent and Stoelinga and Bronkhorst (1988) 4.5 per cent.

As oral surgeons have become increasingly aware of the need to treat keratocysts more aggressively than other jaw cysts, or by the use of special protocols, it is likely that future studies will show a declining frequency of recurrences. It is difficult to ignore the possibility that the variability in reported recurrence rates may, at least partly, be attributable to differences in the surgical techniques used and in the experience of the surgeons. This view is borne out by the experience of Voorsmit, Stoelinga and van Haelst (1981) who reported the results of a follow-up study of two groups of patients treated for keratocysts. In the first group of 52 cases treated between 1959 and 1980, the cysts were treated conservatively by careful enucleation of the entire wall. In the second group of 40 cases treated between 1970 and 1980, the cysts were removed by enucleation along with excision of the mucosa overlying a perforation of the cortical bone which was determined at operation. Before removal, all cysts in this group were treated with Carnoy's solution (see Chapter 18). The recurrence rate in their first group was 13.5 per cent in a 1–21 year follow-up while the recurrence rate in their second group has been 2.5 per cent in a 1–10 year follow-up. Similarly, Forssell, Forssell and Kahnberg (1988) have pointed out that in their series of keratocysts treated before 1975, the recurrence rate was 50 per cent, whereas in the group treated during the period 1975–1980, the recurrence rate had dropped to 22 per cent.

Enlargement

Reference has already been made to Toller's view that keratocysts might possibly be regarded as benign neoplasms. There is, however, not much information about their rate of growth. As they tend to extend along the cancellous component of the bone without producing noteworthy expansion of the cortical plates, they frequently reach a large size, particularly at the angle of mandible and ascending ramus, before they are diagnosed. Although Browne (1971a) was of the opinion that these cysts grow more rapidly than other jaw cysts, Toller's view (1967) was that they grow at a similar rate to other epithelial cysts of the jaws. He suggested that the majority of keratocysts would take about 6 years to recur to a clinically significant size of more than 1 cm diameter but with a wide range, varying from 1 to 25 years. Forssell (1980) has found that the rate of growth of keratocysts varies from 2 to 14 mm a year, with an average of about 7 mm. The growth rate was slow in patients over 50 years of age. The relevant point appears to be, as put by Main (1970b), that although the rate of enlargement of keratocysts may not be greater than that of other jaw cysts, its growth is more unremitting. The reason for this unremitting growth has been investigated by both Main (1970a) and Toller (1971). Main showed that the mitotic value of keratocyst linings ranged from 0 to 19 with a mean of 8.0. This figure was similar to that in the ameloblastoma and in dental lamina, and higher than that found in non-odontogenic cysts which had a mean mitotic value of 2.3, and radicular cysts with a mean mitotic value of 4.5.

Toller estimated mitotic activity by autoradiography following the *in vitro* incubation of cyst linings in tissue culture medium to which had been added tritiated thymidine. The mean labelling indices were 13.0 per cent for a series of 6 keratocysts compared with 1.7 per cent for 5 non-keratocyst jaw cysts. The mean figure for human buccal mucous membrane was 7.0 per cent.

Scharfetter *et al.*(1989) studied the proliferation patterns of the epithelium and connective tissue of a keratocyst by means of autoradiography and DNA cytophotometry in serial sections sampled in numerous areas. These were compared with the proliferation patterns in a radicular cyst studied in the same way. The epithelium of the keratocyst showed a higher rate of proliferation than the radicular cyst, with a mean value of the number of proliferating cells per mm^2 of 4.5 (SD ±3.92), and a range of deviation of 10.35 proliferating cells per mm^2. In the radicular cyst the mean value was 0.51 proliferating cells per mm^2 (SD ±0.42), with a range of deviation of 1.16 proliferating cells per mm^2. The mean marking index (percentage of marked cells out of a total of 770 cells counted per representative area) was also substantially higher in the keratocyst than in the radicular. The authors identified slowly proliferating areas and rapidly proliferating areas in different parts of the cyst wall and in different planes of section. They also demonstrated that the connective tissue wall of the keratocyst showed both slowly and rapidly proliferating areas, whereas the connective tissue wall of the radicular cyst showed a low mean marking index. It was the basal and suprabasal cells of the keratocyst which marked with H^3-thymidine. They concluded that exclusively passive expansion of the cyst connective tissue as a reaction to the growth of the keratocyst was unlikely. They thought that the invasive growth of keratocysts was likely to be the result of active growth of the connective tissue wall. They were unable to answer the question as to whether connective tissue and epithelium proliferate independently of each other or whether proliferating epithelium induces proliferation of the adjacent fibroblasts in an ectomesenchymal interaction. Autoradiography had revealed areas where epithelium and connective tissue had proliferated simultaneously as well as areas where they had not. Microscopic examination of the autoradiographic sections showed that proliferation of neither the epithelium nor the connective tissue of the keratocyst was homogeneous, but irregular and in clusters. Their autoradiographic findings were supported by DNA cytophotometry. In rapidly proliferating areas, the nuclear extinction values were also increased.

Toller (1970b) also considered the role played by the osmolality of the cyst fluid in enlargement of the keratocysts. He showed that there was a mean osmolality of 296 ± 15.6 mosmol (11 cases) compared with a serum osmolality of 282 ± 14.75 mosmol. This difference is statistically significant $P < 0.01$). In view of the low total soluble protein level in keratocysts (Toller, 1970a), he suggested that osmotic differences between sera and cyst fluids are not directly related to proteins in cyst fluids and may be the result of the liberation of the products of cell lysis which may not be proteins. He believed strongly that the raised osmolalities play an important, even if not the sole, role in the expansive growth in the size of the keratocyst as well as other jaw cysts.

Main (1970b), on the other hand, felt that mural growth in the form of epithelial proliferation is the essential process involved in the enlargement of keratocysts and that the evidence for osmotic diffusion is inconclusive. This view was supported by

Browne (1970,1975) and Kramer (1974). They believed that the multilocular and loculated outlines exhibited by some keratocysts are difficult to interpret on the basis of unicentric hydrostatic expansion alone. This form of cyst outline suggests a multicentric pattern of cyst growth brought about by the proliferation of local groups of epithelial cells against the semi-solid cyst contents. Ahlfors, Larsson and Sjögren (1984) also considered that the keratocyst should be regarded as a benign neoplasm. They drew attention to the infolding of the epithelial lining into the capsule and suggested that this was the result of active epithelial proliferation accompanied by collagenolytic activity within the fibrous capsule and resorption of bone. Once this has happened, the intracystic pressure is able to 'level off' the lining in the enlarged bone cavity.

Inflammatory exudate plays a negligible role in its enlargement. Keratocyst fluid contains low quantities of soluble protein composed predominantly of albumin and only relatively small quantities of immunoglobulins (Toller, 1970a; Browne, 1976). Moreover, the cyst walls are usually free of inflammatory cell infiltrate except for occasional foci, and the more or less continuous lining of keratinized epithelium is not a barrier readily penetrable by proteins. Smith, Smith and Browne (1983) confirmed that the fluids of keratocysts contain smaller amounts of protein and that few high molecular weight proteins are present, compared with radicular and dentigerous cysts. This supported the hypothesis that the epithelial wall of the keratocyst is less permeable than that of other odontogenic cysts and that an exclusion barrier to higher molecular weight (greater than approximately 68 000) molecules exists.

Smith, Smith and Browne (1984, 1988a and b) have reported a series of three studies on the presence and role of glycosaminoglycans in odontogenic cysts, including keratocysts. In the first of these studies on cyst fluids, hyaluronic acid showed the highest incidence and abundance in all three cyst types. Appreciable amounts of chondroitin-4-sulphate were also observed, particularly in the radicular cysts, and heparin sulphate showed a higher incidence and abundance in the keratocyst than the other cysts. A considerable proportion of the glycosaminoglycans appeared to be complexed with protein and was released only after proteolytic digestion. They were uncertain about the origin of these macromolecules but concluded that they were probably derived from both the connective tissue and the epithelium of the cyst wall. In their histochemical investigation of odontogenic cyst connective tissue, they demonstrated appreciable amounts of extracellular glycosaminoglycans and proteoglycans in the connective tissue capsules of all three cyst types, predominantly hyaluronic acid, with lesser amounts of sulphated glycosaminoglycans. They observed a subepithelial band of alcianophilia in all cyst types, predominantly in the dentigerous cyst, which was strongest adjacent to the epithelium and extended through the thickness of the epithelium with diminishing intensity. This appeared to be the effect of the presence of heparin sulphate. Mast cells were widespread in the connective tissue of all cyst types, particularly adjacent to the epithelium, and were probably the source of the heparin. They concluded that the major source of the glycosaminoglycans and proteoglycans in cyst fluids is from the ground substance of the connective tissue capsule, released as a result of normal metabolic turnover and inflammatory degradation. Degranulating mast cells release heparin and hydrolytic enzymes and the latter facilitate the breakdown of the glycosaminoglycans and proteoglycans. The epithelial contribution was mainly from goblet cells (Shear, 1960b; Browne, 1972). The authors suggested that the variation between individual cysts depended on the amount of inflammation, the epithelial permeability and the extent of mucous metaplasia.

In their third study (Smith, Smith and Browne, 1988b), they extracted glycosaminoglycans from fresh connective tissue capsules of keratocysts, dentigerous and radicular cysts. In all cyst types, hyaluronic acid was the predominant glycosaminoglycan present, as it was in the cyst fluids. Heparin and chondroitin-4-sulphate were present in substantial amounts. Epithelial permeability, the authors suggested, would probably allow passage of smaller glycosaminoglycan chains into the luminal fluid. The larger chains would probably pass through epithelial discontinuities and through intraepithelial channels (Cohen, 1979). Meurman and Ylipaavalniemi (1982) have shown that these channels are not observed in keratocysts, the epithelium of which is relatively impermeable to high molecular weight substances. Passage of glycosaminoglycans into keratocyst fluid would therefore be, in the view of Smith *et al.*, through areas overlying foci of inflammation, where the normal epithelial structure is replaced by a non-keratinized stratified squamous epithelium. They concluded from their series of studies that the release of these molecules into the luminal fluid could be expected to contribute significantly to its osmotic and hydrostatic pressures and hence to the expansile growth of odontogenic cysts.

Donoff, Harper and Guralnick (1972) have demonstrated the presence of collagenolytic activity on skin collagen in explant and tissue cultures of keratocysts but only when both epithelium and fibrous wall were present in the media. No similar activity was demonstrable in dentigerous cysts. They tentatively proposed that enzymatic mechanisms may be important in the growth of keratocysts.

Uitto and Ylipaavalniemi (1977) demonstrated collagenolytic activity in homogenates of keratocyst and radicular cyst walls. The cyst fluids of both inhibited this collagenolytic activity, but that from the keratocyst to a lesser extent than that from the radicular cyst. They pointed out that the activity of collagenase in tissues is probably controlled by a complex regulatory system and suggested that in cyst tissues this system might exert effects on collagenase activity, thus influencing the expansion of cysts within bone. In a later study from the same laboratory, Sorsa *et al.* (1988) showed that human keratocyst collagenase degraded type I and type II collagens at almost equal rates, but during the same time period no significant degradation of type III collagen occurred, a feature which also characterizes human polymorphonuclear (PMN)-type collagenase. The authors related this PMN collagenase and/or interstitial collagenase with 'PMN-like' characteristics, to connective tissue destruction associated with the growth of keratocysts. The mechanism by which PMN collagenase may contribute to connective tissue destruction in the absence of circulating inflammatory cells in the keratocyst wall, is explained by the authors as possibly the result of degranulation of subcellular compartments of PMNs stimulated by specific keratocyst antigen-induced immunocomplexes and/or by direct contact with the connective tissue being destroyed.

In a histochemical study, Magnusson (1978) demonstrated a high level of leucine aminopeptidase activity in the fibrous capsule of keratocysts. This enzyme has been implicated in the invasiveness of malignant tumours. This finding was confirmed by Chomette *et al.* (1985).

Radiological features

Keratocysts may appear radiologically as small, round or ovoid, radiolucent areas. Frequently, however, the lesions are more extensive. Most of them are well-demarcated with a distinct sclerotic margin as might be expected from

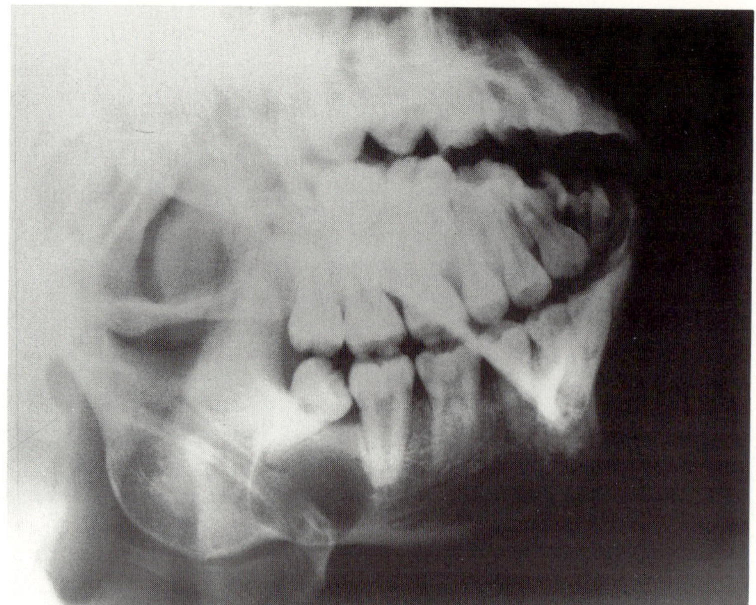

Figure 2.4. Radiograph of a unilocular keratocyst. It has a smooth periphery.

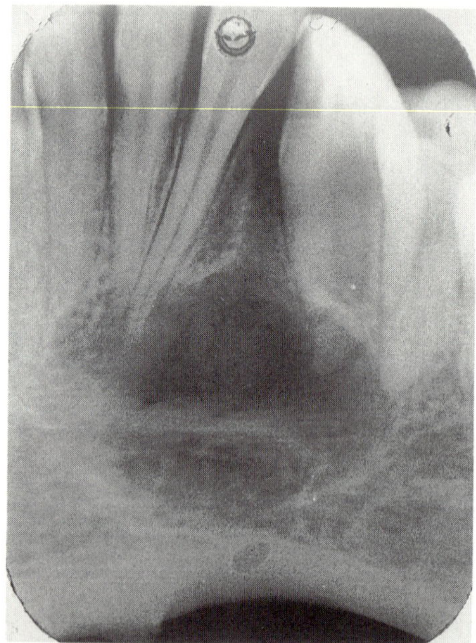

Figure 2.5. Radiograph of a unilocular keratocyst in the anterior region of mandible. The cyst has a smooth periphery.

slowly-enlarging lesions, but part of the border may be diffuse. The majority are unilocular radiolucencies, and many of these have a smooth periphery (**Figures 2.4** and **2.5**). Almost all the maxillary lesions are of this variety and tend to be small as they make their clinical appearance earlier than the mandibular lesions. Some of the unilocular lesions have scalloped margins (**Figure 2.6**) and these may be misinterpreted as multilocular lesions. Almost all of them are found in the mandible. The scalloped margins suggest that unequal growth activity may be taking place in different parts of the cyst lining and this may be observed in occasional gross specimens which are removed intact (**Figure 2.7**). Voorsmit (1984) described this group of keratocysts as multilobular. True multilocular lesions are not uncommon. Browne (1970) found 19 of 83 cysts (23 per cent) to be of this type, all in the mandible, and Forssell (1980) observed a frequency of 25 per cent in a series of 135, also all in the mandible. In the series of Voorsmit (1984), 13 of 103 keratocysts were found to be multilocular at operation. Only one of these was in the maxilla. Forssell has shown that unilocular cysts with a scalloped contour or multilocular cysts are significantly larger than unilocular cysts with a smooth margin. The multilocular variety is particularly liable to be diagnosed as ameloblastoma (**Figure 2.8**). The unilocular and multilocular lesions may involve the body and ascending ramus of the mandible extensively. There may be no expansion of bone at all, but in a substantial proportion of cases, particularly at the angle or in the ramus, expansion may occur (Browne, 1970; McIvor, 1972; Smith and Shear, 1978; Forssell, 1980). Expansion is usually slight but may be considerable in children. Both buccal and lingual expansion occur (Browne, 1970; McIvor, 1972). Voorsmit *et al.* (1981) have found xeroradiography a valuable procedure in demonstrating multilocularity or expansion of bone, but Voorsmit (1984) pointed out that although there may be technical advantages in xeroradiography, the radiation exposure is higher than with a conventional radiograph.

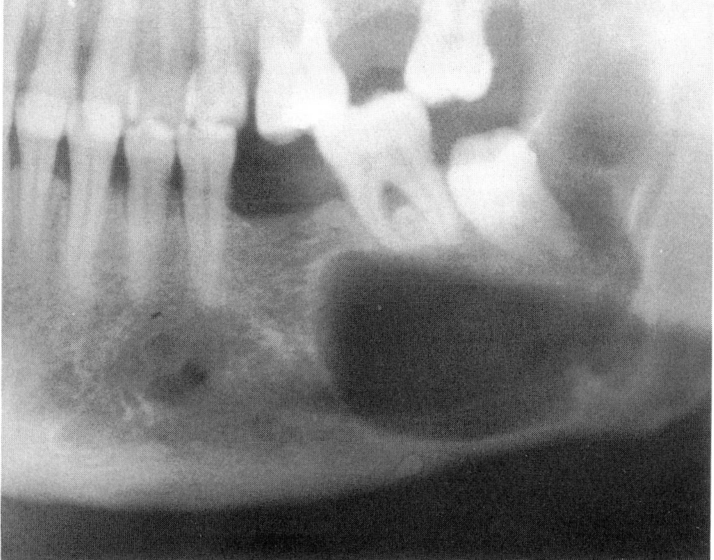

Figure 2.6. Radiograph of a unilocular keratocyst with scalloped margins.

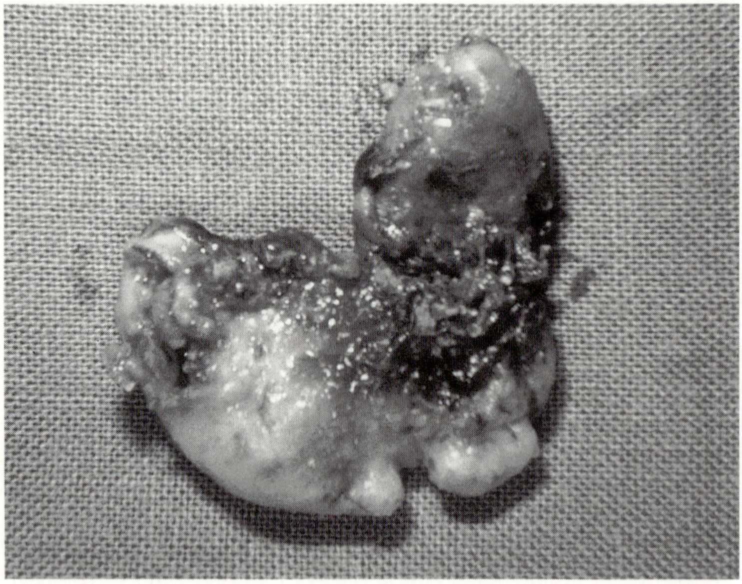

Figure 2.7. Gross specimen of the keratocyst in the radiograph illustrated in Figure 2.6. The cyst was removed intact and the unequal growth responsible for the scalloped margin may be seen.

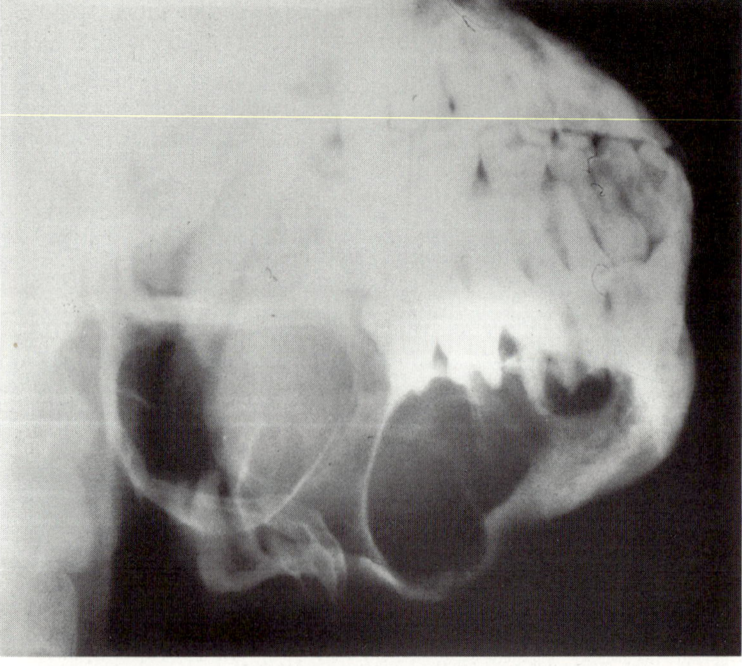

Figure 2.8. Radiograph of a multilocular keratocyst. The multilocularity was confirmed at operation.

Downward displacement of the inferior alveolar canal and resorption of the lower cortical plate of the mandible may be seen as well as perforation of bone (Smith and Shear, 1978; Forssell, 1980; Voorsmit, 1984), and pathological fractures may occasionally occur (Voorsmit, 1984). There may be extensive involvement of the body and ascending ramus of the mandible, with little or no bony expansion. Spitzer and Steinhäuser (1985) suggested that unilocular or multilocular radiolucencies distal to the third molar in the ascending ramus are very probably keratocysts.

Keratocysts may occur in the periapical region of vital standing teeth, giving the appearance of a radicular cyst (Wright, Wysocki and Larder, 1983). They may impede the eruption of related teeth and this results in a 'dentigerous' appearance radiologically (**Figure 2.9**). Forssell (1980) observed a relationship between the cyst and the crown of a tooth in 41 per cent of a series of 135 cases. This association was more frequent in the maxilla. McIvor (1972), however, demonstrated this relationship exclusively in the mandible. Such lesions are frequently misdiagnosed as dentigerous cysts and this has given rise to two misconceptions (**Figure 2.10**). One is that many dentigerous cysts have keratinized epithelial linings similar to those found in keratocysts; and the second is that dentigerous cysts may have an extrafollicular origin (Gillette and Weinmann, 1958). For all this, the point should be made that, very occasionally, the lining of a cyst in a true dentigerous relationship may be identical to that of a keratocyst. It was suggested by Browne (1969) that this occurs when an enlarging keratocyst involves the follicle of an unerupted tooth and fuses with the reduced enamel epithelium. He pointed out that in such cysts the epithelium immediately around the neck of the tooth is not keratinized and shows inflammatory changes in the underlying capsule. This concept has been developed by Altini and Cohen (1980, 1982) who have introduced the term 'follicular primordial cyst' (follicular keratocyst) for this group of lesions. They studied 17 cases in which the cyst lining was typically keratocyst on histological examination but which on macroscopic examination had completely

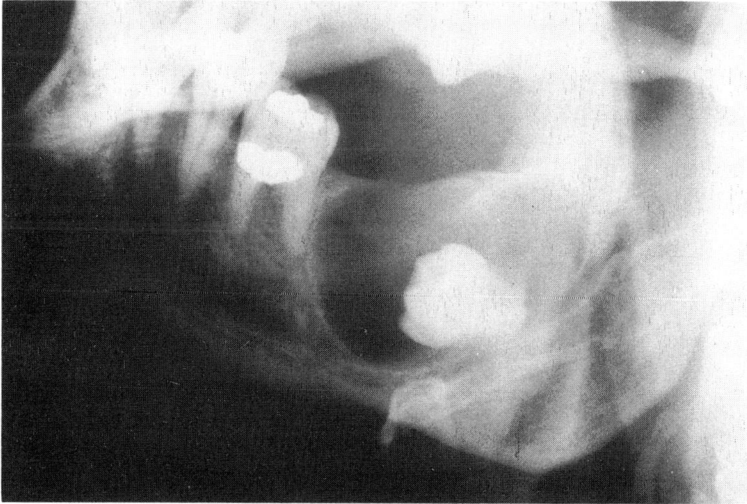

Figure 2.9. Radiograph of a keratocyst which has enveloped an unerupted tooth to produce a 'dentigerous' appearance.

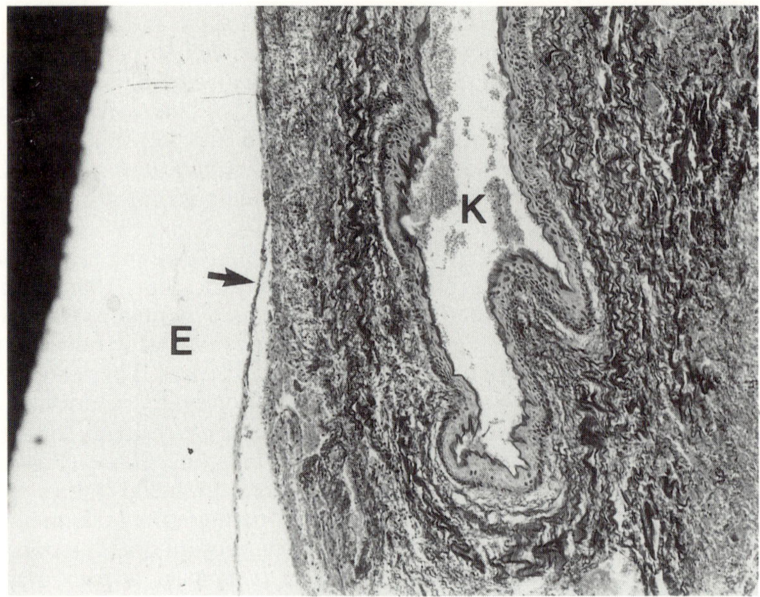

Figure 2.10. Keratocyst (K) which has enveloped an unerupted tooth. Enamel space (E). Reduced enamel epithelium of unerupted tooth indicated with an arrow. (Picromallory; × 50.)

surrounded the crown of the tooth and had been firmly attached to the neck. Eight of their cases occurred in the mandible and nine in the maxilla. Five of the latter were associated with canine teeth, one mandibular case with an unerupted premolar and all the others with third molars. Altini and Cohen postulated that follicular keratocysts might arise following eruption of a tooth into a pre-existing keratocyst cavity in the same way as a tooth erupts into the oral cavity (**Figure 2.11**). Histological study of their series of follicular keratocysts showed that the epithelium which lined that part of the cyst closest to the neck of the tooth was typically reduced enamel epithelium. This epithelium formed an attachment to the neck of the tooth and extended for a short but variable distance. Between this and the typical keratocyst epithelium which lined the remainder of the wall, and fusing with both, was a short segment of non-keratinized, stratified squamous epithelium.

In a later study (Altini and Cohen, 1987), they were able to support their hypothesis in a series of animal experiments. Four weeks after extracting deciduous teeth from both the maxilla and mandible of young Vervet monkeys, recipient sites were prepared by drilling holes in the alveolar bone and small pieces of autogenous palatal mucosa were placed in them. Of 33 implants, cyst formation occurred in 11. These cysts were filled with keratin and lined partly by a thick keratinizing epithelium and partly by a thin non-keratinizing epithelium only a few cell layers thick. In one of the animals killed after 52 weeks, the follicle of an erupting premolar tooth had collided with one of the cysts, the lining of which became incorporated into the follicle, partly replacing the follicular reduced enamel epithelium and forming an integral part of the follicle of the erupting tooth. In some serial sections the implanted epithelium accounted for up to 30 per cent of the epithelial lining of the follicle.

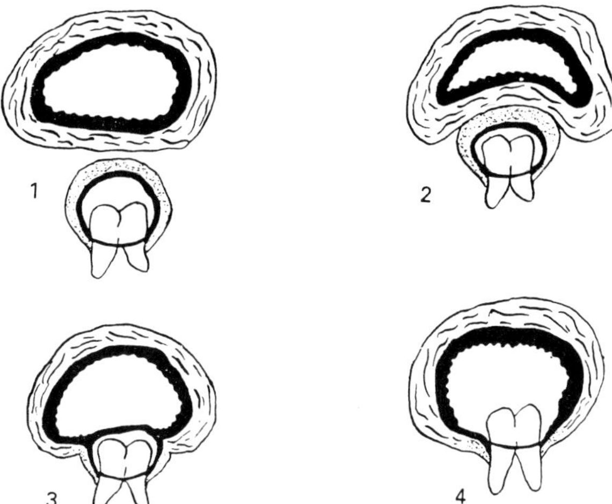

Figure 2.11. Histogenesis of the 'follicular keratocyst' according to Altini and Cohen (1982). A tooth surrounded by its follicle erupts into a keratocyst cavity in the same way as it would erupt into the mouth. (By courtesy of the authors and editor of the *International Journal of Oral Surgery*.)

Main (1970a) has referred to the variety of keratocyst which embraces an adjacent unerupted tooth as 'envelopmental'. Those cysts which form in the place of a normal tooth of the series, he called the 'replacement' variety; and those in the ascending ramus away from the teeth he referred to as 'extraneous'. Main proposed the use of the term 'collateral' for those keratocysts adjacent to the roots of teeth, usually in the mandibular premolar region, which are indistinguishable radiologically from the lateral periodontal cyst (**Figure 2.12**, and **Figure 4.7,** Chapter 4). In Forssell's series (1980) the 'replacement' variety occurred in 7 per cent of 135 cases, and the 'collateral' type in 19 per cent. Occasional cases may occur in the anterior midline of the maxilla and simulate a nasopalatine duct cyst (Brannon, 1976; Woo *et al.*, 1987).

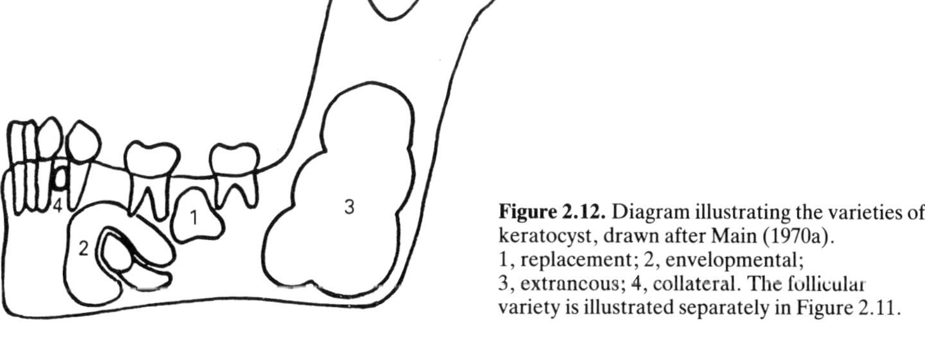

Figure 2.12. Diagram illustrating the varieties of keratocyst, drawn after Main (1970a).
1, replacement; 2, envelopmental;
3, extraneous; 4, collateral. The follicular variety is illustrated separately in Figure 2.11.

Keratocysts may, as they enlarge, produce deflection of roots of teeth. In Voorsmit's study (1984), there was a displacement of unerupted teeth in 33 cases, mostly in the region of the angle of the mandible towards the inferior border of the mandible and occasionally in the ascending ramus and towards the orbital floor. In our own material, root resorption has rarely occurred (Struthers and Shear, 1976), but Forssell (1980) has observed varying degrees of root resorption in 24 per cent of a series of 90 keratocysts associated with roots of adjacent teeth. Forssell pointed out, however, that a large proportion of these showed only a slight degree of resorption. McIvor (1972) noted root resorption in four of a series of 47 cases (8.5 per cent), while Partridge and Towers (1987) observed this in nine of their sample of 82 cases (11 per cent). In a radiological study of 103 keratocysts, Voorsmit (1984) found associated root resorption in only three cases (3.4 per cent).

Postoperative radiological examination is important in the diagnosis of recurrences which depends on the presence of a corticated radiolucency which increases in size on a series of radiographs taken over a period of time (McIvor, 1972). McIvor pointed out that a diagnosis cannot be made with confidence on a single film as the bony defect following surgical removal of the cyst may be indistinguishable from a recurrence.

Keratocysts may present radiologically in the globulomaxillary and median mandibular regions. The question as to whether globulomaxillary and median mandibular cysts in fact exist is controversial and is discussed in Chapter 9.

It is noteworthy that in the rather extensive literature published on the subject of keratocysts over the past 10 years by authors with considerable experience in the diagnosis and treatment of these lesions, very little reference has been made to the use of computed tomography (CT) in their assessment. Voorsmit (1984) described two cases in which this technique was used 'to obtain accurate measurement of the extent of the lesion, exact localization of areas of perforation through the cortex and, particularly, assessment of soft tissue involvement'. He considered that the reliability and accuracy of CT scans in the diagnosis of large mandibular keratocysts was striking and that the technique may be helpful for tumours and cysts of the maxilla, particularly where extension of the lesion to the cranial base is suspected. He described the important features of the technique as lack of image superimposition, preservation of soft tissue detail, selective enlargement of areas of interest, a high degree of accuracy and the possibility of three-dimensional interpretation. On the other hand, resolution of fine details is poorer than with conventional or xerotomography. The high expense of the procedure is referred to, but not the hazards of the radiation exposure.

MacKenzie *et al.*(1985) reported the use of CT in the diagnosis of a keratocyst and emphasized the considerably higher absorbed doses of radiation, particularly to the lens of the eye. In general, these authors stated, the absorbed radiation from CT studies is about 1000 times higher than those associated with a panoramic study. The associated risks, the cost of the examination, and the limits of the CT scan must be weighed against the additional information which can be obtained from the procedure before it is used on an individual patient. Swartz *et al.* (1985) found CT valuable in preoperative diagnosis and surgical management of odontogenic lesions including cysts but made no reference to the higher absorbed doses of radiation.

A report by a joint working party of the National Radiological Protection Board and the Royal College of Radiologists, while stressing the benefits of X-rays in diagnosing disease, commented nevertheless that the avoidable dose of radiation from medicine 'outweighs the combined contribution of all other man-made

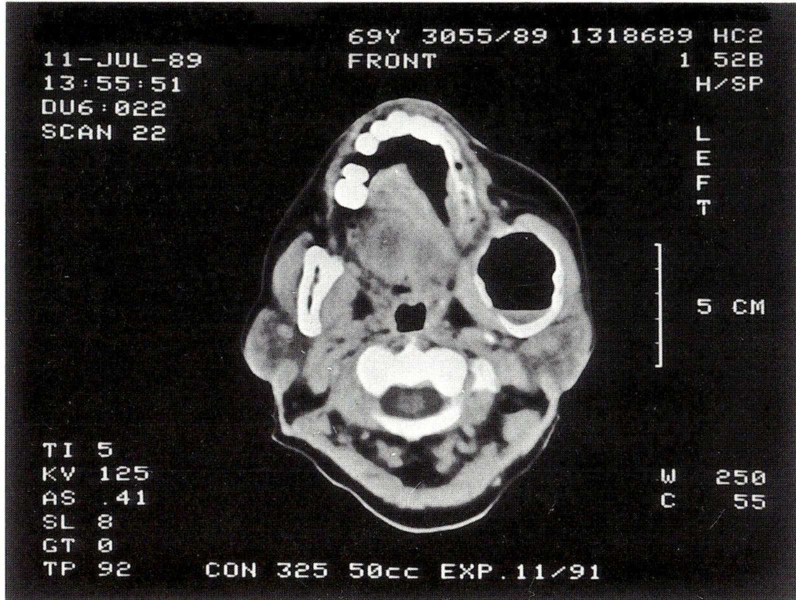

Figure 2.13. Axial CT scan showing a keratocyst in the left ascending ramus. There is buccal and lingual expansion, and thinning of the cortical plate which is breached on the lingual aspect. (By courtesy of Professor J. Lownie.)

sources of population radiation exposure by a factor of three' (Brown, 1990). Data obtained by the Board indicated that CT scans now account for at least 20 per cent of the total effective dose of diagnostic radiation to the population, and the secretary of the working party has suggested that radiologists should be informed of the 'high-dose implications' of CT scans. Wherever possible doctors should use the alternatives to X-ray, mainly ultrasound and magnetic resonance imaging.

Cohen and Mendelsohn (1990), reporting on CT and magnetic resonance (MR) imaging of myxofibroma of the jaws, commented on the advantages of MR over CT, but stated that CT is superior in demonstrating the involvement of the cortical plate of bone.

Figure 2.13 shows a CT of a keratocyst in the left mandible showing expansion of the buccal and lingual cortical plates of bone, and a perforation of the lingual plate.

Pathogenesis

It is generally agreed that the keratocyst is a developmental abnormality arising from odontogenic epithelium. Most of the available evidence points to two main sources of the epithelium from which the cyst is derived: the dental lamina or its remnants (Soskolne and Shear, 1967; Toller, 1967; Browne, 1975; Harris and Toller, 1975; Brannon, 1977; Gardner, Sapp and Wysocki, 1978) and extensions of basal cells from the overlying oral epithelium (Stoelinga, 1971a, 1973, 1976; Stoelinga and Peters, 1973; Stoelinga, Cohen and Morgan, 1975; Ackermann, 1976; Voorsmit *et al.*, 1981). The term 'primordial cyst' was first used by Robinson (1945) to describe a cyst of the jaw which he suggested was derived from the enamel organ in its early stages of development by degeneration of the stellate reticulum before any calcified structures had been laid down. He stated that primordial cysts may occur in single or multiple form arising either from an enamel organ of a single tooth of the regular series or from numerous aberrant dental anlage which become cystic. No histological description of the cyst was given in this paper.

There is still no direct evidence to exclude entirely the possibility of such an origin for keratocysts, but there is also little evidence to support it. Forssell (1980) has pointed out that the frequency of aplasia of the teeth is relatively high when compared with that of keratocysts and that the site distributions of these cysts and supernumerary teeth differ greatly from each other. It is clear from most of the reported series that only a small number of keratocysts (primordial cysts) have developed at a site where a tooth is missing but has not been extracted. The 'replacement' variety of keratocyst described by Main (1970a) would represent one formed in such a way. It is also possible, however, that a 'replacement' cyst might arise from a portion of the dental lamina which was destined to become an enamel organ (the so-called tooth primordium) and that the enamel organ subsequently failed to differentiate. In a series of 130 keratocysts reported by Reff-Eberwein, Donath and Schmitz (1985), only 2 could have arisen in place of a tooth.

As mentioned earlier, evidence derived mainly from the examination of keratocysts from patients with the naevoid basal cell carcinoma syndrome suggests that the cysts may arise directly from dental lamina (Soskolne and Shear, 1967). Satellite microcysts in the walls of the main cysts are often seen apparently arising directly from remnants of the dental lamina (**Figures 2.14** and **2.15**). The stimulus for this phenomenon is not known, but as the naevoid basal cell carcinoma syndrome is transmitted genetically as an autosomal dominant (Gorlin and Goltz, 1960), as the occurrence of multiple keratocysts in patients with the syndrome is a common finding (Meerkotter and Shear, 1964; Woolgar, Rippin and Browne, 1987 a and b; Dominguez and Keszler, 1988), and as multiple keratocysts occur in many patients without other overt features of the syndrome (Ahlfors, Larsson and Sjögren, 1984; Forssell, Forssell and Kahnberg, 1988), it seems likely that there is a predisposition in some individuals to form keratocysts.

Browne (1969) and Rittersma (1972) have suggested that as the naevoid basal cell carcinoma syndrome can appear in varying degrees of completeness, the presence of a cyst without other features of the syndrome may represent the least complete form, but Woolgar, Rippin and Browne (1987b) stated that the results of their study could be interpreted as evidence for or against that hypothesis. The frequent presence of satellite cysts, apparently derived from dental lamina, in the walls of keratocysts, suggested to Browne (1975) that there is a clone of epithelial remnants of the dental lamina which are genetically abnormal and prone to exuberant proliferation.

No one has yet demonstrated a familial tendency to develop keratocysts in the absence of other features of the syndrome, and although it is likely that their occurrence is genetically determined, this has yet to be proved.

The case for the origin of at least some keratocysts from the proliferation of basal cells of the oral epithelium has been put mainly by Stoelinga and his co-workers. In their histological studies they have demonstrated accumulations of epithelial islands in the mucosa superficial to excised keratocysts, especially in the ascending ramus. This phenomenon was particularly notable in cysts removed from patients with the naevoid basal cell carcinoma syndrome. These epithelial islands may sometimes be seen dropping off the basal layer of the surface epithelium and the

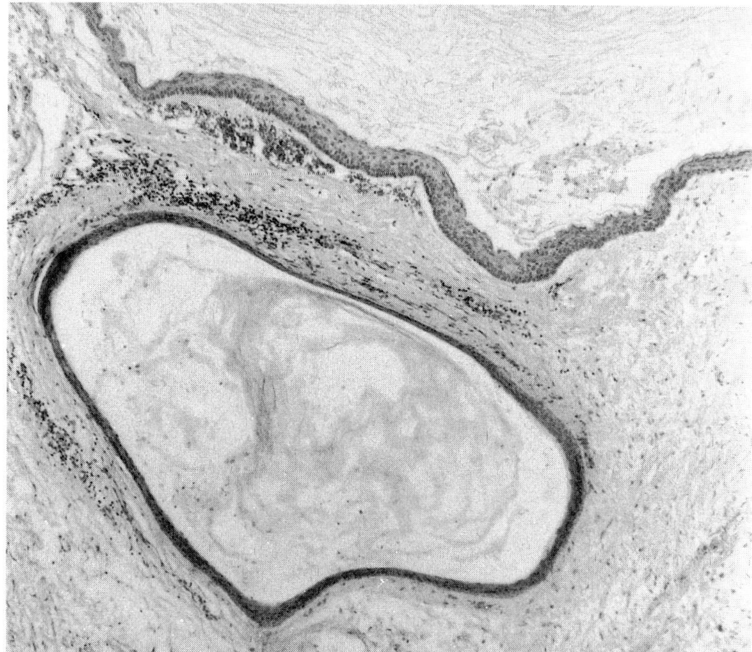

Figure 2.14. Satellite microcyst in the wall of a keratocyst. (H & E; × 60.)

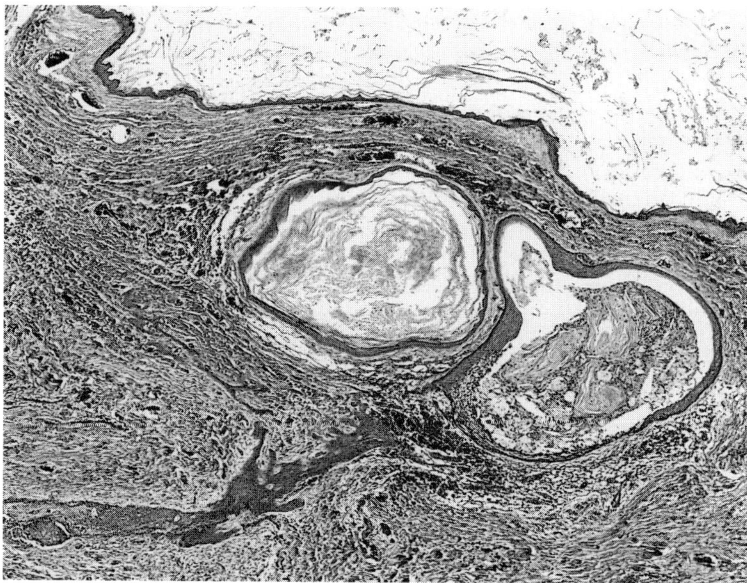

Figure 2.15. Satellite microcysts in the wall of a keratocyst, apparently arising directly from the dental lamina in a patient with the naevoid basal cell carcinoma syndrome. (H & E; × 30.)

cysts may be attached to oral mucosa through fenestrations in the bone. Although acknowledging that remnants of the dental lamina in the tooth-bearing area can probably still be considered as a prominent source for the development of cysts in that region, they stressed that even these are located primarily in the gingiva and that gingival adhesions of these cysts may therefore be expected. Frequently, however, keratocysts are located in the ascending ramus and have no relationship to a tooth follicle or dental lamina. Such cysts, they concluded, may have arisen from basal cell offshoots or basal cell hamartias which originated from the overlying oral mucosa. Shear and Altini (1976) suggested that such basal cell offshoots or hamartias may possibly be induced by residual ectomesenchymal influence in the tooth-bearing areas of the jaws. From the point of view of treatment, Stoelinga and various co-workers have proposed that overlying surface epithelium should be excised together with the cyst as this may avoid recurrences originating from residual epithelial islands and microcysts. They recognized, however, that after such excision, the repaired surface epithelium may have the same potential as the original epithelium for producing cysts.

Ostrofsky (1980) studied serial histological sections of 52 specimens of tissue excised from the retromolar mucosa of patients undergoing surgery for the removal of unerupted third molars. Of these, 39 specimens were found to contain cell nests resembling odontogenic epithelium, deep to the overlying oral epithelium. He concluded that these nests may be the 'hamartias' referred to by Stoelinga but was not able to determine whether they originated from dental lamina or from the basal layer of overlying oral epithelium. He felt, however, that the more mature cell nests may have arisen from dental lamina whereas the immature forms may have been relatively recent offshoots of the basal layer of oral epithelium.

The consistent finding of a keratinized layer in 'true' keratocysts, while this feature is so rarely seen in other jaw cysts, may be related to their origin from primordial odontogenic epithelium which has not yet differentiated and retains the potential inherited from its parent tissue, the stomadeal or oral epithelium (Shear, 1960a; Stoelinga, 1976). It has often been noted that dental lamina can give rise to keratin (Hjørting-Hansen, Andreasen and Robinson, 1969). Dentigerous cysts are lined by reduced enamel epithelium which only very rarely appears to have the capacity for keratinization, and radicular cysts develop from cell rests of Malassez which likewise seem to have very little potential for keratinization.

Atkinson (1972, 1976) has described the histological changes in experimental cysts produced by the transplantation of maxillary molars extracted from 10-day-old C57B1 mice grafted subcutaneously into adult mice of the same strain. After initial degenerative changes in the enamel organ, the reduced enamel epithelium changed to a hyperplastic stratified squamous epithelium in which there was cystic breakdown. This led to the development of cavities lined with a thick parakeratotic stratified squamous epithelium which resembled the lining of an epidermoid cyst. As the cysts enlarged the linings changed to a thin non-keratinized squamous epithelium.

Bartlett, Radden and Reade (1973) transplanted the first maxillary molars of 2-day-old C57B1/10 mice into the subcapsular space of the kidneys of isologous mice. There was no rejection or inflammation. Splits developed and enlarged in the enamel organ epithelium and had developed into keratinizing cysts in the 50-day specimens. No rete ridges or inflammatory cells were present, and the authors regarded the experiment as a model for odontogenic keratocysts despite the absence of other classic features of this lesion. Soskolne, Bab and Sochat (1976) have developed a technique for the production of keratinizing cysts in rat mandibles using autogenous grafts of interdental papilla implanted into prepared cavities. Ramanathan and Philipsen (1981) have done similar studies using intraosseous implants of rat palatal mucosa. Ligthelm (1989) developed an original experimental cyst model in Vervet monkeys and a genetically standardized line of rats (BD–IX–rats). He preformed the cyst walls by wrapping the animals' oral mucosa around a silastic tube with the epithelial surface against the tube. Donor tissue was transplanted into subcutaneous tissues and into prepared cavities in bone. Cysts developed in a very high proportion of the transplants. They initially had the histological appearance of the original epithelium, but the latter became thinner as the cysts enlarged.

Although these models were considered to be useful experimental techniques for the investigation of keratocysts, it should be borne in mind that keratinization is only one of the histological characteristics of keratocysts, and the fact must be faced that these potential models have, as yet, made little contribution to our knowledge of the origin, pathogenesis or behaviour of keratocysts. Virtually all our understanding of this cyst over the past 30 years has been derived from good clinical and experimental studies on human material.

Vedtofte, Holmstrup and Dabelsteen (1982) have transplanted human keratocyst linings into athymic (nude) mice. The cyst epithelium proliferated, and sometimes formed a new cyst in the host tissue. The epithelium retained its typical histological features as long as it was supported by its own connective tissue capsule. Epithelial outgrowths over mouse connective tissue showed an altered morphology. In most specimens the epithelium was keratinized but atrophic and the basal cells were flattened. The possibility that the primary defect in a keratocyst might be in the mesenchymal capsule rather than in the epithelial cells themselves was mooted by Browne in 1975, and other workers have referred to the mesenchymal influence in recurrences (Shear and Altini, 1976; Voorsmit *et al.*, 1981). Stenman *et al.* (1986) grew fresh tissue specimens from three keratocysts and three dentigerous cysts *in vitro*. There was a considerable difference in growth capacity. Within 2 days of explanting the keratocysts there was growth of epithelial cells which reached a peak after 14–16 days, after which growth slowed and stopped after 3–4 weeks. Fibroblast-like cells appeared in the cultures 10–14 days *in vitro* and after 2–3 passages most epithelial cells had disappeared and the cultures consisted mainly of the fibroblast-like cells. The growing epithelial cells showed moderate to high activity of NADH-diaphorase and acid phosphatase, which was most intense close to proliferating fibroblastic cells. These histochemical reactions *in vitro* were similar to those demonstrated in tissue sections of keratocysts compared with other odontogenic cysts (Magnusson, 1978). The authors considered the high levels of enzyme activity in epithelial cells adjacent to the fibroblastic cells of particular interest in view of the findings of Vedtofte, Holmstrup and Dabelsteen (1982), referred to above, and suggested that the close relationship with the mesenchymal cells of the cyst capsule is essential for the maintenance of this metabolic capacity.

El-Labban and Aghabeigi (1990) investigated the blood vessels in keratocysts and dentigerous cysts, both stereologically and ultrastructurally. No significant differences were found between them stereologically, using the volume and surface densities of blood vessels as parameters, suggesting that their overall vascularity may be similar. The ultrastructural study, however, showed considerable differences between blood vessels in the two cyst types. Fenestrated capillaries were found only in keratocysts. Another feature of the keratocyst was degeneration of the epithelial lining, associated with thrombosis. The authors suggested that the fenestrated capillaries in keratocysts and not in dentigerous cysts, might indicate a rapid transfer of fluid to meet the demand of active proliferating epithelium. They also suggested that proliferation of keratocyst epithelium may be promoted by growth factors released from platelets in the thrombosed vessels, as other workers had reported that a platelet homogenate fraction added to culture medium stimulated epidermal cell outgrowth and viability (Hebda *et al.*, 1986).

Pathology

Unless the cyst is small, the linings of keratocysts are rarely received intact in the laboratory. They are usually thin-walled, collapsed and folded. If, however, one is seen intact, the unequal growth which is responsible for the scalloped radiographic margins, may be observed (**Figure 2.7**).

The histological features are characteristic and have been confirmed in numerous publications (Shear, 1960a; Pindborg, Philipsen and Henriksen, 1962; Browne, 1971a; Brannon, 1977; Kramer, Pindborg and Shear, 1992; and others). The cysts are lined by a regular keratinized stratified squamous epithelium which is usually about 5–8 cell layers thick and without rete ridges (**Figure 2.16**). The form of keratinization is exclusively parakeratotic in about 80–90 per cent of cases, but is sometimes orthokeratotic (**Figure 2.17**) and both forms are found in different parts of some cysts (Brannon, 1977; Cohen and Shear, 1980; Voorsmit, 1984). A stratum granulosum is associated with the orthokeratin layer in some but not all cases. The parakeratotic layers often have a corrugated surface. There is a well-defined, often palisaded, basal layer consisting of columnar or cuboidal cells or a mixture of both.

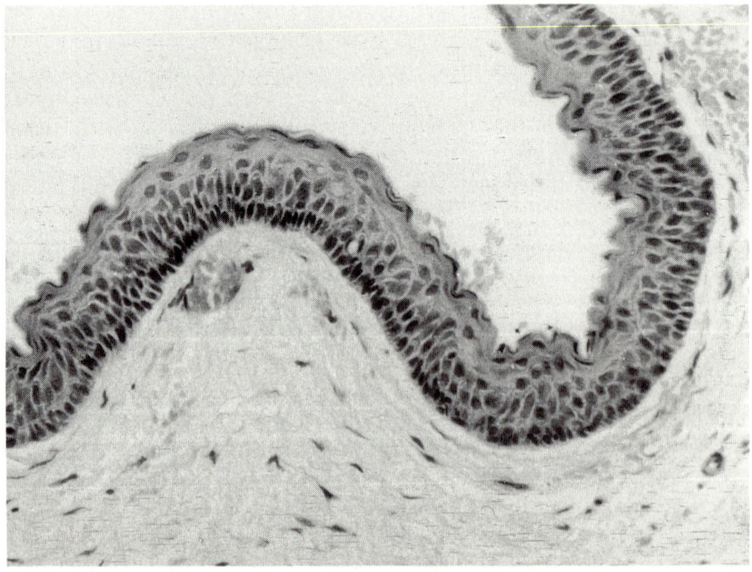

Figure 2.16. Keratocyst lined by parakeratinized stratified squamous epithelium. (H & E; × 270.)

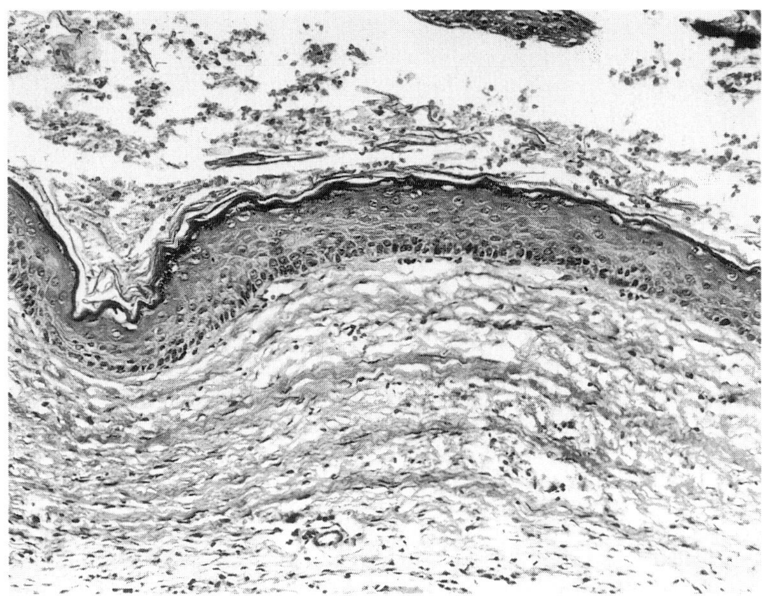

Figure 2.17. Keratocyst lined by orthokeratinized stratified squamous epithelium. (H & E; × 175.)

Cuboidal basal cells occur relatively more frequently in relation to the orthokeratinized linings (Cohen and Shear, 1980). Flattened basal cells may also be found in some orthokeratinized linings (Wright, 1981; Siar and Ng, 1988). The nuclei of the columnar basal cells in the parakeratotic linings tend to be orientated away from the basement membrane and in the majority of cases are intensely basophilic. This is a particularly important feature in distinguishing 'true' keratocysts from other keratinizing jaw cysts (Forssell and Sainio, 1979). Desquamated keratin is present in many of the cyst cavities. The cells superficial to the basal layer are polyhedral and often exhibit intracellular oedema. Mitotic figures are found in the basal layer but more frequently in the suprabasal layers (Browne, 1971a), and mitotic activity is significantly greater in keratocysts from patients with the naevoid basal cell carcinoma syndrome than from patients without (Woolgar, Rippin and Browne, 1987a). Some linings (**Figures 2.18, 2.19** and **2.20**) show features of epithelial dysplasia (Rud and Pindborg, 1969) and some workers, while stressing that malignant transformation in jaw cysts is extremely rare, have made the point that keratinizing cysts appear to have a greater tendency to such change than others (Toller, 1967). Browne and Gough (1972) proposed that keratin metaplasia in an otherwise non-keratinized odontogenic cyst may indicate carcinomatous potential, a view supported by van der Waal *et al.* (1985) who reported a well-documented case of a keratocyst which underwent change to a squamous cell carcinoma. Browne and Gough observed, however, that there is little evidence that the keratocyst is associated with malignant change more commonly than other types of odontogenic cyst. Ahlfors, Larsson and Sjögren (1984) found four examples with epithelial dysplasia in their series of 319 keratocysts but there was no case in which a carcinoma developed. MacLeod and Soames (1988) reported a case of a keratocyst which showed areas of epithelial

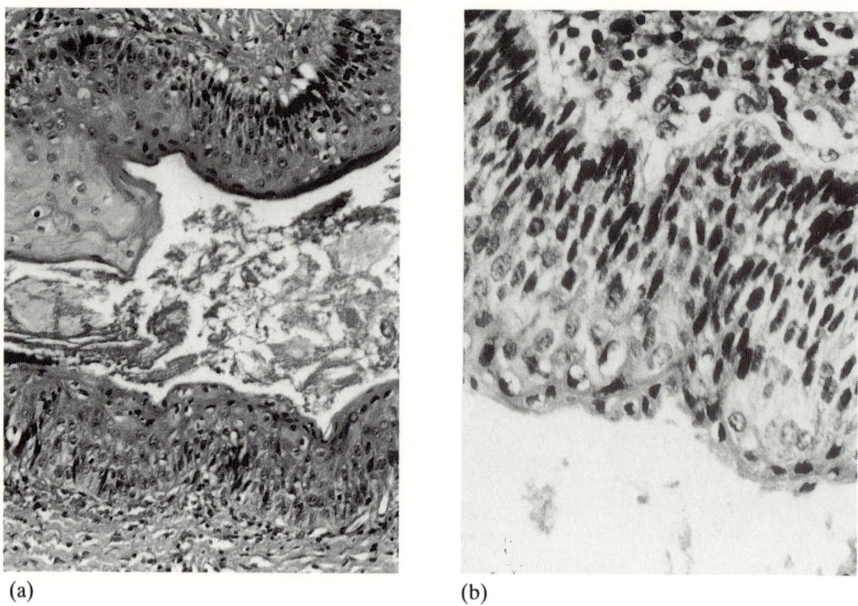

Figure 2.18 (a) Keratocyst lining with epithelial dysplasia. (H & E; × 85). (b) A different area of the cyst illustrated in Figure 2.18(a) showing the epithelial dysplasia. (H & E; × 310.)

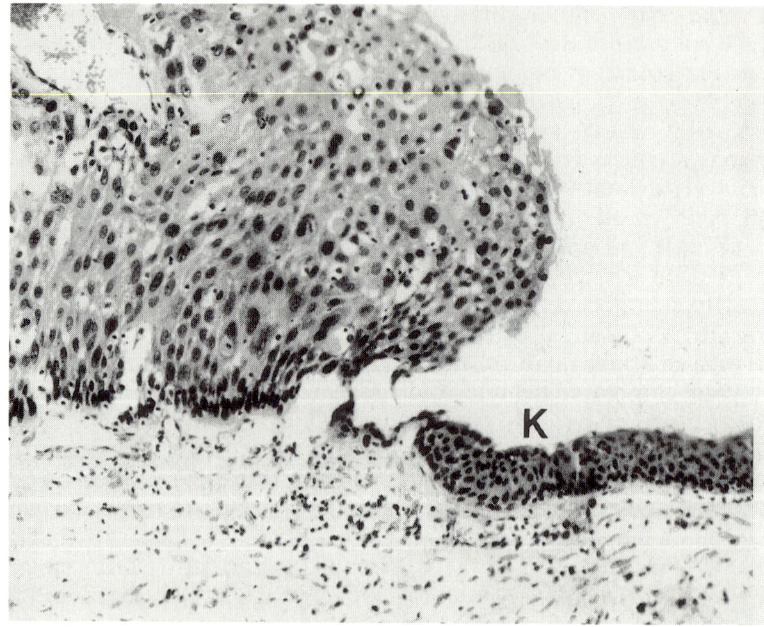

Figure 2.19. Keratocyst lining (K) showing severe epithelial dysplasia. (Section lent by Professor J. J. Pindborg.) (H & E; × 120.)

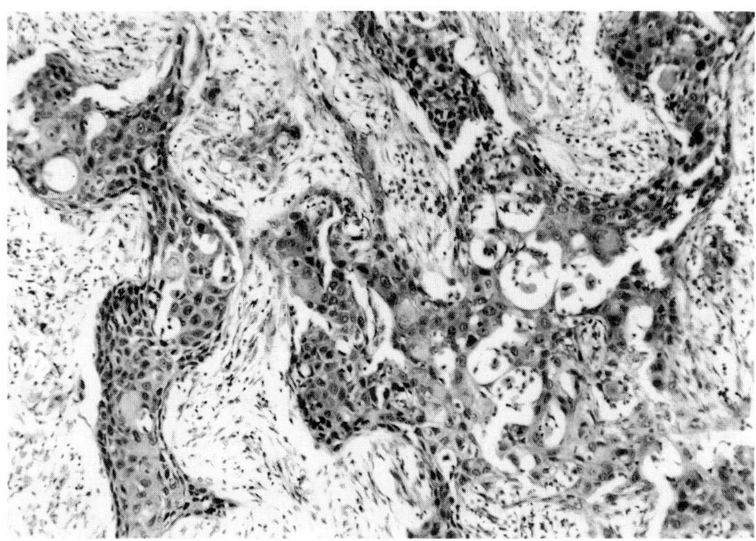

Figure 2.20. Infiltrating squamous carcinoma in another area of the cyst illustrated in Figure 2.18. (H & E; × 85.)

dysplasia and transformation to an infiltrating well-differentiated squamous carcinoma.

Using techniques that allow flow cytometry to be performed on tissue stored in paraffin wax, High, Quirke and Hume (1987) examined the DNA content of cells from a keratocyst which underwent epithelial dysplasia and malignant transformation. They showed that the DNA distribution in control keratocysts had a single large peak on the left-hand-side of the channel number scale, representing cells in the G0/G1 phase that are diploid (2N) value. A smaller and less well defined peak was seen to the right and represents cells that had passed through S-phase and were in G2 or mitosis (M) and have twice as much DNA (4N). Those cells intermediate in position were in DNA-synthesis (S-phase) at the time of staining. The keratocyst with epithelial dysplasia had a large additional peak to the right of the diploid G0/G1 peak and represents a DNA aneuploid G0/G1 component which has a DNA index of 2.0. The subsequent carcinoma demonstrates a smaller but significant DNA-aneuploid G0/G1 peak, also with a DNA index of 2.0. The authors were hesitant to suggest that the presence of aneuploidy in a single case may predict the future biological behaviour of these lesions, but as the measurement of DNA-aneuploidy from paraffin-embedded sections can now be performed easily and routinely, there is considerable scope for further study.

Cox, Eveson and Scully (1991) extracted DNA from a keratocyst and detected human papilloma virus (HPV) type 16 DNA sequences. They resisted the temptation to propose that HPV 16 infection may give rise to this group of lesions with a higher malignant potential. Their alternative proposal was that as HPV 16 is also found in a high percentage of keratinizing oral mucosal lesions, with HPV replication presumed to be dependent on differentiating epithelial cells for the completion of the virus life cycle, certain conditions such as keratosis, squamous carcinoma and cystic lesions such as in their case, may merely provide the correct type of differentiating cell in which a previously latent HPV may replicate.

Brannon (1977) pointed out that orthokeratinization was uncommon in keratocysts of patients with the naevoid basal cell carcinoma syndrome or of patients with multiple cysts and suggested that orthokeratinized cysts did not often recur. Wright (1981) confirmed the low recurrence rate of orthokeratinized cysts and suggested that these be regarded as a distinct entity. In the series of Ahlfors, Larsson and Sjögren (1984), all orthokeratinized cysts were single and none had recurred; nor had any of the cases of Siar and Ng (1988). Brannon (1977), Wright (1981), Voorsmit (1984) and Siar and Ng (1988) have all commented on the frequent association between orthokeratinized cysts and the crowns of unerupted teeth, and the relatively less aggressive behaviour of some of these may be because they are keratinized dentigerous cysts and not 'true' keratocysts. Ultrastructural differences between parakeratinized and orthokeratinized varieties have been demonstrated by Wysocki and Sapp (1975).

Vedtofte and Dabelsteen (1975) have studied the expression of blood group antigens A and B in eight ameloblastomas, 16 keratocysts from patients with the naevoid basal cell carcinoma syndrome, 11 keratocysts from patients without the syndrome, and 12 non-keratinizing odontogenic cysts, using a double layer immunofluorescence staining technique. All ameloblastomas reacted negatively, three cysts from the patients with the naevoid basal cell carcinoma syndrome reacted negatively and the keratocysts from patients without the syndrome, as well as the non-keratinizing odontogenic cysts, all gave a positive reaction. This is of interest in view of other studies (Dabelsteen and Fulling, 1971) which showed that there was a loss of blood group antigens A and B in dysplastic epithelium compared with normal oral epithelium. In a study similar to that of Vedtofte and Dabelsteen (1975), Wright (1979a) demonstrated a positive reaction for blood group antigens in all of four keratocysts of unspecified origin in patients with blood group A. He pointed out, however, that in all positive cases, positive areas alternated with negative areas and only between 5 and 50 per cent of all the squamous epithelium present showed localization of blood group A substance. In a later study, Vedtofte, Pindborg and Hakomori (1985) repeated some of the experiments done in the 1975 investigation. They demonstrated A, B and H type 2 antigens in keratocysts and in dentigerous and radicular cysts. They did not, however, detect *N*-acetyl lactosamine in the keratocysts as they did in the non-keratinized cysts. They emphasized the need to examine extensive areas of the cyst linings in order to ensure accurate sampling. None of these cell surface carbohydrates was demonstrable in a series of ameloblastomas, and the authors suggested that these immunohistochemical methods were useful in distinguishing the tumour from odontogenic cysts.

In a histochemical study of the cell membrane carbohydrate components in paraffin sections of keratocysts using horseradish peroxidase-conjugated lectins, Aguirre *et al.* (1989) demonstrated strong intra- and intercellular staining in the spinous and keratinized layers of three-quarters of their specimens using *Concanavalin ensiforme* (Con A) following periodic acid oxidation. The basal cells stained only at their bases. Con A lectin binds the neutral sugars D-glucose and D-mannose. This Con A binding after periodate oxidation is attributed by the authors either to an unmasking of mannose hydroxyl groups, or to unmasking of glycogen. In a parallel study on a series of ameloblastomas, Aguirre *et al.* (1989) showed a higher concentration of receptors for Con A and periodic acid–Con A in this tumour than in keratocysts. Saku *et al.* (1991) demonstrated that the lectins *Ulex europaeus* agglutinin I (UEA-I) and *Bandeirea simplicifolia* agglutinin I

(BSA-I) bound to the epithelial linings of keratocysts, dentigerous cysts and radicular cysts, but not to the epithelial component of ameloblastomas. They suggested that this could be useful for the differential diagnosis of cystic ameloblastomas and simple epithelial-lined cysts of the jaws.

The fibrous capsule of the keratocyst is usually thin with relatively few cells widely separated by a stroma which is often rich in mucopolysaccharide and resembles mesenchymal connective tissue (**Figure 2.16**). Inflammatory cells are very infrequent but there may be a mild infiltration of lymphocytes and monocytes. In the presence of an intense inflammatory process, the adjacent epithelium loses its keratinized surface, may thicken and develop rete processes or may ulcerate (**Figure 2.21**). In a series of 112 keratocysts examined to study the relationship between inflammation and the epithelial cyst lining, Rodu, Tate and Martinez (1987) showed that inflammation without the aforementioned changes in the epithelium was found in 10 cases (8.9 per cent). Conversely, no cysts were seen with such epithelial changes in the absence of inflammation. Hyalinization is sometimes seen in the capsules of cysts removed from older patients (Browne, 1971a). In 11 per cent of Brannon's large series, the cyst linings were intimately associated with surrounding soft tissues such as skeletal muscle, salivary gland and oral mucosa.

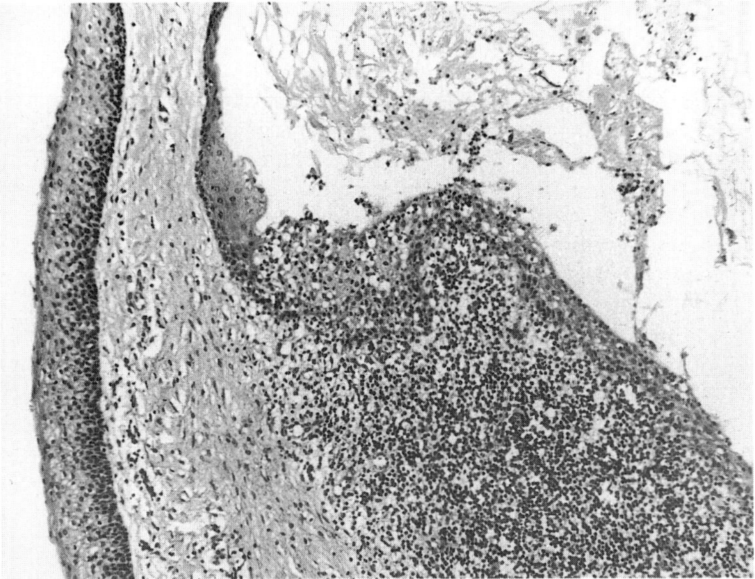

Figure 2.21. Inflamed portion of the wall of a keratocyst. (H & E; × 75.)

The attachment between epithelium and the connective tissue capsule tends to be weak and in many areas separation occurs. The collapsed and folded thin-walled cysts may give an erroneous impression of multilocularity in histological sections.

At intervals there are 'infoldings' of the epithelial lining into the fibrous cyst wall with resultant inlets of the lumen or crypts (Ahlfors, Larsson and Sjögren, 1984). That these are not merely folds of the lining following collapse of the wall on removal of the cyst, can be gauged from the fact that the cyst capsules are narrower at these locations than elsewhere and that the subepithelial collagen bundles follow the curvature of the fold while the main collagen bundles are arranged circumferentially. The authors considered that the infoldings may be the result of cyst epithelium being pushed into the capsule by active proliferation.

Satellite cysts, epithelial rests and proliferating dental lamina are sometimes seen in the cyst capsules, particularly in patients with multiple cysts and with the naevoid basal cell carcinoma syndrome (**Figure 2.15**). Although the epithelial linings of the cysts in the syndrome patients usually show the classic features of keratocysts, Waldron (1969) has described some histological variants. In some of his syndrome cases the epithelial linings were considerably thicker than in classic cases and showed prominent nests of basaloid cells budding off from the cyst linings. Detailed histological studies on the frequency of satellite cysts, basal budding, odontogenic rests, epithelial islands and 'ameloblastomatoid' features in patients with solitary and multiple keratocysts associated and unassociated with the naevoid basal cell carcinoma syndrome, have been reported by Ahlfors, Larsson and Sjögren (1984), Woolgar, Rippin and Browne (1987a and c), and Dominguez and Keszler (1988).

Ahlfors, Larsson and Sjögren demonstrated budding of the basal layer in 25 per cent of their pooled sample and much more frequently in patients with multiple cysts or with the syndrome, than in patients with postoperative recurrences; whereas Woolgar, Rippin and Browne found no significant difference in the frequency of basal budding between cysts which did not recur, primary cysts which eventually recurred, their first recurrences, and cysts in patients with the syndrome. Ahlfors, Larsson and Sjögren found islands or remnants of odontogenic epithelium in the fibrous capsule in 23 per cent of their sample with a substantially higher frequency in patients with multiple cysts and the syndrome and Woolgar, Rippin and Browne reported a significantly higher frequency of odontogenic rests and solid islands in their patients with the syndrome, but not between their control and recurrent samples. Dominguez and Keszler also found a significantly higher frequency of intramural odontogenic epithelium in their syndrome sample. Ahlfors, Larsson and Sjögren found satellite cysts frequently in the walls of those cysts in patients with the syndrome (50 per cent) and where there were multiple cysts (27 per cent), but only very rarely otherwise. Woolgar, Rippin and Browne observed satellite cysts significantly more frequently in patients with the syndrome (54 per cent) than in their control sample of keratocysts, as did Dominguez and Keszler. Woolgar, Rippin and Browne demonstrated solid proliferating islands of odontogenic epithelium significantly more frequently in the syndrome patients than in the controls but not between their control and recurrent samples. In the studies of both Ahlfors, Larsson and Sjögren and Woolgar, Rippin and Browne, ameloblastomatoid formations were occasionally observed; in the latter study, only in patients with the syndrome. None of these workers has reported ameloblastomatous change in keratocysts. Ahlfors, Larsson and Sjögren described the presence of suprabasilar clefts in the epithelial linings which were found more frequently in the recurrent, multiple and syndrome-associated cysts. They interpreted the split as a preparation artefact, but as they had only rarely observed them in other types of jaw cyst, considered that their frequent presence in cysts from patients who were prone to develop them may reflect an intrinsic property of the cyst epithelium.

Melanin pigmentation has occasionally been observed in the epithelial linings of keratocysts (Browne, 1971a; Macleod, Fanibunda and Soames, 1985).

Mucous metaplasia, hyaline bodies (Rushton, 1955) and cholesterol clefts are sometimes present in the walls of keratocysts (Browne, 1971a; Brannon, 1977; Voorsmit, 1984; Woolgar, Rippin and Browne, 1987a). Jensen *et al.* (1979) observed odontogenic epithelial cell nests embedded in nerve bundles in the fibrous capsules of two keratocysts. Their ultrastructural studies confirmed that these were epithelial and not the neuro-epithelial organ of Chievitz. They emphasized that such epithelial islands in nerve bundles should not be misinterpreted as neural invasion by carcinoma.

Mast cells were found to be present in substantial numbers in keratocyst walls, as well as in the walls of dentigerous and radicular cyst walls (Smith, Smith and Basu, 1989). The highest concentration was in the subepithelial zone where the count was 5.71 (SD $\pm$3.52) per microscopic field, the latter being defined as the area encompassed by a 1 cm^2 graticule. Mast cells were also observed in the epithelial linings, which the authors suggested implies a chemotactic stimulus to mast cells in odontogenic cysts, attracting them to the epithelial lining or luminal fluid contents. This work on mast cells followed three previous studies by the same group on glycosaminoglycans in keratocysts, dentigerous and radicular cysts (Smith, Smith and Browne, 1984, 1988a and b) which have been referred to earlier in this chapter in the section on enlargement of keratocysts.

Ultrastructural studies of keratocysts have been reported by Hansen and Kobayasi (1970b), Wysocki and Sapp (1975), Philipsen *et al.* (1976), Wilson and Ross (1978), Voorsmit (1984) and Herbener *et al.* (1991). Scanning electron microscopy of the parakeratinized forms showed a complex series of elevations and depressions on the cell surfaces; whereas scanning electron microscopy of the orthokeratinized variety revealed a uniform, flat surface covered with a thick layer of leafy squames of orthokeratin with no evidence of surface corrugations or deep epithelial infoldings (Wysocki and Sapp, 1975). Transmission electron micrographs of the surface of parakeratinized epithelium confirmed the presence of the cytoplasmic interdigitations and desmosomal junctions which give rise to the complex surface morphology. The orthokeratinized cysts showed a loose attachment between superficial shreds of orthokeratin and a compact layer of underlying keratin.

Using a series of 12 cysts from patients with the naevoid basal cell carcinoma syndrome as their material for an ultrastructural study, Philipsen *et al.* (1976) demonstrated that juxta-epithelially, deep to the lamina densa, the collagen showed signs of dissolution and often disappeared completely. They suggested that this process of collagenolysis might be produced by a collagenase or other proteases and it appears to be this phenomenon which is responsible for the ready separation of keratocyst epithelium from its supporting capsule. Tonofilaments occurred in increasing numbers from the basal towards the superficial layers, but unlike the situation in keratinizing oral epithelium, cytoplasmic organelles such as mitochondria, endoplasmic reticulum and Golgi apparatus showed no significant changes in structure or number through the strata towards the keratinized cell layers. This was interpreted as indicating that the cells of the stratum spinosum should be regarded as rather poorly differentiated. A feature of the cells of the stratum spinosum, was the presence of considerable amounts of glycogen, a characteristic which was also observed by Wilson and Ross (1978), Voorsmit (1984) and Herbener *et al.* (1991).

There has been considerable interest recently in immunohistochemical techniques that can be used to improve the accuracy of histopathological diagnosis. Immunohistochemical staining with monoclonal antibodies was used by Hormia *et al.* (1987) to study and compare the cytokeratin content of odontogenic cysts, normal gingival epithelium and ameloblastomas. They described cytokeratins as major structural proteins of all epithelial cells. Those identified in human tissues are coded for by two distinct gene families: Types I and II keratins. The cytokeratin filaments of epithelial cells appear to be heteropolymers of these two classes of proteins and any epithelium will therefore express at least two, but usually several, cytokeratins in a tissue-specific manner. Their results showed that keratocysts, radicular cysts and dentigerous cysts have distinct profiles of cytokeratin polypeptides and that with the exception of some dentigerous cysts, they all lack large cytokeratins typical of keratinizing squamous epithelia. With immunofluorescence microscopy, PKK2 (indicating the presence of cytokeratin polypeptides 7, 17 and 19) and KA1 (which reacts with cytokeratins in stratified squamous epithelium) antibodies reacted with all cell layers in keratocyst epithelia. With K_S 8.12 antibody (which reacts with cytokeratins 13 and 16) the suprabasal cell layers were positive. PKK1 and K_M 4.62 antibodies (which reacts with cytokeratin 19) gave a strong fluorescence confined to the basal cells and a few suprabasal cell layers. These reactions were similar to those in gingival epithelium. The authors concluded that epithelial cells in keratocysts thus appear to undergo a gradual maturation as they migrate to the upper cell layers, whereas in radicular and dentigerous cysts, no basal to apical differentiation was seen with these antibodies. A surprising finding in their study was the absence of cytokeratin polypeptides typical of keratinizing epithelia, namely, numbers 1, 9, and 10/11, in all keratocyst epithelia as judged by two monoclonal antibodies which react with these cytokeratins: KA5, and K_K 8.60. These keratins are typical of mature keratinocytes and their absence indicates, the authors suggested, that no true keratinization takes place in keratocysts. They concluded therefore that the presence of true keratinization is not a distinguishing feature of keratocysts. A more reliable marker, they suggested, is the presence of a cellular maturation gradient which can be detected histologically by an accentuated basal cell layer and immunohistochemically by the presence of distinct cytokeratin polypeptides in the basal epithelial cells of keratocysts.

Matthews, Mason and Browne (1988) examined 50 odontogenic cysts using an enhanced indirect immunoperoxidase method to investigate the expression of keratins, epithelial membrane antigen (EMA), carcinoembryonic antigen (CEA) and rat liver antigen (RLA) by their epithelial linings. In addition, proliferating cells within the epithelium were studied using the monoclonal antibody Ki67. As far as the keratins are concerned, antibodies having a wide keratin specificity (CK1 and AE1-3) showed homogeneous staining of the epithelial linings of all cysts with the exception of some isolated surface cells and goblet cells in some radicular and dentigerous cysts. The anti-stratified squamous epithelium antibody (RPN 1161) showed a consistent patchy reactivity pattern in all cyst linings but occasionally homogeneous staining of all cell layers was evident.

Using monospecific antibodies, keratin 19 was detected in the epithelial linings of all cyst specimens and was normally expressed by the majority of epithelial cells, irrespective of their level within the epithelium and/or differentiation. In contrast to the findings of Hormia *et al.* (1987), keratins associated with cornified epithelia (keratins 10/11) were detected in the upper suprabasal layers in 17 of their sample of 18 keratocysts. Matthews, Mason and Browne ascribed the conflicting results to differences in the techniques used, and advocated the application of monoclonal antibodies to dry cryostat sections. They suggested that the apparently keratocyst 'specific' profile (keratin 19, 10/11 positivity) is dependent on cellular differentiation rather than histogenesis or cyst type. Keratin profiles are therefore unlikely to distinguish between an inflamed keratocyst which has lost its typical histological appearance, and other odontogenic cysts which have keratinized epithelial linings as a result of metaplasia. The epithelial linings of all cyst specimens were positive with antibodies specific for keratin 13 and an epitope shared between keratins 13 and 16.

The authors found that expression of CEA and EMA by keratocyst epithelium was usually restricted to weak, patchy staining of the epithelial surface and superficial cell layers. Areas of keratocyst epithelium showing disordered structure often exhibited cytoplasmic staining of most cells, especially for EMA. RLA was expressed by the majority of suprabasal cells in all cyst linings and occasionally by all layers. Proliferating cells, detected by positive nuclear staining with Ki67, were present in the epithelial linings of all cysts, but keratocysts contained the highest number of them, most of which were located in lower suprabasal layers. Cytoplasmic staining occurred in the basal cells of keratocysts, similar to that found in oral epithelium. They concluded by indicating that expressions of keratins 7, 8, 10/11 and 18, CEA and EMA by the epithelial linings of odontogenic cysts is related to differentiation rather than cyst type and that both keratin 13 and 19 may provide useful markers for odontogenic epithelium as they have also been detected in ameloblastomas and in odontogenic epithelial cell rests.

Howell *et al.* (1988) demonstrated CEA immunoreactivity of varying staining intensity in all seven keratocysts examined in their study of odontogenic tumours and cysts. Both radicular cysts investigated, gave a negative reaction. There was, however, a reduction in the staining intensity and the number of positive cases in the keratocyst sample when absorbed anti-CEA antiserum was used to obviate non-specific reactivity, which suggests that their results were not inconsistent with those of Matthews, Mason and Browne (1988).

In an abstract, Morgan, Seddon and Lane (1988) reported that in their sample of keratocysts, dentigerous and radicular cysts, all the epithelia expressed keratins 4, 13, 14 and 19, and keratocysts expressed keratins 1, 10 and 16 in the upper layers.

These immunohistochemical studies are interesting and it is important that they be pursued because they are providing fundamental information about the tissues being investigated. Thus far, the diagnostic potential appears to be limited, and the variability of the results from different laboratories suggests that there needs to be further refinement and standardization of the methodology.

The consistent histological appearance of keratocyst epithelium, suggested to Shuler and Shriver (1987) that a specific set of genetic events might be responsible for its particular pattern of differentiation. As the pattern of expression of keratin genes had been shown to be closely linked to the differentiation of epithelium, and that specific subsets of the keratin gene family are found in specific epithelial tissues, they examined the specific keratin proteins in the lining epithelium of keratocysts by electrophoretic and immunologic methods in order to determine whether the unique histologic appearance is reflected in a reproducible pattern of keratin proteins. Such a precise pattern of molecular differentiation, they thought, could reflect the presence of specific local factors responsible for the classic pattern of epithelial differentiation.

Their studies were done on three fresh keratocyst specimens. Normal oral mucosa and maxillary sinus lining were used to obtain keratins for comparison. Polyacrylamide gel electrophoresis resolved identical patterns of proteins in the cytoskeletal extracts from the three cysts, which were in the keratin molecular weight range (40 to 70 kilodaltons). All three keratocysts had proteins with molecular weights of 46, 48, 50, 52, 54, 58 and 59 kD in this range. The qualitative and quantitative distribution of this group of seven proteins was identical for all three extracts. The 46, 48, 52, and 58 kD species were the major proteins present in this molecular weight range. Maxillary sinus lining protein extracts had only three proteins (46, 50 and 60 kD), and normal oral mucosal extracts had six proteins (50, 52, 58, 60, 62, and 67 kD) in a similar molecular weight range. Immunoblot analysis of the proteins with the antikeratin AE1 and AE3 monoclonal antibody, demonstrated that the previously identified proteins had keratin antigenicity. A positive reaction was observed for all seven proteins previously identified, but with variable intensity. The 46 and 58 kD major proteins were strongly labelled, while the 48 and 52 kD proteins were positive but less reactive. The 50 kD protein was more strongly reactive than would have been predicted by the silver staining. These findings were consistent with other studies which had linked epithelial differentiation and keratin gene expression and suggested a common pattern of gene expression underlying the characteristic histological pattern of the keratocyst. Further studies on other odontogenic cysts are required to determine whether this pattern of keratins is unique for parakeratinized keratocysts. Their finding of 50 and 58 kD keratins is consistent with previous studies that show that these keratins are specific for stratified squamous epithelium. The lack of keratins of molecular weights in excess of 60 kD is compatible with the hypothesis that these are found only in orthokeratinized epithelium and the orthokeratinized variant of the keratocyst might be expected to have a different set of keratin proteins, and consistent with the findings of Hormia *et al.* (1987), reported above.

Estimation of the soluble protein level in aspirated cyst fluid may be a valuable aid in the preoperative diagnosis of keratocysts. Toller (1970a) has shown that fluids from keratinizing cysts have soluble protein levels below 3.5 g per 100 ml (mean 2.2 g per 100 ml), whereas the values for non-keratinizing cysts were in the range 5.0–11.0 g per 100 ml with a mean of 7.1 g per 100 ml. Electrophoretic studies corroborated the finding that keratinizing cysts are very low in soluble proteins and Toller felt that a protein level of less than 4.0 g per 100 ml indicated a diagnosis of keratocyst. A value of over 5.0 g per 100 ml, however, would suggest a radicular, dentigerous or fissural cyst, or even an ameloblastoma. He postulated that fully keratinized linings are impervious to all proteins whereas the usual type of radicular or dentigerous cyst wall will at least slowly transmit the smaller proteins. In the presence of a fairly pronounced inflammatory reaction in a keratocyst wall, the degree of keratinization over these areas will be altered and this is likely to increase the permeability of the lining and result in a soluble protein level in the fluid higher than in the uninflamed keratinizing cysts. Toller's estimates of protein levels in cyst fluids have been confirmed by Ylipaavalniemi, Tuompo and Calonius (1976a). These workers considered that the inflammatory process itself influenced the protein content of the cyst fluid, not merely the nature of the epithelial lining.

Kramer suggested in 1970 that a preoperative diagnosis of keratocyst might be made by aspirating cyst fluid and demonstrating keratinized squames in a stained film. In a later study, Kramer and Toller (1973) reported on the combined use of exfoliative cytology and protein estimations in the preoperative diagnosis of these cysts. In some instances, when aspirates were sent in the post, a period of up to 2 days had elapsed before smears were prepared, but whenever practicable smears should be done as soon as possible after sampling. Smears are made by placing a drop of fluid on a clean glass slide and spreading with the edge of a dry coverslip. Two smears of each specimen are allowed to air-dry and are stained respectively with haematoxylin-eosin and by the rhodamine B fluorescence method (Clausen and Dabelsteen, 1969). A third is allowed to dry to a tacky state and fixed in a solution containing 75 per cent ethyl alcohol and 3 per cent acetic acid prior to staining with the Papanicolaou procedure.

Kramer and Toller examined a total of 56 jaw cysts and of these subsequent histological examination showed that 21 were keratocysts, 32 were simple cysts and three were cystic neoplasms. Examination for squames gave the correct result, namely keratocyst or not keratocyst, in 47 of the 56 cases. When this cytological procedure was combined with protein estimation of cyst fluid, the correct diagnosis was reached in all 21 keratocysts. There were six false positives among the other cysts and squames were also found in the fluid from a cystic carcinoma.

They found that examination of the exfoliative cytology smears achieves comparable diagnostic accuracy with each of the three staining methods and that this accuracy was similar to that achieved by use of the protein estimations. Although none of the methods gives complete accuracy, the number of incorrect diagnoses is reduced if smears stained by two or three methods and protein estimations are performed on each case. The smear technique requires very little material and this can almost always be aspirated even if the cyst contents are thick.

These findings have been confirmed by Smith, Smith and Browne (1986) who recommended the bromocresol green dye-binding method for albumin and the glyoxylic acid method for globulins because they do not appear to suffer from the non-specific colour interference or turbidity seen in the biuret method. They also advised that the the use of positive displacement pipettes is essential for accurate sampling of cyst fluid rather than air displacement pipettes because of the mucinous nature of some fluids. Fluid aspirates from their sample of 18 keratocysts showed very much lower levels of albumin, total globulins and total protein (4.70 ± 0.73 g per 100 ml). The higher proportion of albumin relative to total globulins in the keratocyst is reflected in the higher albumin:globulin ratio observed. They advised that protein analysis, qualitative protein electrophoresis and smears can be carried out on an aspirate of volume as small as 100 μl. In their experience, the combination of protein analysis and the demonstration of epithelial squames in the smear resulted in accurate diagnosis of the keratocyst in virtually every case.Voorsmit (1984) reported a diagnostic accuracy of 100 per cent when the combined techniques were used, using a total protein level in the cyst fluid of less than 4.8 g per 100 ml as an indication that the lesion is a keratocyst.

Kuusela *et al.* (1982) demonstrated an antigen in the fluid of keratocysts which was not present in the fluids of other cyst types nor in plasma or saliva. A double-antibody fluoresence technique localized the antigen to the epithelial cells of the keratocyst and they called it keratocyst antigen (KCA). In a later study from the same group, Kuusela, Ylipaavalniemi and Thesleff (1986) showed that KCA existed in keratocyst fluid as a 60–68 kD polypeptide with an isoelectric point of p*I* 6.8. Immunoblotting analysis of various isolated keratins revealed a typical polypeptide pattern of each keratin when anti-KCA antiserum was used for staining. These findings suggested that KCA and keratin are related molecules and that KCA may be a soluble component of keratin. They proposed that the keratin may become soluble in the cyst fluid by proteolysis and moreover, that the relationship of keratin and KCA would enable the use of commercially available antikeratin antibodies in the detection of KCA in the cyst fluids, thus making it possible to distinguish keratocysts prior to surgery.

In the search for either a single protein or group of proteins that is characteristic of a particular cell type, Douglas and Craig (1986) used immunological techniques to search for components of non-serum origin in cyst fluids. Separate antisera were raised against keratocyst, dentigerous cyst and radicular cyst fluids and used to analyse a range of fluids from cysts of known type. Samples were subjected to crossed immunoelectrophoresis into homologous antiserum through an intermediate gel containing antibody to whole human serum in order to screen out serum derived components. Their investigation identified the presence of a major antigen in the fluid aspirated from the fluid of keratocysts. This seemed to be of epithelial origin, but was not a keratin. It was present in all the keratocyst fluids assayed, despite total soluble protein concentrations ranging from 1.86–22.0 g per 100 ml. This antigen, which they named antigen X, was later identified as lactoferrin, a secretory substance present in the azurophilic granules of polymorphonuclear leucocytes and body secretions but not in serum (Douglas and Craig, 1987). They were unable to explain why lactoferrin consistently accumulates in keratocyst fluids. Its presence could not be attributed solely to the presence of inflammation, which is rare in keratocysts compared with radicular cysts, and lactoferrin was only occasionally found in the cavity fluids of the latter. They speculated that lactoferrin may be derived from the keratocyst epithelium, but preliminary attempts at immunoperoxidase localization of the substance in formalin-fixed keratocyst linings had been disappointing. Finally, they suggested that the polymorphonuclear leucocytes that do infiltrate the cyst wall act as the source of the lactoferrin in the fluid and, as it is unable to diffuse away into the surrounding tissues because of the relative impermeability of the keratocyst to proteins, its concentration may increase with time.

In the third of their series of papers on the subject, Douglas and Craig (1989) used a competitive enzyme linked immunosorbent assay (ELISA) to measure the concentration of lactoferrin in fluids from keratocysts, dentigerous and radicular cysts. Keratocyst fluids contained significantly higher concentrations of lactoferrin than fluids from the other two cyst types, but the range of values obtained within each group was large, and the lactoferrin concentration cannot therefore be regarded as an absolute marker for keratocysts. The lactoferrin concentration correlated very strongly with the numbers of neutrophils present in keratocyst fluids, assessed in smears, but not with fluids from dentigerous and radicular cysts. The authors suggested that neutrophils are the source of lactoferrin in the three cyst types and developed the idea mooted in their earlier paper, that the relatively impermeable nature of the keratocyst lining probably accounts for the particularly high concentrations of lactoferrin found in their fluids. The molecular weight of lactoferrin is in the range 77–85 kD and its ability to diffuse through the keratocyst lining is likely to be impeded. Speculating further on the presence of neutrophils in keratocyst fluids, the authors suggested that they may be a response to the keratin in the cyst lining, possibly mediated by interleukin-1 (IL-1) which is chemotactic to neutrophils. Much work remains to be done to pursue these interesting ideas.

As it is so important from the point of view of treatment of keratocysts that a correct preoperative diagnosis be established, these diagnostic procedures can be of considerable value.

Toller and Holborow (1969) examined 15 jaw cyst fluids by immunoelectrophoresis and found that cysts with keratinized epithelial linings had the lowest levels of immunoglobulins. Smith *et al.* (1987), in a study of immunoglobulin-producing cells in human odontogenic cysts, found that IgG-containing plasma cells were the predominant species in all cyst types with a much lower percentage of IgA- and few IgM-containing plasma cells. There were significantly fewer IgG and significantly more IgA plasma cells observed in the keratocysts than in the radicular and dentigerous cysts. IgA plasma cells appear to represent a significantly higher proportion of the total plasma cell population in keratocysts than in radicular and dentigerous cysts, although IgG cells still predominate. Generally, IgG plasma cells predominate in areas of diffuse chronic inflammation and the raised proportion of IgA plasma cells in the keratocyst may, the authors speculate, reflect the focal nature of the inflammatory infiltrate. They also found intense extracellular staining for IgG in the capsule and this they thought would support the view that the IgGs in odontogenic cyst fluids may be derived from local synthesis in the cyst capsules as well as from the inflammatory exudate. Further consideration of this subject will be found in Chapter 11.

Browne, Rowles and Smith (1984) found crystalline deposits in aspirated fluid of 38 per cent of keratocysts examined, compared with 10 per cent of radicular cysts and no dentigerous cysts. There was a high incidence of the crystalline calcium phosphates, hydroxyapatite and whitlockite in both types of cyst. Calcium and magnesium levels were within normal ranges for serum, but the levels of inorganic phosphate were considerably raised in the keratocysts and slightly elevated in the radicular cysts. The higher levels of these ions in the cyst fluids may possibly be responsible for the higher frequency of deposits in their walls.

Treatment

In view of the now well-known tendency for the keratocyst to recur, its treatment has given rise to much discussion among oral surgeons and is considered in detail in Chapter 18.

Chapter 3

Gingival cyst and midpalatal raphe cyst of infants

The gingival cyst and the midpalatal raphe cyst of infants are conveniently discussed together because of clinical features which they share, although the first is of odontogenic origin and the latter of developmental non-odontogenic origin. In view of their different histogeneses, they are separated in the classification.

Clinical features

The frequency of gingival cysts is high in newborn infants but they are rarely seen after 3 months of age. It is apparent that most of them undergo involution and disappear, or rupture through the surface epithelium and exfoliate, as very few are submitted for pathological examination. Monteleone and McLellan (1964) and Fromm (1967) have done extensive clinical surveys of newborn infants to look for nodules in the mouth, frequently referred to as Bohn's nodules or Epstein's pearls. There is some confusion about the two eponyms and their relation to gingival cysts. It would appear that Epstein's pearls are those which occur along the mid-palatine raphe and are not of odontogenic origin, whereas Bohn's nodules are found on the buccal or lingual aspects of the dental ridges. Fromm (1967) pointed out moreover that Bohn was writing about remnants of mucous glands and had called them 'mucous gland cysts'. Gingival cysts, according to Fromm, are found only on the crests of the maxillary and mandibular dental ridges. For all this, the three terms are frequently used synonymously.

Monteleone and McLellan found nodules in the midpalatine raphe region of 79 per cent of black infants and 85 per cent of white infants. The incidence in Fromm's study was 76 per cent, most of which were along the midpalatal raphe at the junction of hard and soft palates. They were found less frequently along the maxillary dental ridge and least of all along the crest of the mandibular ridge. The nodules were 2–3 mm in diameter. Some infants had only one cyst, some had many, but usually there were five or six. Very few infants had more than one or two along the dental ridges. They are white or cream-coloured (**Figure 3.1**). Their absence from the soft palate was explained by Burdi (1968) whose embryological studies suggested that a consolidation of the soft palate and uvula takes place not by fusion but by subepithelial mesenchymal merging of bilateral primordia without direct apposition and breakdown of epithelium.

Common as they are in infants, gingival cysts are extremely rare over 3 months of age. Saunders (1972), however, has reported a case in a 3-month-old child and some occur in adults although these are of a different nature and are discussed in Chapter 4.

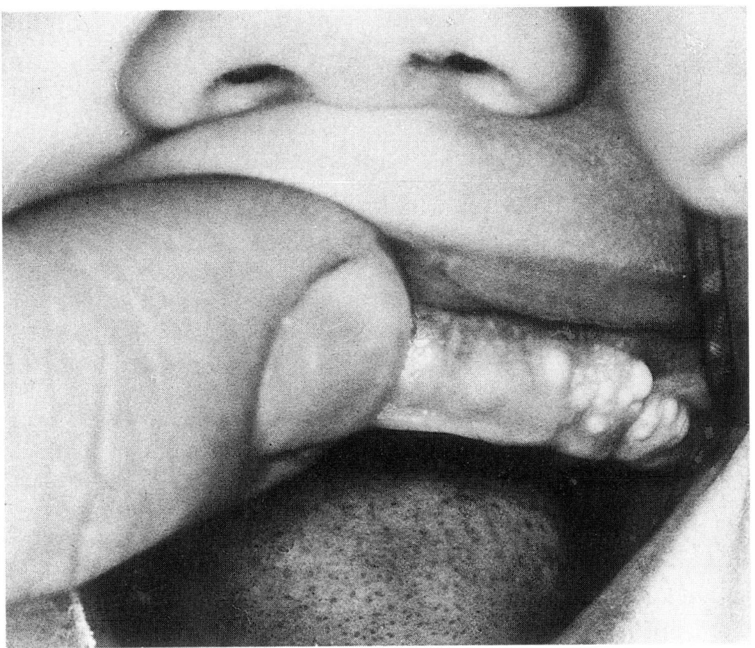

Figure 3.1. Gingival cysts in an infant. (By courtesy of Professor J. J. Pindborg.)

Pathogenesis

There is general agreement that gingival cysts in infants arise from the dental lamina. Stout, Lunin and Calonius (1968) studied epithelial remnants in fetal, infant and adult material. In human fetuses aged between 10 and 12 weeks there was evidence of small amounts of keratin formation in fragmented portions of dental lamina. By late in the 12th week the dental laminae were fragmented and many fragments showed keratin cyst formation (**Figure 3.2**). They found epithelial remnants or gingival cysts in the maxillae of 109 infants ranging in age from birth to 4 years who were examined at autopsy. In their adult material, only one of 266 subjects had a cyst although epithelial nests were demonstrated in 90.

The epithelial remnants of the dental lamina, the so-called glands of Serres, have the capacity, from as early a stage in development as 10 weeks *in utero*, to proliferate, keratinize and form small cysts. Moskow and Bloom (1983) noted in human fetal material that as tooth development progresses, but prior to separation of the tooth germ from the oral epithelium, a proliferative tendency was often noted in the dental lamina with the formation of multiple areas of distinct microcyst formation and keratin production. In the morphodifferentiation (late bell) stage of tooth development, according to Moskow and Bloom, disintegration of the dental lamina begins to occur and numerous islands and strands of odontogenic epithelium are seen in the corium between the tooth germ and the oral epithelium, remote from the developing alveolar process. Those dental lamina remnants which had already evolved into small cysts, expanded rapidly at this stage (15–20 week embryos) and there was thinning of the overlying oral epithelium.

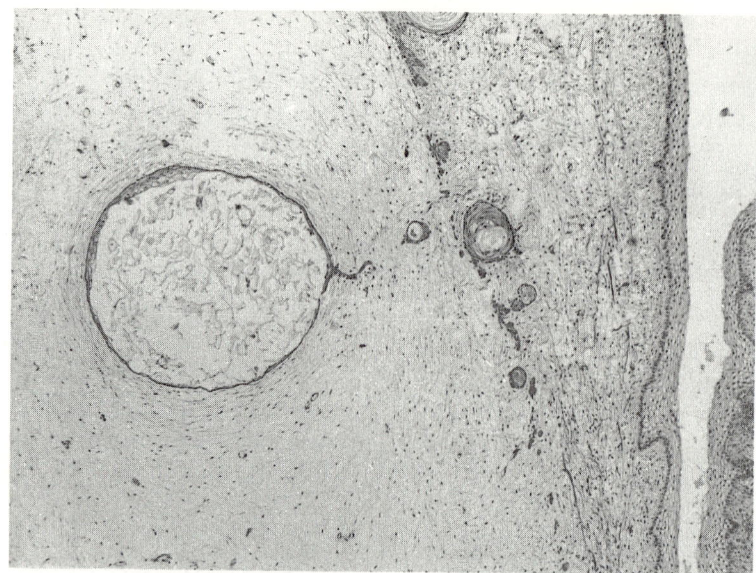

Figure 3.2. Fragmentation of dental lamina with formation of microcysts containing keratin in the developing alveolus of a human embryo of crown–rump length 135 mm. (Section lent by Professor C. W. van Wyk.) (Van Gieson; × 50.)

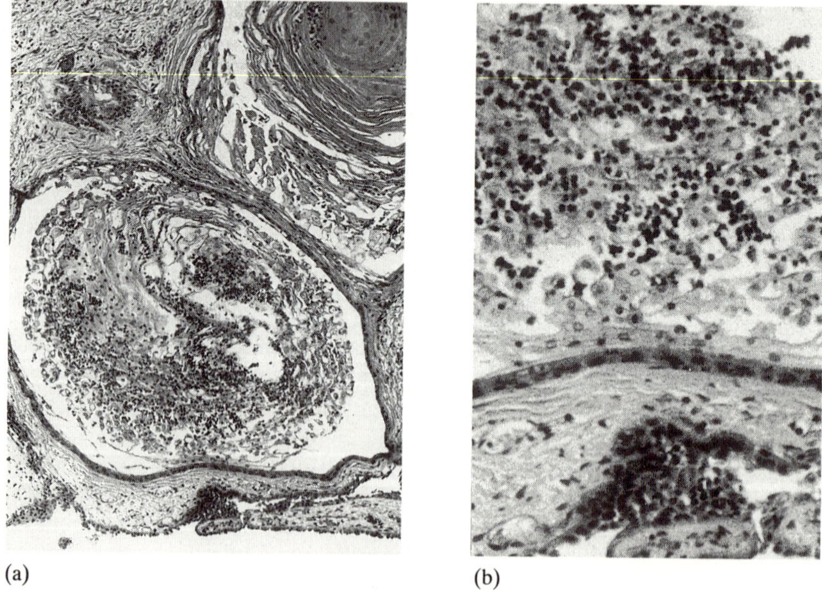

(a) (b)

Figure 3.3. (a) Gingival cyst in an infant. Epithelial-lined clefts extend between cyst and surface. (Section lent by Professor W. G. Shafer.) (H & E; × 27.) (b) Higher magnification of portion of the gingival cyst illustrated in (a). (H & E; × 150.)

Some of the gingival cysts probably open onto the surface leaving clefts (**Figure 3.3**); others may be involved by developing teeth. Some degenerate and disappear, the keratin and debris being digested by giant cells. Saunders (1972) reported that when he incised the mucosa over one of these cysts the contents were ejected, suggesting that they might be under pressure. Very few, as previously mentioned, become clinical problems.

The cysts along the midpalatal raphe have a different origin. They arise from epithelial inclusions at the line of fusion of the palatal folds and the nasal processes. This is normally completed by the end of the fourth month. After birth the epithelial inclusions usually atrophy and become resorbed. Some may however produce keratin-containing microcysts (**Figure 3.3**) which extend to the surface and rupture during the first few months after birth. Burke *et al.* (1966) confirmed the presence of frequent palatine raphe cysts but suggested the possibility that they may represent abortive glandular differentiation leading to cyst formation.

In a meticulous study on serial sections of 32 human heads, approximately 8–22 weeks of fetal age, Moreillon and Schroeder (1982) showed that keratinizing microcysts which develop from the dental lamina increase in number from the 12th to the 22nd week with a maximum of 190 cysts per fetus. Not more than 20 midpalatal raphe cysts were found in any fetus by week 14 and they do not increase in frequency with time. These authors' observations suggested that as the cysts developed, their epithelium differentiated, fused with the oral epithelium and their contents were discharged.

It is of considerable importance to note that the ability of the dental lamina to proliferate in the course of development of the gingival cyst of infants, is of limited potential, quite unlike that of the keratocyst in which a common pattern of gene

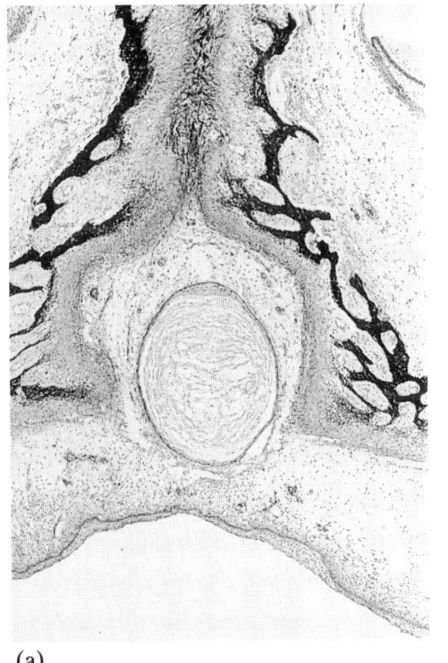

(a)

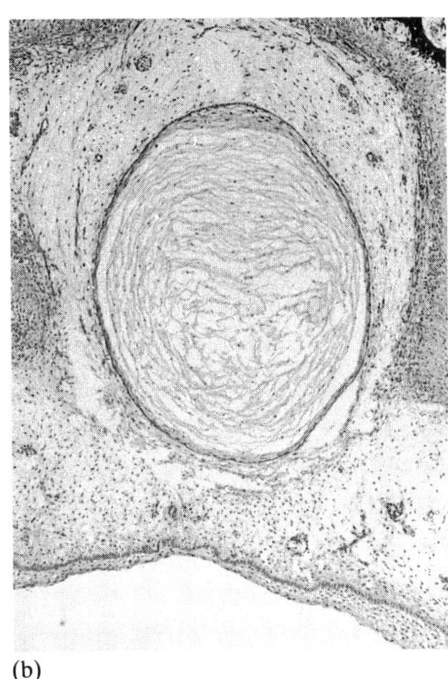

(b)

Figure 3.4. (a) Midpalatal raphe cyst in a human embryo or crown–rump length 135 mm. (Section lent by Professor C. W. van Wyk.) (Van Gieson; × 20.) (b) Higher magnification of midpalatal raphe cyst illustrated in (a). (H & E; × 45.)

expression appears to underlie the characteristic histological pattern (Shuler and Shriver, 1987), and possibly therefore, its behaviour. The subsequent growth and behaviour of the two lesions are decidedly different, despite their common origin.

Pathology

The cysts are round or ovoid and may have a smooth or an undulating outline in histological sections. There is a thin lining of stratified squamous epithelium with a parakeratotic surface and keratin fills the cyst cavity, usually in concentric laminations containing flattened cell nuclei (Moskow and Bloom, 1983). The basal cells are flat, unlike those in the keratocyst. Epithelial-lined clefts may develop between the cyst and the surface oral epithelium. As a result of pressure from the cyst, the oral epithelium may be atrophic (**Figure 3.3**). Midpalatal raphe cysts have a similar histological appearance (**Figure 3.4**).

Garlick *et al.* (1989) have described a congenital gingival cyst 1 cm in diameter, with the histological features of a gingival cyst of adults, but I have not encountered any similar reports.

Treatment

There is no indication for any treatment of gingival cysts or of midpalatal raphe cysts in infants.

Chapter 4

Gingival cyst of adults, lateral periodontal cyst, botryoid odontogenic cyst and glandular (sialo-)odontogenic cyst

There is a great deal of confusion about the relationship between the gingival cyst of adults and the lateral periodontal cyst, much of which appears to have arisen because both types of cyst have a predilection for occurrence in the canine and premolar area of the mandible. The pathogenesis of these cysts, particularly with regard to the cells of origin, is also far from clear. This confusion is further complicated by the fact that many cysts in the lateral periodontal position are really keratocysts (Soskolne and Shear, 1967), while others are of inflammatory origin arising adjacent to an accessory root canal in the presence of a necrotic pulp, or by infection through the gingival crevice. Bhaskar (1965) grouped the gingival and lateral periodontal cysts together as gingival cysts and considered that they both arise from extraosseous odontogenic epithelium although 13 of his 29 cases showed circumscribed radiolucencies indicative of lateral periodontal cysts. He believed that the radiolucencies were the result of cup-shaped depressions on the periosteal surfaces of the cortical plates produced by enlargement of the gingival cysts. Wysocki *et al.* (1980) postulated, on the basis of the clinical and morphological similarities between the two cysts, that they have a common histogenesis and that they represent the intraosseous and extraosseous manifestations of the same lesion. Shear and Pindborg (1975) regarded them as distinct lesions, as did Buchner and Hansen (1979) who suggested, however, that they were probably of the same epithelial origin.

The gingival cysts may certainly occur without bone involvement and may produce a gingival swelling, although usually they go unnoticed and most of them have been detected in the course of histological examination of large numbers of gingival biopsies (Moskow, 1966). Ritchey and Orban (1953) discovered six such cysts in 350 gingival biopsies. It is improbable, though not impossible, that a cyst originating in the gingival soft tissues could enlarge sufficiently to produce a radiologically obvious bone erosion without producing any gingival swelling. Yet many lateral periodontal cysts are discovered on routine radiological examination in the absence of any clinical symptoms or signs (Moskow *et al.*, 1970; Gold and Sliwkowski, 1973; Fantasia, 1979). These are likely to have arisen within the periodontal ligament and eroded outwards. In the case of lesions which have produced both gingival swelling and a radiolucency, a faint shadow indicates a surface depression and hence a gingival cyst (**Figure 4.1**). Where the radiolucency is dark and sharply demarcated then communication with the periodontium is indicated and the lesion is more likely to be a lateral periodontal cyst which has eroded outwards (see **Figure 4.11**). These assumptions, based on the radiological

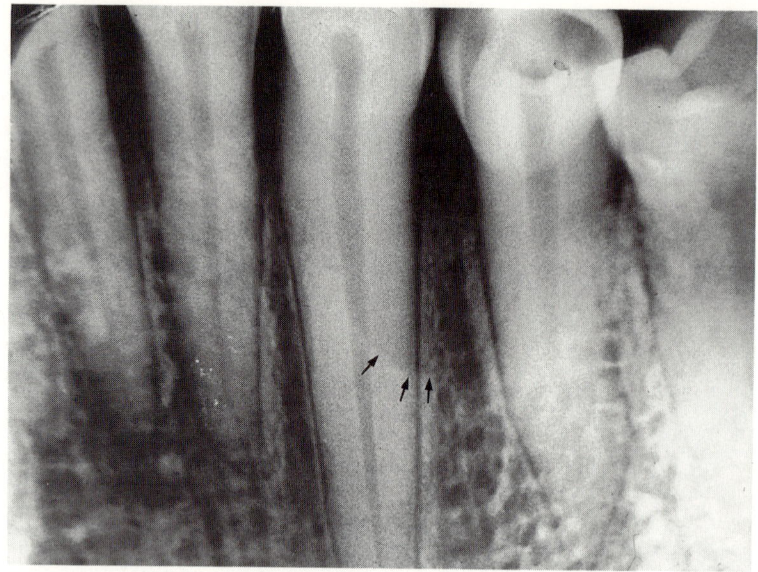

Figure 4.1. Gingival cyst in an adult. There is a faint radiographic shadow (arrowed) indicative of surface bone erosion.

features, can be confirmed by surgical exploration when the lesion is being removed.

Gingival cyst of adults

Clinical features

As most published studies have, until fairly recently, combined gingival and lateral periodontal cysts, meaningful clinical data have been difficult to obtain. Relatively few cases have been recorded in our own archives and most publications on the subject have reported only single cases or small series. This suggests that there may, in the past, have been a lack of awareness of the lesion among clinicians, a situation which appears to be changing. Furthermore, many gingival cysts may not enlarge sufficiently to produce symptoms.

Reeve and Levy (1968) reported four cases and Buchner and Hansen (1979) published a series of 33 cases of gingival cyst of adults. Only soft tissue lesions of the gingiva with no bony involvement, or only superficial bone erosion on surgical exploration, were included in the latter study. Of their 33 cases, seven were found to be epidermoid cysts or keratocysts on histological examination and are best excluded if a critical assessment of the gingival cyst of adults is to be done. Wysocki *et al.* (1980) have reported another 10 examples. Nxumalo and Shear (1990, 1992) studied a series of 14 cases of their own and pooled their clinical data with those in the cases reported above. Epidermoid cysts of the gingiva and those with typical keratocyst linings were excluded from their investigation.

Frequency

In our own material, only 14 of the series of 2616 cysts of the jaws (0.5 per cent) were gingival cysts of adults (**Table 2.1**, p. 6). The true frequency is probably higher than this as some cases are probably not submitted to the pathologist because so little tissue might have been retrieved at surgery. In the study of Buchner and Hansen (1979), the 33 cases were retrieved from 21 503 surgical specimens over an 11-year period.

Age

Most cases of gingival cyst of the adult occur in the fifth and sixth decades. The age distribution of 40 cases including 10 of our own, four reported by Reeve and Levy (1968) and 26 by Buchner and Hansen (1979) is shown in **Figure 4.2**. This number

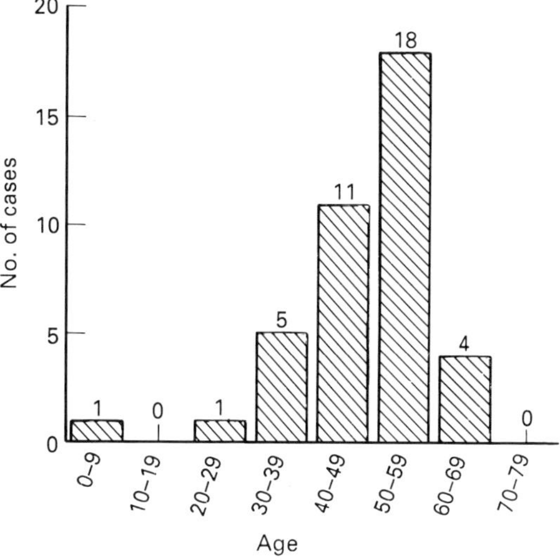

Figure 4.2. Age distribution of 40 patients with gingival cysts of the adult.

excludes the seven cases of Buchner and Hansen which showed the histological features of epidermoid cysts or keratocysts. Dr Buchner kindly provided me with the additional information. In the series of 10 cases reported by Wysocki *et al.* (1980) the patients ranged in age from 41 to 75 with a mean of 50.7 and a median of 47 years.

Sex

Three of the four patients in the sample of Reeve and Levy (1968) were females, and of the 26 histologically confirmed cases reported by Buchner and Hansen (1979), 17 (65 per cent) involved females and nine (35 per cent) were in males. Five of the patients in the series of Wysocki *et al.* (1980) were males, four were females and the sex of one was not known. Seven of our patients were males and seven were females. In view of the considerable variation in sex distribution reported in the four studies, pooling of the data would not be justified.

Site

Gingival cysts of adults occur much more frequently in the mandible than in the maxilla, and particularly in the premolar-canine region of the mandible. Of the four cases of Reeve and Levy (1968) three were between the mandibular canine and premolar teeth, while one was between a mandibular lateral and canine. In the report of Buchner and Hansen (1979) 19 of 26 cases (73 per cent) were in the mandible and 17 of these were adjacent to a premolar or canine. Of their seven maxillary cases, six were associated with the premolars or canines. Seven of the series of Wysocki *et al.* (1980) were in the premolar-canine-incisor area of the mandible, one in the lateral incisor area of the maxilla, and the location of two was unknown. Eight of our cases involved the mandible and six the maxilla, and all but one were adjacent to a premolar or canine tooth. One maxillary case was associated with a molar.

Clinical presentation

The patient may give a history of a slowly enlarging, painless swelling. The cysts are well-circumscribed swellings, usually less then 1 cm in diameter and may occur in the attached gingiva or the interdental papilla, invariably on the facial aspect. The surface is smooth and may be the colour of normal gingiva or bluish (**Figure 4.3**). I have seen one case, however, which was red and on histological examination was filled with blood, presumably as a result of recent trauma. The lesions are soft and fluctuant and the adjacent teeth are usually vital. During surgical exploration slight erosion on the surface of the bone may be observed without extension to the periodontium.

Radiological features

There may be no radiographic change or only a faint round shadow indicative of superficial bone erosion (**Figure 4.1**). Of 46 cases diagnosed as gingival cysts in the study of Moskow *et al.* (1970), 19 showed radiolucencies but only two of 33 cases showed this change in the report of Buchner and Hansen (1979).

Pathogenesis

A number of suggestions have been made about the pathogenesis of the gingival cyst in adults. It was originally proposed that they may arise from odontogenic epithelial cell nests; or by traumatic implantation of surface epithelium; or by cystic degeneration of deep projections of surface epithelium (Ritchey and Orban, 1953). It has also been postulated that, very rarely, they may be derived from glandular elements (Traeger, 1961).

The most favoured theory of origin is from odontogenic epithelial cell nests derived from the dental lamina although Shafer, Hine and Levy (1983) felt that cysts arising from traumatic implantation of surface epithelium may occur. Reference has already been made to the frequency with which remnants of the dental lamina, many of them forming microcysts, are found in the gingiva of infants. In a study of 266 specimens of adult human gingiva, Stout, Lunin and Calonius (1968) demonstrated epithelial nests in 90 and a true cyst in one. They found no evidence of traumatic implantation or heterotopic glandular tissue. Many

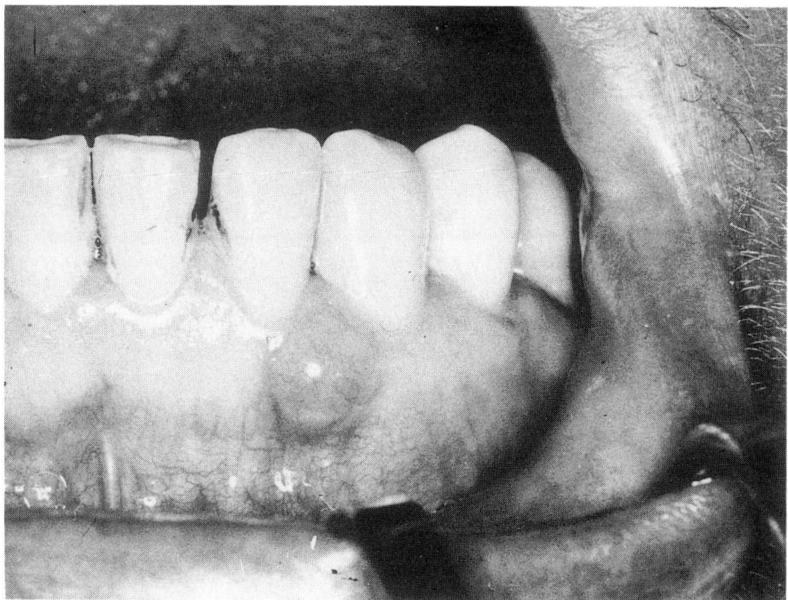

Figure 4.3. Gingival cyst in an adult. (By courtesy of J. J. Pindborg.)

of the epithelial remnants which they observed resembled the cell rests of Malassez. Hodson (1962) found epithelial residues in the anterior incisor areas in 58 per cent of 26 autopsies and in 14 per cent of 58 edentulous third molar regions. In a number of cases cell nests were found in the connective tissue of the gum without any specific relation to the surface epithelium. Unfortunately, for purposes of the present discussion, Hodson did not examine mandibular premolar regions. There is no clear explanation as to what the stimulus for the proliferation of these nests and their subsequent cystic breakdown might be, but it is certainly not an inflammatory stimulus, which produces well-recognized effects on odontogenic epithelium in radicular cysts, as are described in Chapter 11. Wysocki *et al.* (1980), who favour origin of these cysts from the dental lamina, have suggested that either unicystic or polycystic forms may develop depending on whether single or multiple enlarged epithelial cell nests of the dental lamina break down.

With the publication of convincing evidence that some gingival cysts of adults are lined by epithelium identical to that seen in lateral periodontal cysts (Moskow and Weinstein, 1975; Buchner and Hansen, 1979; Wysocki *et al.*, 1980) it is necessary to try to reconcile their respective histogeneses. In material which we were able to study (Nxumalo and Shear, 1990; 1992) we observed in a number of cases that the epithelial cyst lining extends to the deep aspect of the specimen where it lies close to, and is even possibly in continuity with, the junctional epithelium (**Figure 4.4**). This same phenomenon can be seen in Figure 1 of the paper by Buchner and Hansen (1979). This has suggested the possibility that at least some examples of gingival cyst of the adult may arise from junctional epithelium (previously called epithelial attachment), which in its turn is derived from reduced enamel epithelium (Schroeder, 1976). This view is reinforced by the frequent occurrence of lining epithelium in these cysts which closely resembles the reduced enamel epithelium

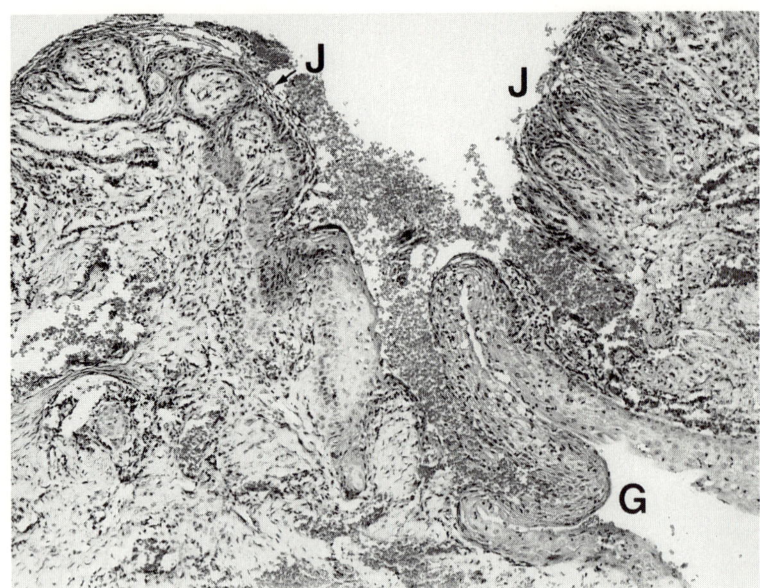

Figure 4.4. The epithelial lining of a gingival cyst of adults (G) lying contiguous to the junctional epithelium (J) of an adjacent tooth. (H & E; × 80.)

found in dentigerous cysts (**Figure 4.7**). Furthermore, the regular observation of epithelial atrophy (**Figure 4.8**), the tenuous attachment of of the epithelium to the connective tissue wall of the cyst (**Figure 4.9**), and the occasional presence of low columnar cells on the surface of the epithelium which suggest derivation from ameloblasts (**Figure 4.8**) lead to the conclusion that the epithelial lining is likely to originate from postfunctional reduced enamel epithelium.

Of the remaining theories, origin from basal cell extensions of overlying epithelium, or from remnants of the dental lamina, or from the cell nests of Malassez are theoretical possibilities, but I do not feel comfortable with them because the gingival cyst of adults is so different histologically from other cysts derived from these structures. Like other authors (Buchner and Hansen, 1979; Wysocki *et al.*, 1980) I am impressed by the numerous similarities between the gingival cyst of adults and the lateral periodontal cyst, both clinically and histologically. This accords with the view that what is now recognized as the typical gingival cyst of adults and the lateral periodontal cyst may arise from the same source. The lateral periodontal cyst would then develop from reduced enamel epithelium before eruption of the tooth and the gingival cyst of adults from reduced enamel epithelium (junctional epithelium) after eruption of the tooth (**Figure 4.5**). Origin from postfunctional epithelium, such as reduced enamel epithelium, would help to explain the unaggressive nature of the gingival cyst of adults and the lateral periodontal cyst compared with the keratocyst.

The multicystic form which is found in both the gingival cyst of adults and in the lateral periodontal cyst and the rarer botryoid form of the lateral periodontal cyst (**Figures 4.16**, **4.17**) may arise from epithelial plaques which are pinched off from the mother cyst (**Figures 4.14**, **4.15**), a suggestion first proposed by Weathers and Waldron (1973). If, however, the dental lamina theory is correct, then the satellite

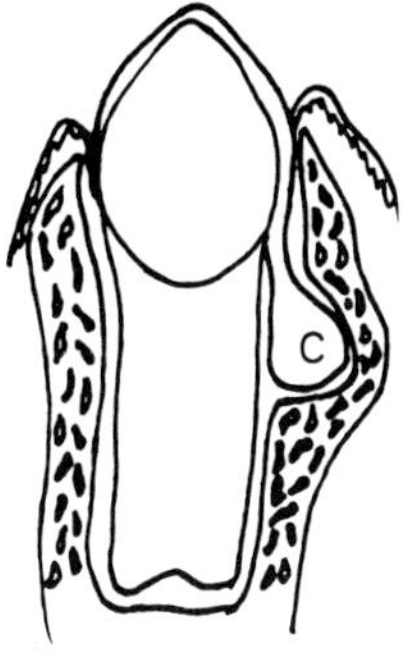

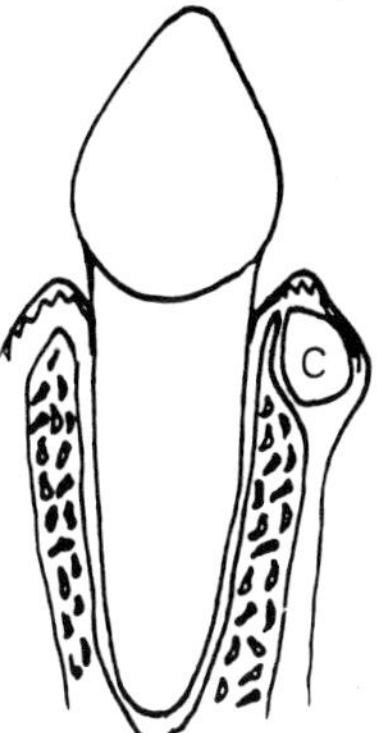

Figure 4.5. Diagram illustrating possible histogenesis of the lateral periodontal cyst (left) and the gingival cyst of adults (right). The lateral periodontal cyst is formed from the reduced enamel epithelium by dilatation of the follicle before eruption of the tooth, whereas the gingival cyst of adults is derived from junctional epithelium after eruption of the tooth.

cysts would undoubtedly be derived from these remnants. The stimulus which leads to the development of these cysts is clearly not inflammatory, and further work at a molecular level is required in order to postulate a genetic origin.

This hypothesis refers to those gingival cysts which are lined predominantly by a thin, non-keratinized epithelium which resembles reduced enamel epithelium and may show localized epithelial thickenings or plaques. The epidermoid and keratocyst varieties described by Buchner and Hansen (1979) have different pathogeneses. The epidermoid variety appears to be derived from cell remnants of the dental lamina which have survived into adult life and has developed in a manner similar to that of the gingival cyst of infants. The pathogenesis of the keratocyst has been dealt with in Chapter 2.

Histology

Gingival cysts in the adult have a variable histological pattern. They are usually small. Some have an extremely thin epithelium, closely resembling reduced enamel epithelium, with one to three layers of flat to cuboidal cells containing darkly-staining nuclei (**Figures 4.6**, **4.7**). In others the epithelial lining may be of a rather thicker stratified squamous nature without rete ridges (**Figures 4.6**, **4.8**). Many of the epithelial cells have pyknotic nuclei and show perinuclear cytoplasmic vacuolation. Others are atrophic and only 'ghost' outlines remain (**Figure 4.8**). In some cysts localized epithelial thickenings or plaques occur. Some are relatively small and flat, whereas others are more prominent. Some protrude into the cyst lumen, and some extend into the fibrous cyst wall. The cells in the plaques frequently have a whorled configuration. Some are compact and fusiform, whereas others are swollen and clear, the so-called 'water-clear' cells (Bhaskar, 1965; Buchner and Hansen, 1979; Wysocki *et al.*, 1980).

These epithelial plaques are identical to those which have been described in lateral periodontal cysts (Shear and Pindborg, 1975), (**Figures 4.13**, **4.14**, **4.15**), and this is one of the reasons why some workers have concluded that the two cysts originate from the same epithelium (Buchner and Hansen, 1979; Wysocki *et al.*,

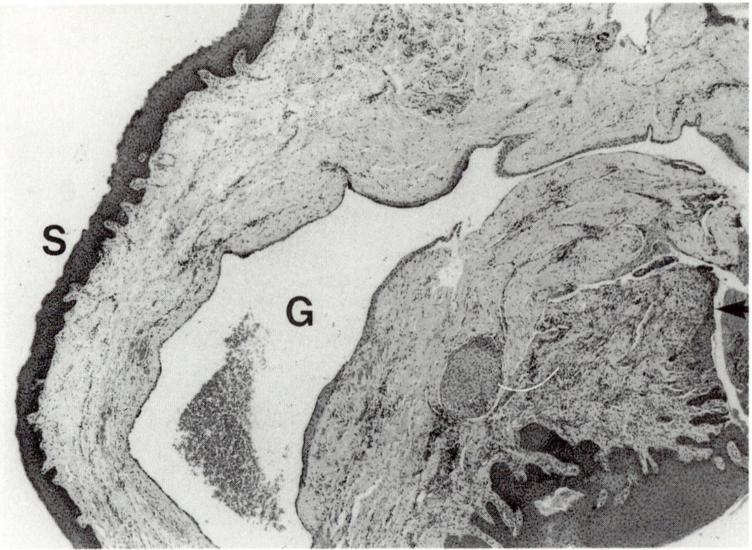

Figure 4.6. Gingival cyst of adults. The cyst (G) lies deep to gingival epithelium (S). It is lined partly by a thin epithelial lining 1–2 cell layers wide and partly by a thicker stratified squamous epithelium. This lining extends to junctional epithelium (arrow). An epithelial island lies between the cyst and the crevicular epithelium. (H & E; × 20.)

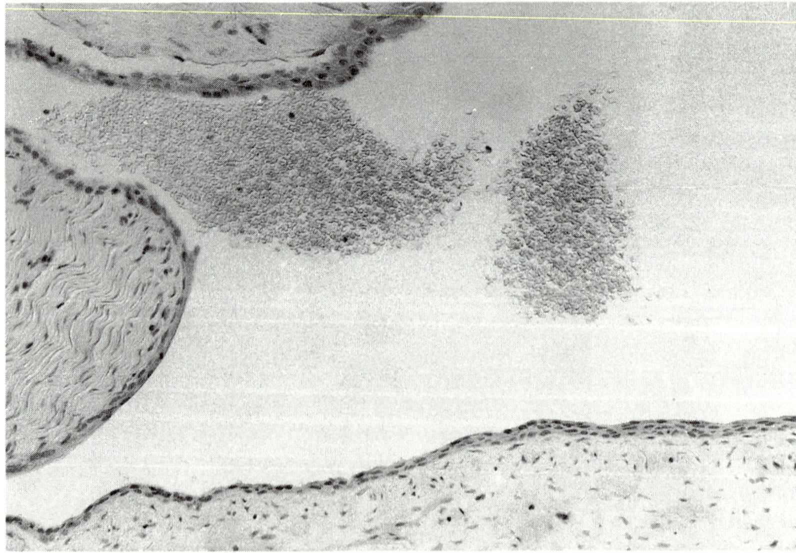

Figure 4.7. Gingival cyst of adults. This cyst is lined in part by a thin epithelium, 1–3 layers wide, closely resembling reduced enamel epithelium. (H & E; × 144.)

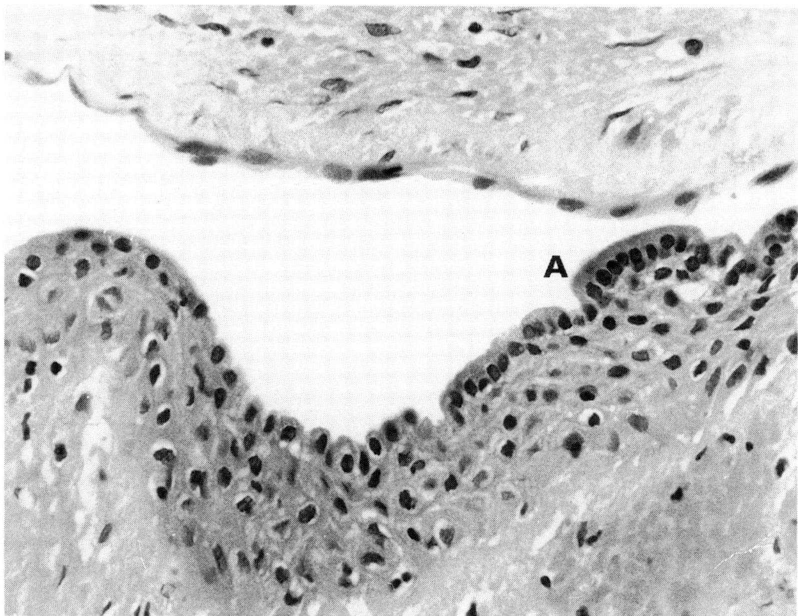

Figure 4.8. Gingival cyst of adults lined partly by a non-keratinized stratified squamous epithelium. Nuclei are pyknotic and shrunken and have disappeared from many cells, leaving ghost outlines of cells. Some cells show perinuclear haloes. In parts, the surface epithelial cells are low columnar (A) and suggest origin from the ameloblasts. (H & E; × 360.)

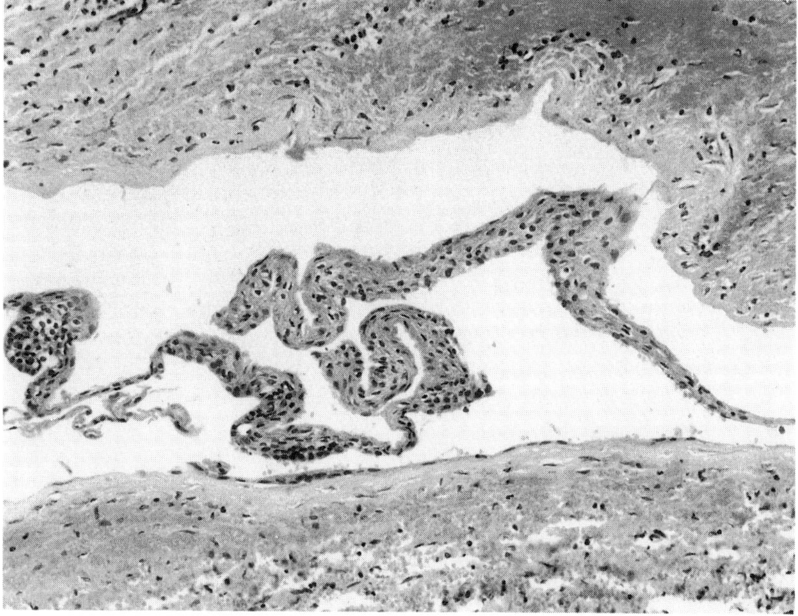

Figure 4.9. Gingival cyst of adults. Epithelial attachment to the cyst wall is tenuous and peels away in parts, leaving epithelial discontinuities. (H & E; × 144.)

1980). The attachment of the epithelium to the underlying connective tissue is tenuous and easily peels off, leaving epithelial discontinuities (**Figure 4.9**). Occasionally, low columnar cells have been observed on the surface of the epithelium, suggesting origin from ameloblasts (**Figure 4.8**) and reinforcing the impression that the lining is derived from reduced enamel epithelium. In a number of instances, the epithelial lining could be traced to, or close to, the junctional epithelium in serial sections (**Figures 4.4**, **4.6**).

The fibrous connective tissue wall is usually relatively uninflamed except close to the junctional epithelium where a chronic inflammatory cell infiltrate may occur; and rarely may contain small epithelial islands. The lesion is usually unicystic, but occasional multicystic variants are encountered. We found one such example in our series of 14 cases.

The histological variant described by Buchner and Hansen (1979) in which the cyst is lined by a keratinized stratified squamous epithelium and the lumen contains keratin, closely resembles the gingival cyst of infants histologically. It appears to be of dental lamina origin and to have followed a similar histogenesis. Two other specimens in their series were lined by epithelium identical to keratocyst epithelium and should be diagnosed as such despite having an apparently classic gingival cyst picture clinically.

Treatment

The gingival cyst is removed by local surgical excision and in the majority of cases there is no tendency for recurrence. Caution must however be observed if the pathologist reports a multicystic or botryoid variety and this is referred to again later in this chapter. The surgical treatment of cysts of the soft tissues is considered in Chapter 18.

Lateral periodontal cyst

The designation 'lateral periodontal cyst' is confined to those cysts which occur in the lateral periodontal position and in which an inflammatory aetiology and a diagnosis of collateral keratocyst have been excluded on clinical and histological grounds (Shear and Pindborg, 1975). As mentioned before, many publications on the subject have not distinguished between the lateral periodontal cyst and the gingival cyst of adults. Others have pooled data relating to the lateral periodontal cyst with cysts in that position of inflammatory origin and with collateral keratocysts (Fantasia, 1979; Eliasson, Isacsson and Köndell, 1989). Few publications on the subject have appeared since the previous edition of this book and clinical information about the lesion is therefore still relatively sparse.

Clinical features

Frequency

Eighteen cases of lateral periodontal cyst have been registered in our department between 1958 and 1989, representing 0.7 per cent of the 2616 cysts of the jaws seen during that period (**Table 2.1**). Of some significance, however, is the fact these were recorded during the 17-year period 1973–89, indicating that prior to this a number of cases were probably going unrecognized.

Age

The ages of 15 of our series of 18 patients ranged from 19–67 years with a mean of 52 years. All but two of our patients were in the 40–69 age group. In the series of 39 cases studied by Wysocki *et al.* (1980), the patients ranged in age from 22 to 85 years with a mean of 50 and a median of 53 years. In the sample of 37 cases reported by Cohen *et al.* (1984), the ages of the patients ranged from 21 to 82 years with a mean of 54 years. There was a prominent peak distribution in the sixth decade. Rasmusson, Magnusson and Borrman (1991) included 32 examples in 31 patients in their study. Their patients ranged in age from 26–77 with a mean of 55 years and a peak in the sixth decade. The age distribution of our 15 patients, pooled with those of Cohen *et al.* (1984) and Rasmusson, Magnusson and Borrman (1991) is shown in **Figure 4.10**.

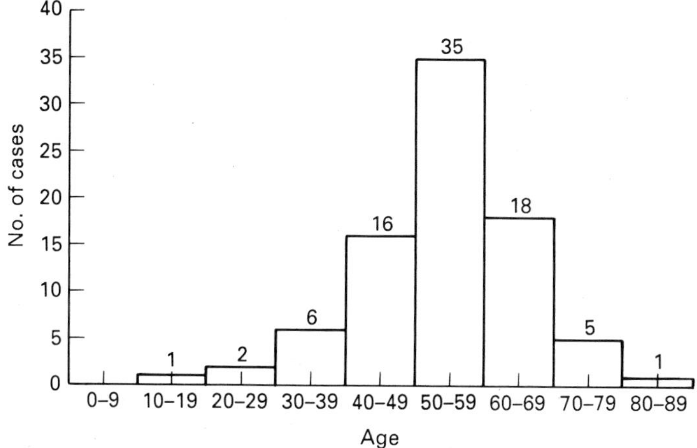

Figure 4.10. Age distribution of 84 patients with lateral periodontal cysts. Our data pooled with those of Cohen *et al.* (1984) and Rasmusson, Magnusson and Borrman (1991).

Sex

Wysocki *et al.* (1980) observed a male preponderance of 26 to 11 females. There was an equal sex distribution in the sample reported by Cohen *et al.* (1984) and of our 18 patients, 10 were males and eight were females. Rasmusson, Magnusson and Borrman (1991) found 22 lesions in men (69 per cent) and 10 in women (31 per cent).

Site

The most frequent location of lateral periodontal cysts reported in the literature is the mandibular premolar area, followed by the anterior region of the maxilla. In the study by Wysocki *et al.* (1980), 26 of the 39 cases (67 per cent) occurred in the premolar-canine-incisor region of the mandible and seven of these were located between the first and second premolars. In Fantasia's series (1979) all 12 cases which fulfilled the criteria for diagnosis as developmental lateral periodontal cysts occurred adjacent to the premolar or canine teeth of the mandible. In the study of

Cohen *et al.* (1984), 78 per cent of cases occurred in the mandible, all of which were anterior to the first permanent molar and most were between the premolars. In the sample of Rasmusson, Magnusson and Borrman (1991), 28 of the cysts (88 per cent) were found in the mandible and four in the maxilla (12 per cent). All were in the premolar-cuspid-incisor area. In our material, surprisingly, the distribution was somewhat different. Although all our cases occurred anterior to the first permanent molars, 10 of 18 cases (56 per cent) were found in the maxilla, all of which were clustered anterior to the first premolar teeth.

Clinical presentation

Lateral periodontal cysts may be symptomless and are discovered fortuitously during routine radiological examination of the teeth. Sometimes a gingival swelling may occur on the facial aspect and it is this type of case which must be differentiated from a gingival cyst, particularly as some lesions are described as blue fluctuant swellings. Pain was a symptom in a number of our cases and in those of Cohen *et al.*(1984), as was tenderness on palpation (Eliasson, Isacsson and Köndell, 1989). One case produced a swelling 3 cm in diameter which was depicted as 'springy with egg shell crackling' while another was described as having a gelatinous feel. The associated teeth will be vital unless they happen to have been otherwise involved.

Radiological features

Radiographs of the lateral periodontal cyst show a round or oval well-circumscribed radiolucent area, usually with a sclerotic margin. The cysts lie somewhere between the apex and the cervical margin of the tooth (**Figure 4.11**). Resorption of the adjacent root has not been reported. Most of them are less than 1 cm in diameter except the botryoid variety which may be larger and multilocular

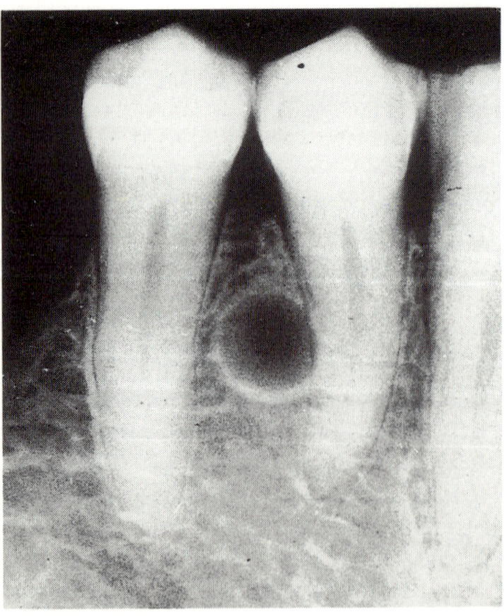

Figure 4.11. Radiograph of a lateral periodontal cyst between the mandibular premolar teeth. Keratocysts also sometimes occur in this situation and in such cases are indistinguishable radiologically from lateral periodontal cysts. (Previously published (1975) in *Scand. J. Dent. Res.* **83**, 103–110, and reproduced here by courtesy of the Editor.)

(Kaugars, 1986; Greer and Johnson, 1988). Rasmusson, Magnusson and Borrman (1991) provided some useful data about the sizes of the lesions in their sample. At the time of treatment, they ranged from 2.5–15 mm in diameter but most were in the range 3–7 mm. In only four cysts did the diameter exceed 10 mm. In some of their cases radiographs from previous examinations were available. The longest follow-up was 14 years during which the diameter of the cyst increased from 9 to 17 mm. They estimated from the four cysts in which such data were available that the mean growth was 0.7 mm per year. The collateral variety of keratocyst may have an identical radiological appearance and the distinction is usually not made until the histological examination.

Pathogenesis

Standish and Shafer (1958) commented that the lateral periodontal cyst was of varied aetiology but that the term 'lateral periodontal cyst' should be used to indicate all cysts developing in the anatomical region of the lateral periodontium. In view of this varied aetiology, however, they suggested that the term should be qualified to indicate whether the cyst's origin is pulp infection, infection through the gingival crevice or idiopathic stimulation of cell nests. It is now widely accepted, however, that the term 'lateral periodontal cyst' should be confined to cysts in the lateral periodontal position in which an inflammatory aetiology and a diagnosis of gingival cyst of the adult and collateral keratocyst have been excluded on clinical and histological grounds (Shear and Pindborg, 1975; Wysocki *et al.*, 1980; Cohen *et al.*, 1984).

Although there can be little doubt that lateral periodontal cysts are of odontogenic origin, there is, as with many other odontogenic lesions, considerable doubt about which odontogenic epithelium they arise from. Proof of origin from any particular source is lacking and any hypotheses must therefore be based on presumptive evidence. Histological studies show that they are usually devoid of inflammatory cell infiltration except at a distance from the lining and it is reasonable therefore to regard them as being of developmental origin.

Assuming then that the lateral periodontal cyst is a distinct entity of developmental odontogenic origin, from which epithelium does it arise? There seem to be three possibilities: reduced enamel epithelium, remnants of dental lamina and cell rests of Malassez. As will be seen from a description of the histological features, the cyst is lined for the most part by a narrow non-keratinized epithelium which resembles reduced enamel epithelium. As such, the proposal that it arises initially as a dentigerous cyst developing by expansion of the follicle along the lateral surface of the crown (Shafer, Hine and Levy, 1983) is an attractive one. **Figure 5.6** (p. 81) is a radiograph of such a phenomenon, which is usually referred to as a lateral dentigerous cyst. If tooth eruption is normal, the expanded follicle may finally lie on the lateral aspect of the root, as illustrated diagrammatically in **Figure 4.12**. This hypothesis is supported by the fact that lateral periodontal cysts tend to occur in areas where dentigerous cysts are likely to be associated with vertically impacted teeth such as mandibular premolars and maxillary incisors and canines. In this respect it is of interest that epithelial plaques similar to those seen in the lateral periodontal cyst are sometimes found in dentigerous cysts. Further support for origin of lateral periodontal cysts from reduced enamel epithelium comes from immunocytochemical studies (Hormia *et al.*, 1987; Heikinheimo *et al.*, 1989). The former group investigated the cytokeratin composition of the cyst

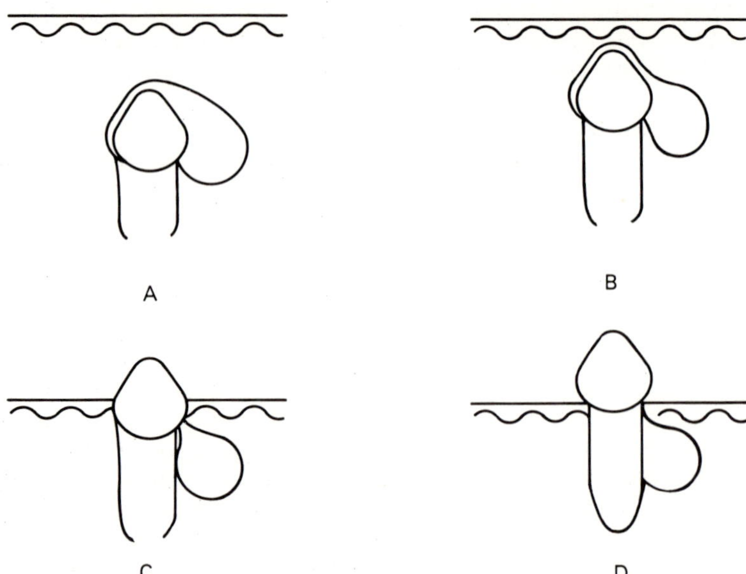

Figure 4.12. Diagram illustrating the possible pathogenesis of the lateral periodontal cyst. At [A] there is expansion of the follicle on the lateral surface of the crown of an unerupted tooth. At this stage a radiograph would show a lateral dentigerous cyst. At <B–D> the tooth erupts leaving the expanded follicle behind. (Previously published (1975) in *Scand. J. Dent. Res.* **83**, 103–110, and reproduced here by courtesy of the Editor.)

epithelium in a case of a botryoid variety of lateral periodontal cyst and found that cytokeratin no. 18 was strongly expressed; whereas the former workers have reported that this cytokeratin is present in some dentigerous cysts but not in other types of odontogenic cyst.

Wysocki *et al.* (1980) have proposed that the lateral periodontal cyst, like the gingival cyst of adults, arises from clear cell rests of dental lamina. They suggested that unicystic forms arise through cystic change in a single dental lamina rest and polycystic lesions develop if concomitant changes occur in several adjacent cell rests. They postulated that the limited growth potential of the lateral periodontal cyst compared with the keratocyst, which is also of dental lamina origin, is that the former arises from postfunctional cells of the dental lamina whereas the latter presumably arises from that part of the dental lamina still possessing marked growth potential. In support of their hypothesis, Wysocki *et al.* placed a lot of emphasis on the fact that glycogen-containing clear-cell rests of the dental lamina may sometimes be demonstrated, and that similar cells also occur in parts of the lining of lateral periodontal cysts, as well as in the epithelial plaques which are a feature of their linings. They also pointed to the occasional presence of glycogen-rich clear-cell rests of what they interpreted as dental lamina in the wall of the cysts. As will be pointed out later in this chapter, the epithelial plaques are not comprised of clear cells *de novo*, but start rather as fusiform cells with scanty cytoplasm arising by localized proliferation of basal cells. I have also suggested, in my discussion of the pathogenesis of the gingival cyst of adults, that what were described by Wysocki *et al.* as rests of dental lamina in these cyst walls, may in fact be 'pinched-off' epithelial plaques. I share with Wysocki *et al.* (1980) the view that the lateral periodontal cyst and the gingival cyst of adults have a common ancestry (**Figure 4.9**) and the argument on this point has been pursued earlier in this chapter.

The third possibility is origin from the cell nests of Malassez. Other than the fact that the rests of Malassez occur in the periodontium and that they are well-positioned for a lateral periodontal cyst, this is not a theory which has received very much support.

Histology

Most commonly the lateral periodontal cyst is lined by a thin, non-keratinizing layer of squamous or cuboidal epithelium usually ranging from one to five cell layers wide, which resembles the reduced enamel epithelium (**Figure 4.13**). The epithelial cells are sometimes separated by intercellular fluid. Their nuclei are small and pyknotic. Wysocki *et al.* (1980) also described the occasional presence of conspicuous, sometimes numerous, glycogen-rich clear cells in the epithelial linings. In a recent histological study in our own department on 20 cases, Altini and Shear (1992) confirmed the presence of glycogen in about two-thirds of them, either in the lining epithelium or in the plaques, or both. It was not found exclusively in the clear cells, many of which showed no positivity, but also occurred in the superficial layers of the squamous and cuboidal cells of the lining epithelium.

Sometimes the epithelial lining may be of a more distinctly stratified squamous nature, but when the characteristic features of a keratocyst are observed, then as

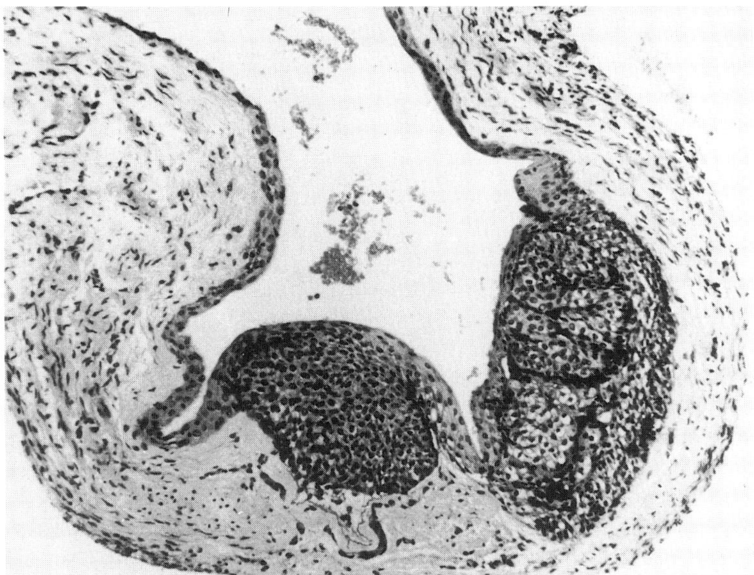

Figure 4.13. Lateral periodontal cyst which in part has a thin, non-keratinized, stratified squamous epithelial lining resembling reduced enamel epithelium. Two epithelial plaques are seen. The one on the right is convoluted as in stage [F] in Figure 4.15. (H & E; × 75.) (Previously published (1975) in *Scand. J. Dent. Res.* **83**, 103–110, and reproduced here by courtesy of the Editor.)

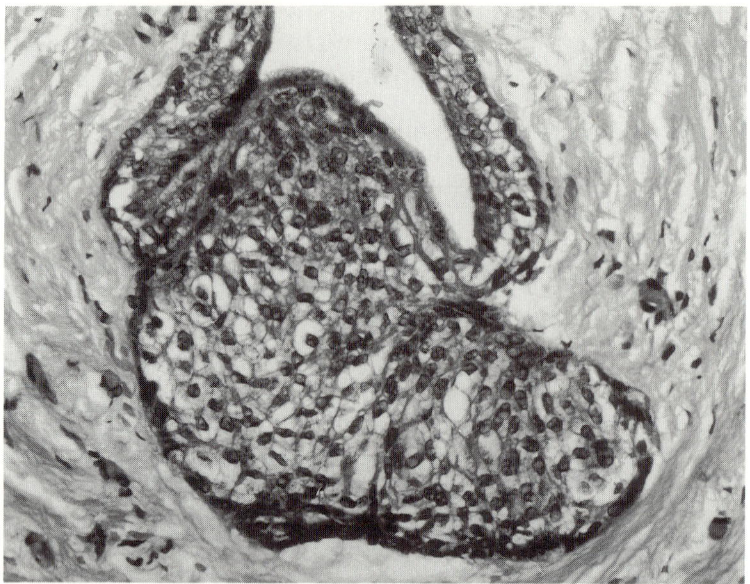

Figure 4.14. Epithelial plaque in a lateral periodontal cyst. This is represented diagrammatically by stage [E] in Figure 4.15. (H & E; × 235.) (Previously published (1975) in *Scand. J. Dent. Res.* **83**, 103–110, and reproduced here by courtesy of the Editor.)

indicated earlier, this should be the diagnosis rather than lateral periodontal cyst. Indeed, Gold and Sliwkowski (1973) have shown in their study that such collateral keratocysts cysts have, as one would expect, a definite tendency to recur following surgical removal.

An interesting feature which is seen in many lateral periodontal cysts is the presence of what appear to be localized plaques or thickenings of the epithelial lining (**Figures 4.13**, **4.14**, **4.15**). Some of these are small whereas others are larger and extend into the surrounding cyst wall as well as producing mural bulges which protrude into the cyst cavity. Some cysts contain a number of the plaques. The cells of the plaque are sometimes fusiform with their long axes parallel to the basement membrane; frequently they are large and clear, with small pyknotic nuclei, and Wysocki *et al.*(1980) have shown that these contain glycogen.

Examination of histological material at the light microscope level, and particularly study of serial sections, indicates the possible mode of formation of these plaques (Shear and Pindborg, 1975). The usual sequence (**Figure 4.15**) is that there appears to be proliferation of the flat basal cells which produces a slight localized thickening of the epithelium.

At this stage the thickened epithelium consists predominantly of darkly staining fusiform basal cells. This early plaque may extend into the fibrous wall of the cyst or bulge into the lumen. The plaque increases in size both by further basal cell proliferation and by swelling of these epithelial cells. At this stage there is a more pronounced bulging into the lumen and also into the wall. The bulbous nature of the thickening into the wall sometimes leads to undermining of the adjacent cyst lining. Complex convolutions of the epithelium may be seen in the larger plaques.

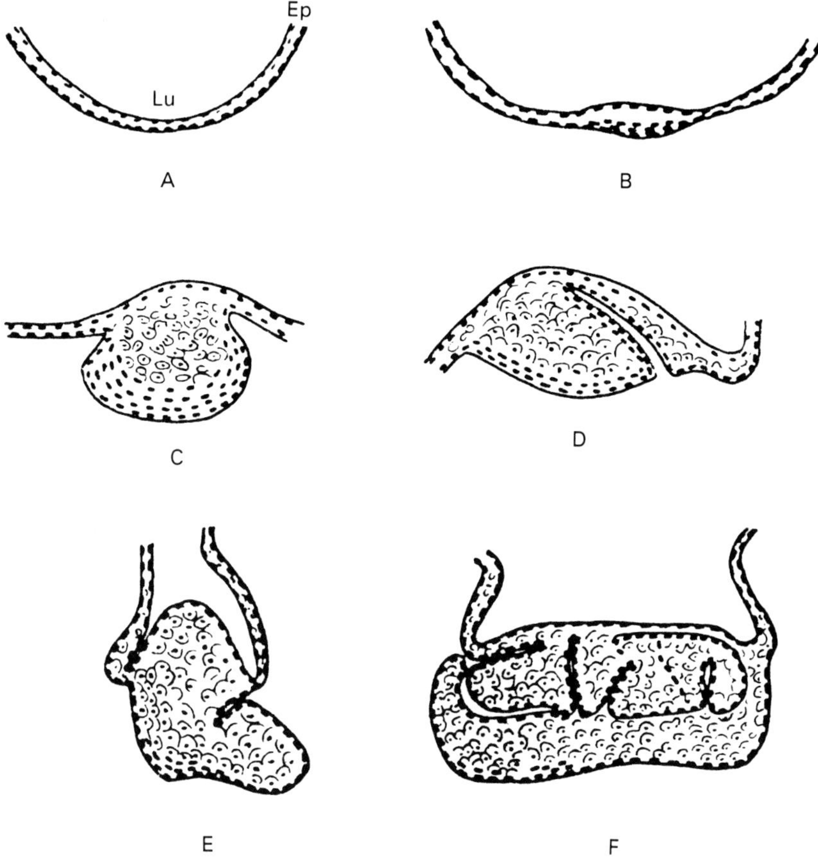

Figure 4.15. Diagram illustrating the possible mode of formation of epithelial plaques by localized proliferation of cells. [A], cyst lined by thin epithelium resembling reduced enamel epithelium. [B], early epithelial thickening by basal cell proliferation. [C], basal cells continue to proliferate. Superficial cells swell by accumulation of intracellular fluid. [D] and [E], basal cell proliferation ceases or slows down. Superficial cells waterlogged and swollen. Plaque protrudes into cyst cavity and cyst wall where it can undermine and raise adjacent cyst lining. [F], epithelial plaque can form convolutions. Protrusions into cyst wall in [C–F] may be pinched off and develop into daughter cysts, leading to the formation of the botryoid variety. [L_u], cyst lumen. [E_p], epithelial lining.

Occasionally the cells of the plaque may differentiate and take on a distinctly spinous appearance.

What produces these localized epithelial proliferations is not known. They do however seem to be a spontaneous process which tends to occur in reduced enamel epithelium and probably also in other lesions of odontogenic epithelium. It is possible that the thickenings represent another of the many examples of odontogenic epithelium recapitulating ontogeny under pathological conditions. In this instance, the process seems to be similar to that which takes place during the early stages of tooth development, when there is thickening of stomadeal ectoderm to form the dental lamina.

In their histological study of 20 cases, Altini and Shear (1992) recognized two groups of lateral periodontal cyst: the unicystic (nine cases, 45 per cent); and the multicystic (11 cases, 55 per cent). Some of the multicystic lesions (six of our series) consisted of two or more cystic spaces contained within a single round or ovoid capsule, whereas others (five of our series) were larger and more irregular, having a distinctly botryoid appearance, consisting of several cystic spaces of varying size separated by fibrous tissue. Most of the lesions were small, varying from 5–15 mm in diameter, whereas the botryoid variety were substantially larger, one of the cases having measured 50 mm.

While the unicystic and multicystic varieties shared similar histological features, the botryoid type may occasionally show somewhat different characteristics which will be described in a separate section later in this chapter. All varieties of lateral periodontal cyst may have small epithelial nests or follicles in the fibrous wall. These are often closely associated with the epithelial plaques and there is some histological evidence to suggest that they may arise from them.

The epithelial linings may separate to differing degrees from the fibrous cyst wall and there are occasional areas of juxta-epithelial hyalinized collagen. The fibrous cyst wall shows a variable chronic inflammatory cell infiltrate and is usually remarkably free of inflammation.

In a histochemical study on the linings of their sample, Rasmusson, Magnusson and Borrman (1991) demonstrated positive reactions for $NADH_2$ and $NADPH_2$-diaphorase, glutamate dehydrogenase and lactate dehydrogenase in the epithelium while the reaction for acid and alkaline phosphatase was very weak. They observed the same reactions in the epithelial islands in the cyst walls. They pointed out that these reactions differed from those in keratocysts which exhibit a high level of acid phosphatase activity in the epithelium.

Grand and Marwah (1964) have reported a lateral periodontal cyst in the epithelial lining of which were melanin-containing cells. Gold and Christ (1970) have described what they referred to as a granular-cell odontogenic cyst which had the clinical and radiological features of a lateral periodontal cyst. Histologically, the epithelial lining cells had undergone extensive granular cell change, as had some of the odontogenic epithelial islands in the cyst wall. They commented on the similarity between these cells and those found in the granular cell ameloblasoma. Buchner (1973) reported another example of a granular cell odontogenic cyst and his specimen had features which suggested the diagnosis of unicystic granular cell ameloblastoma. The case of Gold and Christ recurred 18 years later as a follicular ameloblastoma, with no histological evidence of granular cells (Abaza, Gold and Lally, 1989), and the latter authors concluded that the original lesion was probably a unicystic granular cell ameloblastoma.

Treatment

Provided that the lesion is unilocular on radiological examination, the lateral periodontal cyst is treated by surgical enucleation. Attempts should be made to avoid sacrificing the associated tooth, but this may not always be possible. A number of reports have been published which indicate that the botryoid variety has a predilection for recurrence, and this feature is dealt with in the next section of this chapter. It is not yet clear from the literature whether the encapsulated multicystic lateral periodontal cyst has the same tendency to recur following simple enucleation. Eight of 10 recurrent cases reported by Greer and Johnson (1988) were unilocular radiologically but multilocular histologically. Until we have further information about the behaviour of the encapsulated multilocular variety, clinicians are advised to follow these cases for a number of years. (See also Chapter 18.)

Botryoid odontogenic cyst

Weathers and Waldron (1973) reported two examples of a multilocular cystic lesion of the jaws for which they proposed the term 'botryoid odontogenic cyst' because the gross specimen resembled a cluster of grapes. Since their original description,

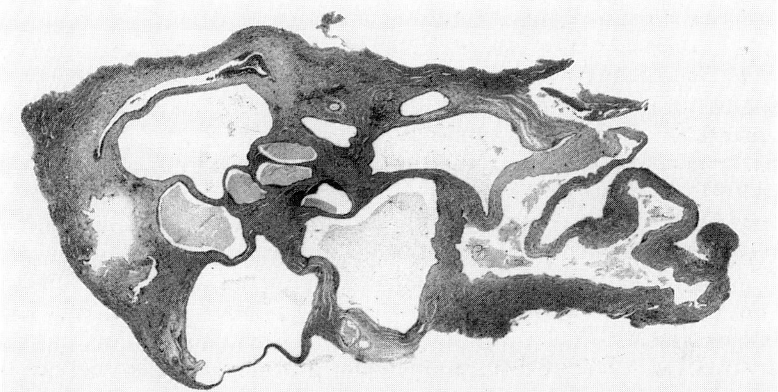

Figure 4.16. Botryoid odontogenic cyst developing from a lateral periodontal cyst. (H & E; × 10.)

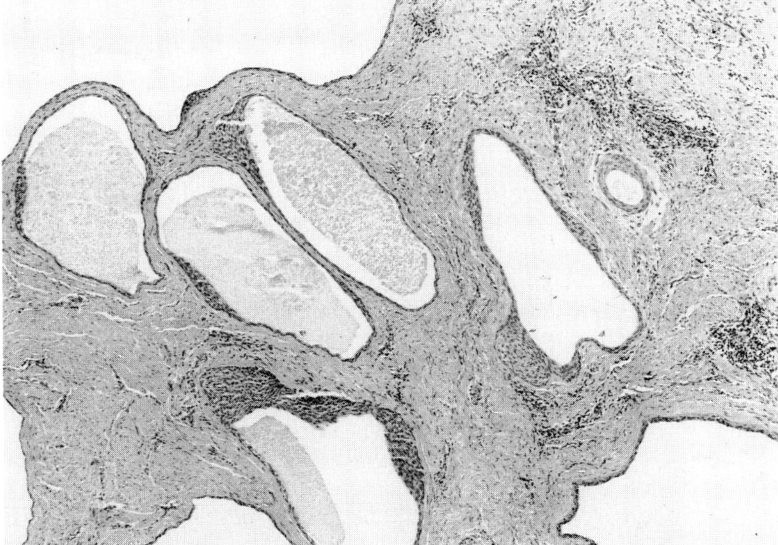

Figure 4.17. Botryoid odontogenic cyst. Higher magnification of lesion illustrated in Figure 4.16. The daughter microcysts also show epithelial plaques which in turn could be pinched off to form granddaughter cysts. (H & E; × 50.)

botryoid odontogenic cysts have been widely regarded as variants of the lateral periodontal cyst and publications on the subject have not distinguished them from the smaller multicystic lateral periodontal cysts. Microscopically, (**Figures 4.16, 4.17**) the lesion is similar to the lateral periodontal cyst but exhibits some differences. The lesion is multilocular with thin fibrous connective tissue septa. The cyst cavities are of varying size, with the smaller ones tending to be orientated towards the larger ones. The cyst cavities are sometimes lined by a thin non-keratinized epithelium of, for the most part, 1–2 layers of flat cells but in two of our four cases the cysts are lined in some areas by a somewhat thicker stratified squamous epithelium. In many of the cysts there are foci of plaque-like thickenings, most of them consisting of flat fusiform cells. Weathers and Waldron suggested that these plaques may possibly be the source of new cyst locules, an opinion with which I concur. In the two of our cases referred to above, clear cells are unusual both in the lining epithelium and in the plaques. There is an increase in the nucleo-cytoplasmic ratio in much of the epithelium with resultant crowding of the cells, the nuclei of which are pyknotic.

Some years elapsed after the publication of the article by Weathers and Waldron before any further papers appeared on this variety of lateral periodontal cyst. Kaugars (1986) reported three cases, one which occurred in the midline of the mandible, one between the mandibular premolars and one in an edentulous mandible. The three patients were all in their fifties. All the lesions produced multilocular radiolucencies on radiological examination. Two of the lesions are reported to have enucleated easily. All showed the same histological features, as described above. Kaugars suggested that a lesion that is radiologically or histologically multilocular would have an increased risk of recurrence or persistence and recommended that patients treated for a botryoid odontogenic cyst should be followed periodically.

Greer and Johnson (1988) reported 10 cases. The ages of the patients ranged from 26 to 66 years with a mean of 46 years; eight of the 10 lesions were in the mandible, predominantly the anterior region; 8 showed unilocular radiolucencies and two were multilocular, ranging in size from 0.4–4.5 cm. Three of the cases represented recurrences, 8, 10 and 10 years respectively, after previous surgery, and the authors supported Kaugar's concern that patients must be followed-up. All cases showed the same histological features already described, and all 10 were multicystic. The plaques were compared by means of light and electron microscopy with the convoluted zones seen in three adenomatoid odontogenic tumours, and in two cases were found to be remarkably similar. This observation is of interest because early adenomatoid odontogenic tumours can be shown to arise in the epithelial linings of dentigerous cysts, particularly those related to maxillary canine teeth. In view of this finding, and their opinion that the botryoid odontogenic cyst may arise from the stratum intermedium, it is surprising that Greer and Johnson reject the possibility of origin from reduced enamel epithelium. Where does stratum intermedium go if not into reduced enamel epithelium?

Further documentation of the tendency for the botryoid odontogenic cyst to recur is provided in papers by Phelan *et al.* (1988), Heikinheimo *et al.* (1989) and Machado de Sousa *et al.* (1990). Heikinheimo *et al.* (1989) also undertook an immunocytochemical comparison of the cytokeratin expression of the cyst epithelium from their case with that of the overlying epithelium. Simple cytokeratin no. 18 was strongly expressed, an observation of some interest as this cytokeratin has previously been reported to be present in some dentigerous cysts but not in other types of odontogenic cyst (Hormia *et al.*, 1987). Cytokeratin no. 19, which is a major component of odontogenic epithelia, was distinctly expressed in all epithelial cells of their cyst. The cyst lining also showed features of non-keratinizing epithelia, as seen in some odontogenic cysts as well as in tooth germs.

The publications referred to above have not distinguished between the smaller apparently encapsulated multilocular lateral periodontal cysts and the frankly botryoid variety, which do not appear to be entirely synonymous. It would be useful to discriminate between the two in prospective clinicopathological studies as this will help us to determine whether there is a difference in behaviour between them. It must be regarded as a theoretical possibility that the multicystic variety can develop into a botryoid type by continued expansion of individual cysts.

Three of our cases of the botryoid variety also share some features with the glandular odontogenic cyst, in that they have epithelial crypts and superficial low columnar cells, although no mucous cells were demonstrated. This raises the question of whether the glandular odontogenic cyst forms part of the clinicopathological spectrum of the lateral periodontal cyst. For this reason, it is discussed in a separate section of this chapter.

Treatment

It is clear from the numerous reports of recurrences that the botryoid odontogenic cyst requires careful excision and that attempts at conservative enucleation have not been successful. As indicated earlier it is yet to be determined whether the smaller apparently encapsulated multicystic variety has the same tendency to recurrence. Until there is clarification on this point, cases must be carefully followed for a number of years.

Glandular odontogenic cyst (sialo-odontogenic cyst; mucoepidermoid odontogenic cyst)

A cyst with fairly typical histological features which has some characteristics in common with the lateral periodontal cyst and the botryoid odontogenic cyst, has recently been reported (Padayachee and Van Wyk, 1987; Gardner *et al.*, 1988) and discussed at the meeting of the International Association of Oral Pathologists in 1984. In view of its partial resemblance to these two lesions, and its possible relationship to them, this cyst is being presented in the same chapter. Waldron and Koh (1990) have discussed it in connection with the central mucoepidermoid tumour of the jaws and Ficarra, Chou and Panzoni (1990) reported a case in which a diagnosis of low-grade mucoepidermoid carcinoma had been made.

The name of the cyst is not yet established. The term most descriptive of the lesion is probably ‘mucoepidermoid odontogenic cyst’ because of the presence of both secretory elements and stratified squamous epithelium (Sadeghi *et al.*, 1991). The use of this name might, however, lead to confusion with the mucoepidermoid carcinoma, and is therefore unlikely to find favour.

Padayachee and Van Wyk (1987) reported two cases which resembled both the botryoid odontogenic cyst and the central mucoepidermoid tumour of the jaws but, after a careful analysis, concluded that they differed sufficiently to warrant separation as an entity. They indicated that the typical features of the cyst are that it is intrabony and multilocular radiologically; that it can recur if not adequately excised; that it is multicystic, with the cystic spaces lined by a non-keratinized epithelium akin to reduced enamel epithelium, with epithelial thickenings or plaques; that mucous and cylindrical cells form an integral part of the epithelial component; and that mucinous material within the cystic spaces is a prominent feature.

Gardner *et al.* (1988), who favoured the name 'glandular odontogenic cyst', suggested also that its histological features and biological behaviour are sufficiently distinct for it to be regarded as an entity. They reported eight cases, from which they felt that they could draw certain conclusions about its biological behaviour. It apparently occurs over a wide age range, in either jaw, and has the propensity to grow to a large size and to recur. One of their cases, however, grew very slowly and remained small. Radiologically, some of their cases showed unilocular radiolucencies with either smooth or scalloped margins, while others were distinctly multilocular. They gave a detailed account of the histological features of their series.

Patron, Colmonero and Larrauri (1991) reported three new cases and summarized the data from 13 cases. The age range was 19–85 years, nine of the 13 cases were in men and 10 occurred in the mandible. Radiologically the lesions have been well defined with a unilocular or multilocular pattern but without specific diagnostic features. Three of 10 cases that have been followed-up have recurred.

The radiograph illustrated in **Figure 4.18** shows a unilocular radiolucent area with a smooth corticated margin between the maxillary lateral and canine teeth, the roots of which are displaced.

I have had the opportunity of studying histological sections of a few cases. The microscopic features are variable. The cyst may be lined in parts by a non-keratinized stratified squamous epithelium with a chronic inflammatory

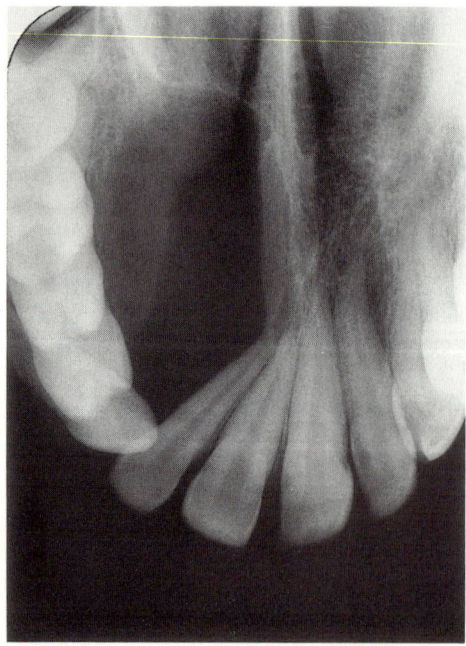

Figure 4.18. Radiograph of a glandular odontogenic cyst. There is a large unilocular radiolucent area with a smooth corticated margin. These features are non-specific. (By courtesy of Professor E. J. Raubenheimer.)

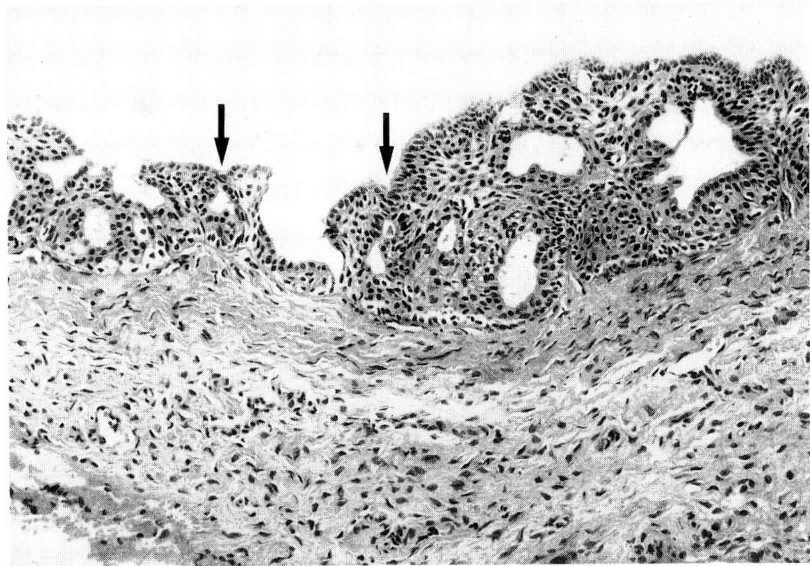

Figure 4.19. Glandular odontogenic cyst. In this area, columnar and cuboidal cells lie on the surface of the epithelium and extend into, and line, the intraepithelial crypts. The openings onto the surface (arrowed) give the epithelium a corrugated appearance. (H & E; × 148.) (Section lent by Dr R. Morency.)

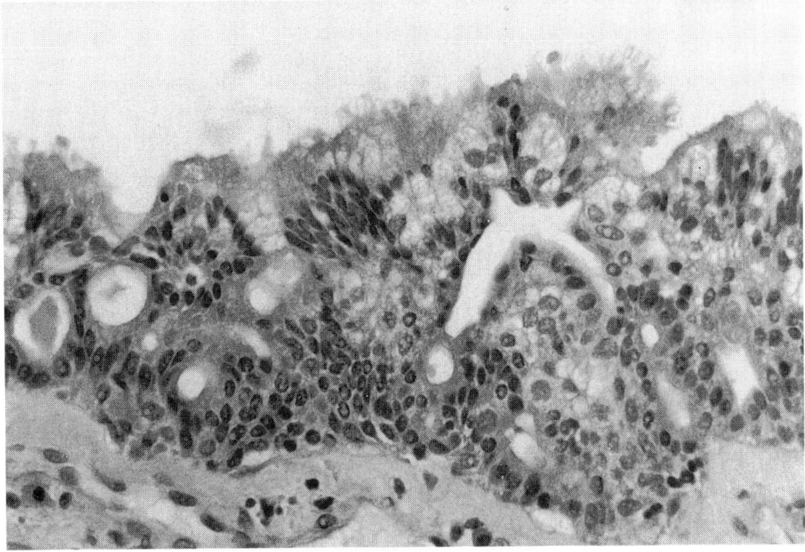

Figure 4.20. Glandular odontogenic cyst. In this field there are cilia, goblet cells and crypts. In transverse section the crypts appear to be pools. (H & E; × 360.)

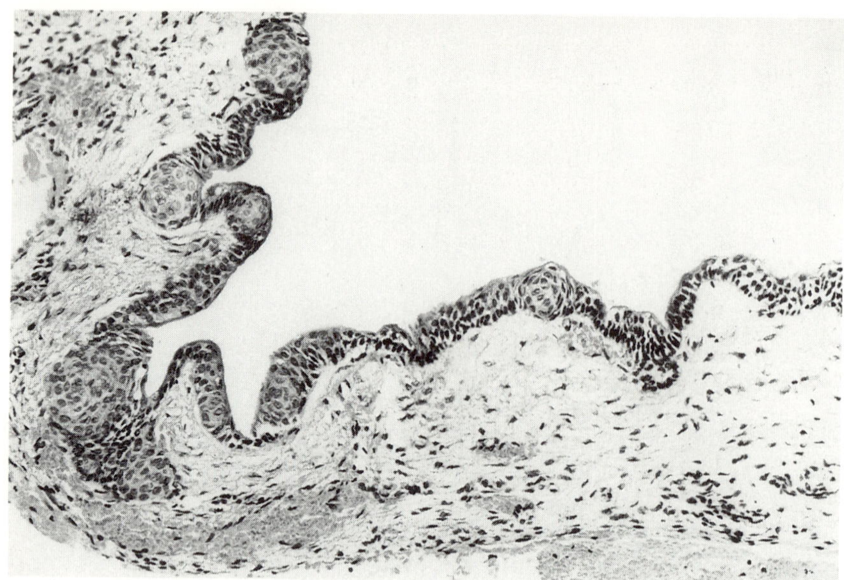

Figure 4.21. Glandular odontogenic cyst. This area is lined by a thin non-keratinized epithelium resembling reduced enamel epithelium. Numerous epithelial plaques may be seen. (H & E; × 148.) (Section lent by Dr R. Morency.)

infiltration of the connective tissue wall, the same as is found in a radicular cyst. The diagnosis is made when the superficial layer of the epithelial lining consists of columnar or cuboidal cells (**Figure 4.19**), occasionally with cilia (**Figure 4.20**), and the epithelium has a glandular or pseudoglandular structure, with intraepithelial crypts or microcysts or pools lined by cells similar to those on the surface (**Figures 4.19, 4.20**). In certain planes of section, these microcysts may be seen to open onto the surface of the epithelium through openings or crypts, giving the epithelium a papillary or corrugated surface (**Figures 4.19**). They are sometimes empty and sometimes contain a structureless eosinophilic material which gives a positive mucicarmine reaction. Numerous goblet cells may be be present, mainly in the superficial part of the epithelium (**Figure 4.20**). Occasionally the epithelium is thinner, similar to reduced enamel epithelium. Epithelial thickenings or plaques may be present in either this thin epithelium (**Figure 4.21**) or in the stratified squamous epithelium. The plaques, which are identical to those in the gingival cyst of adults, the lateral periodontal cyst and the botryoid odontogenic cyst, may either protrude into the cyst cavity or extend into the connective tissue wall. Islands of odontogenic epithelium and even microcysts may be present in the connective tissue wall of the cyst. Irregular calcifications may be present in the connective tissue wall.

Takeda (1991) observed similar epithelial microcysts, which he called duct-like structures, in the odontogenic epithelium of a compound odontoma.

Treatment

Despite the paucity of documented examples of this cyst, the available information suggests that, like the botryoid odontogenic cyst, it should be carefully excised rather than enucleated in order to obviate recurrence.

Chapter 5

Dentigerous (follicular) cyst

A dentigerous cyst is one which encloses the crown of an unerupted tooth by expansion of its follicle, and is attached to the neck (**Figure 5.1**). It is important that this definition be applied strictly and that the diagnosis of dentigerous cyst is not made uncritically on radiographic evidence alone, otherwise keratocysts of the envelopmental variety (Main, 1970a), follicular keratocysts (Altini and Cohen, 1982, 1987) and unilocular ameloblastomas involving adjacent unerupted teeth, are liable to be misdiagnosed as dentigerous cysts.

Clinical features

Frequency

In the 32-year period 1958–89, 433 of 2616 jaw cysts recorded in our department (**Table 2.1**, p. 6) have been dentigerous cysts (16.6 per cent). This means that we

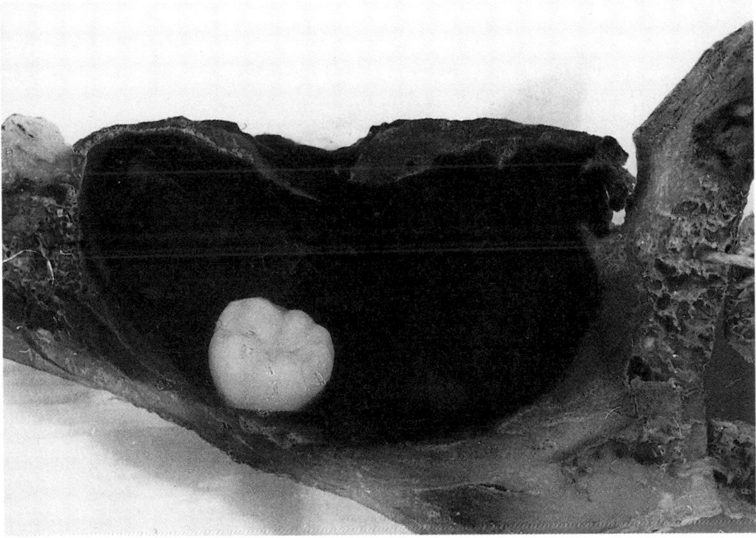

Figure 5.1. Gross specimen of a dentigerous cyst involving the mandibular third molar tooth.

are seeing about 14 cases a year and, as our material is drawn from a number of sources, individual surgeons and departments are apparently dealing with far fewer than this number each year. In a study of the incidence of dentigerous cysts on the Witwatersrand (Shear and Singh, 1978), it was shown that the age-standardized incidence rates for dentigerous cysts, standardized against a world standard population, per million per year, were 1.18, 1.22, 9.92 and 7.26 for black males, black females, white males and white females, respectively (**Table 5.1**).

Table 5.1 Age-standardized incidence rates of dentigerous cysts on the Witwatersrand, 1965–74, standardized against standard European, World and African populations (from Shear and Singh, 1978)

	Per million per year		
	European	*World*	*African*
Black male	1.09	1.18	1.22
Black female	1.18	1.22	1.39
White male	9.93	9.92	10.83
White female	7.30	7.26	8.04

Age

The age distribution of 206 patients in our series is shown in **Figure 5.2**. The age-specific morbidity rates for black and white males and females on the Witwatersrand are shown in **Table 5.2**. Although dentigerous cysts occur in the first decade more commonly than do other jaw cysts, the frequency in that period is

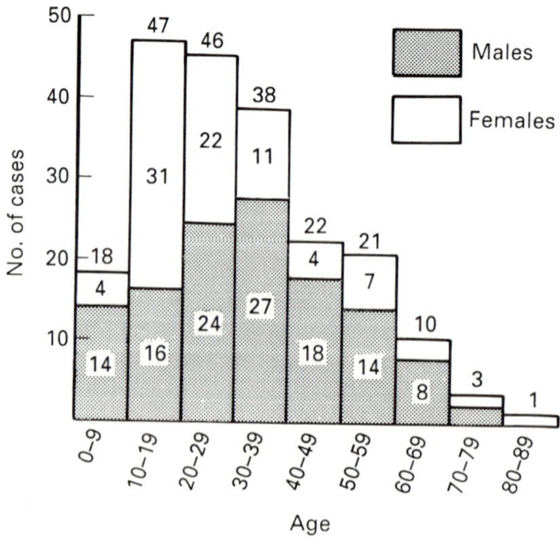

Figure 5.2. Age distribution of 206 patients with dentigerous cysts.

Table 5.2 Average annual incidence rates for dentigerous cyst in the Witwatersrand area, South Africa, 1965–74

	Average annual incidence per million by age group (years)							
	0–9	*10–19*	*20–29*	*30–39*	*40–49*	*50–64*	*65–74*	*75+*
Black male	0.64	1.94	2.62	0	0.85	1.27	0	0
Black female	0.69	1.47	1.57	1.90	2.71	0	0	0
White male	7.51	6.83	14.90	15.39	10.87	11.58	0	0
White female	1.95	12.04	9.41	10.46	7.29	6.46	0	8.90

decade more commonly than do other jaw cysts, the frequency in that period is nevertheless lower than in the subsequent three decades. This is because the lower wisdom teeth and the maxillary permanent canines, which are the teeth most frequently involved in dentigerous cysts are at an early stage of development (**Figure 5.3**). Of 17 cases in the first decade, for which the tooth of origin was known, the mandibular first premolar was involved in six, the mandibular second premolar in four, the first permanent molar twice, and the maxillary permanent central, lateral, canine and premolars were each involved once. In the second decade, there is a substantially higher frequency than in the first, most of the cysts

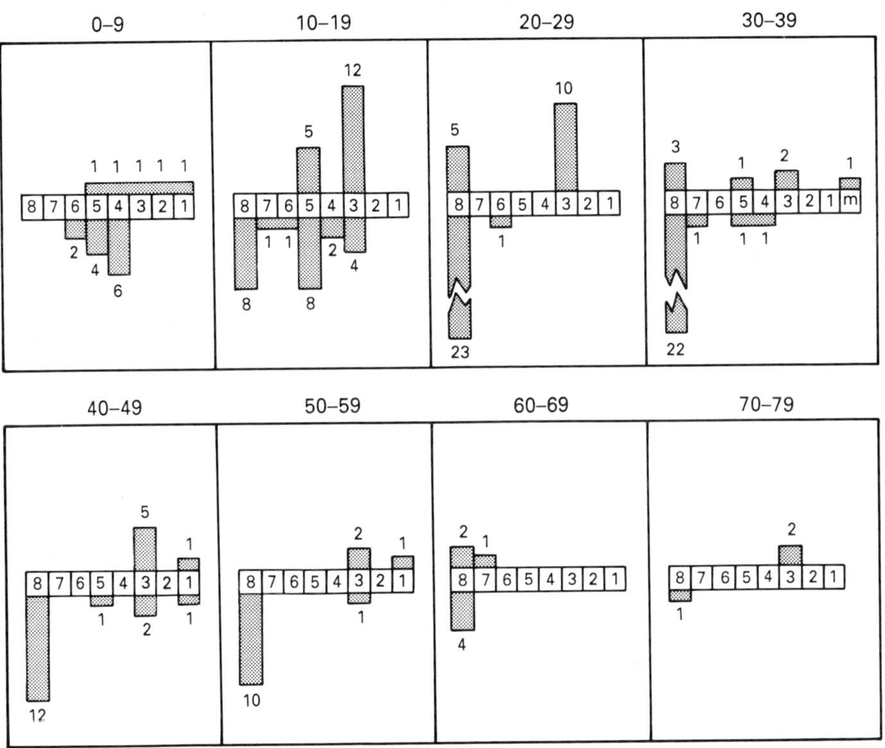

Figure 5.3. Teeth involved by dentigerous cysts in different decades.

involving the maxillary permanent canine, the mandibular wisdom tooth and the upper and lower second premolars. The third and fourth decades show the peak involvement of the lower wisdom teeth and it is during the third decade that the upper wisdom tooth becomes involved for the first time. During the subsequent decades there is a gradual decline in frequency with the mandibular wisdoms and maxillary permanent canines most often involved.

It is interesting to observe that the age distribution in our South African sample is similar to that of Mourshed's (1964c) United States group and that of Roggan and Donath (1985) from Germany, whereas the British material of Browne (1972) and Killey, Kay and Seward (1977) showed a peak frequency at a later age. A difference in age distribution of radicular cysts between British and South African samples has also been observed and is commented on under that heading. In our studies the peak incidence for white females is found at a younger age than other groups (**Table 5.2**).

Sex (Tables 5.2 and 5.3)

The frequency of dentigerous cysts is significantly greater in males than females ($P < 0.001$). In a sample of 218 of our patients with this cyst, 134 (62 per cent) were males and 84 (38 per cent) females, a male:female ratio of 1.6:1. These figures are almost identical to those of Mourshed's United States sample and that of Roggan and Donath, although the series of both Browne and Killey *et al.* showed an even greater male preponderance. Our age-standardized incidence rates show a male preponderance of a similar order of magnitude for whites but not for blacks (**Table 5.1**).

Table 5.3 Sex distribution of black and white patients with dentigerous cysts

	Male	*Female*	*Total*	*M:F ratio*
Black	28	10	38 (25%)	2.8:1
White	106	74	180 (75%)	1.4:1
Total	134 (62%)	84 (38%)	218	1.6:1
W:B ratio	3.8:1	7.4:1	4.7:1	

Although there might be a tendency to assume that the less frequent occurrence in females results from their having a lower prevalence of unerupted teeth, this assumption is not entirely borne out by data such as that collected by Mourshed (1964a) and Brown *et al.* (1982). In surveys of large series of radiographs, both groups found that there was no sex difference in the frequency of unerupted teeth. In the study of Brown *et al.* (1982), however, there was a difference in the frequency of impactions between black males and females ($P < 0.001$) although there was no significant difference between males and females either in whites or in the total sample. These data suggest that there is another factor, as yet not identified but possibly innate, which may influence the development of dentigerous cysts other than the mere physical fact of their origin in unerupted teeth.

Race (Tables 5.1, 5.2 and 5.3)

In our material there is a very much higher frequency of dentigerous cysts in whites than in blacks. Of 218 patients, 180 were whites and 38 were blacks, a ratio of 4.7:1. The age-standardized study confirms the higher incidence among whites in the population sampled and it seems that blacks have a lesser tendency than whites to develop dentigerous cysts. In Mourshed's series, there was also a very considerable preponderance of white patients compared with blacks, but Mourshed discounted this on the grounds that the biopsy service at his school deals predominantly with material from white patients.

If, however, the difference in racial incidence is a real one, then the reason for this must be sought either in differences in the frequency of impacted teeth or in the unidentified factor which may be responsible for the greater preponderance in males than females, or in both. In a study on the Witwatersrand of 576 patients with impacted teeth observed in a series of 1853 radiographs (Brown *et al.*, 1982), white patients had a higher frequency of impactions (455 or 34.8 per cent of the white sample) than black patients (121 or 22.2 per cent of the black sample). This difference is highly significant statistically (corrected $\chi^2 = 28.19$; $P < 0.0001$) and is likely to be a factor influencing the higher frequency of dentigerous cysts in white patients.

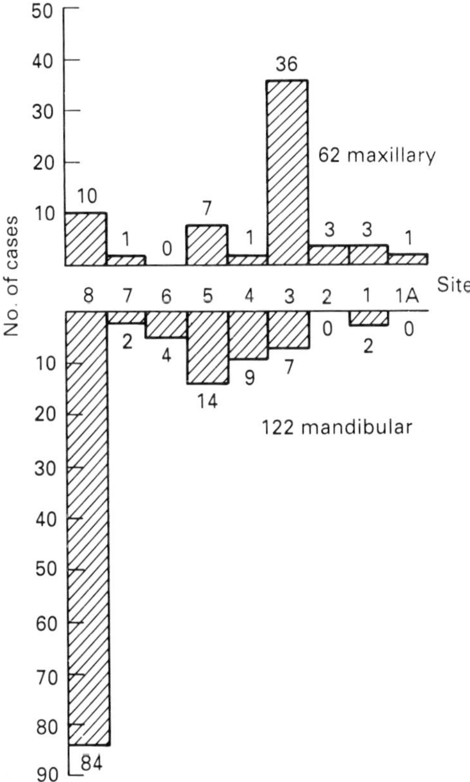

Figure 5.4. Anatomical distribution of 184 dentigerous cysts.

Site

The anatomical distribution of 184 dentigerous cysts, in relation to tooth involved, is shown in **Figure 5.4** and this has already been discussed with regard to the age distribution. A very substantial majority involve the mandibular third molar. The maxillary permanent canine is next in order of frequency of involvement, followed by the mandibular premolars and the maxillary third molar. A similar distribution was reported by Roggan and Donath (1985).

Lustmann and Bodner (1988) reported on dentigerous cysts associated with supernumerary teeth. In a review of 42 such cases from his own material and those reported in the literature, he found that about 90 per cent were associated with a maxillary mesiodens. Kaugars, Miller and Abbey (1989) documented the occurrence of dentigerous cysts associated with a substantial number (27.6 per cent) of a series of 351 odontomas.

Clinical presentation

Like keratocysts, dentigerous cysts may grow to a large size before they are diagnosed. Most of them are discovered on radiographs when these are taken because a tooth has failed to erupt, or a tooth is missing, or because teeth are tilted or are otherwise out of alignment. Many patients first become aware of the cysts because of slowly enlarging swellings, and this is the common form of presentation with edentulous patients in whose jaws unerupted teeth have inadvertently been retained. Dentigerous cysts may occasionally be painful particularly if infected. Although patients may give a history of a slowly-enlarging swelling, Seward (1964) has shown radiologically that lesions 4–5 cm in diameter may develop in 3–4 years.

Radiological features

Radiographs show unilocular radiolucent areas associated with the crowns of unerupted teeth. The cysts have well-defined sclerotic margins unless they become infected. Occasionally trabeculations may be seen and this may give an erroneous impression of multilocularity. The unerupted teeth may be impacted as a result of inadequate space in the dental arch or as a result of malpositioning such as by a horizontally impacted mandibular third molar or an inverted tooth. Supernumerary teeth may develop dentigerous cysts (Mourshed, 1964b; Lustmann and Bodner, 1988).

Three radiological variations of the dentigerous cyst may be observed. In the central variety (**Figure 5.5**) the crown is enveloped symmetrically. In these instances, pressure is applied to the crown of the tooth and may push it away from its direction of eruption. In this way, mandibular third molars may be found at the lower border of the mandible (**Figure 5.1**) or in the ascending ramus and a maxillary canine may be forced into the maxillary sinus as far as the floor of the orbit. A maxillary incisor may be found below the floor of the nose (**Figure 5.5**). The lateral type of dentigerous cyst (**Figures 5.6** and **5.7**) is a radiographic appearance which results from dilatation of the follicle on one aspect of the crown. This type is commonly seen when an impacted mandibular third molar is partially erupted so that its superior aspect is exposed (**Figure 5.6**). The so-called circumferential dentigerous cyst in which the entire tooth appears to be enveloped by cyst (**Figure 5.7**) results when the follicle expands in the manner illustrated in

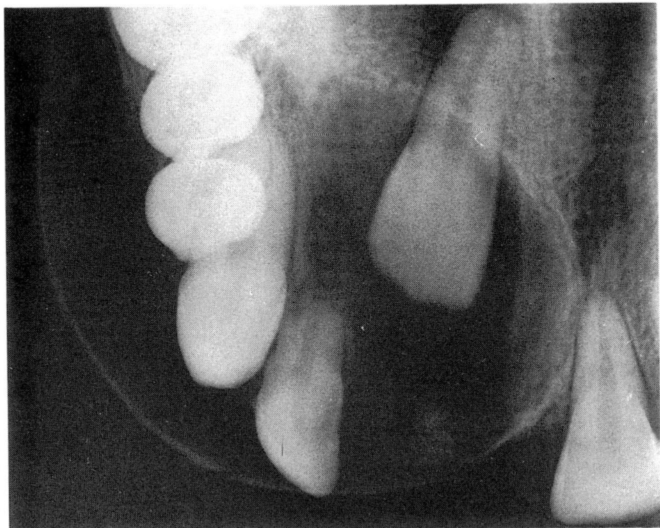

Figure 5.5. Radiograph of a central type of dentigerous cyst involving a maxillary central incisor tooth. (By courtesy of Dr M. Copelyn.)

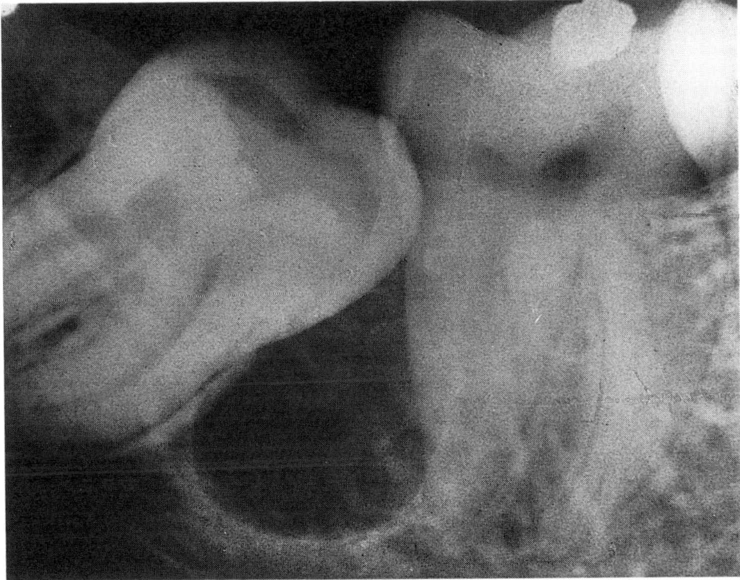

Figure 5.6. Radiograph of a lateral type dentigerous cyst.

Figure 5.8C. It is important that this variety be differentiated from the envelopmental type of keratocyst.

Some unerupted teeth have a slightly dilated follicle in the pre-eruptive phase. This does not signify a cyst, nor even necessarily a potential cyst unless the pericoronal width is at least 3–4 mm.

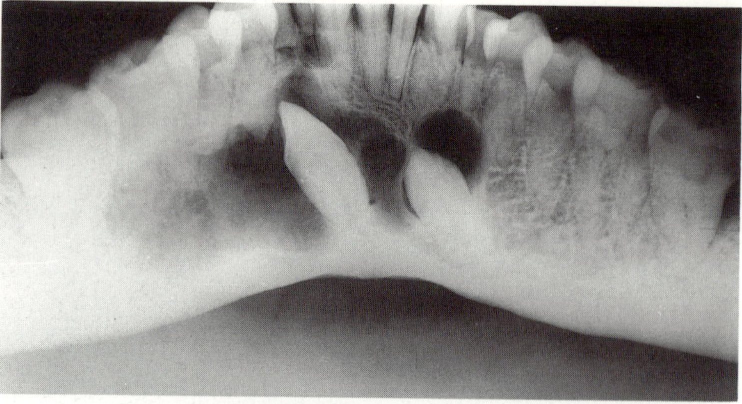

Figure 5.7. Status X-radiograph of two dentigerous cysts. The cyst on the right is a lateral type; that on the left is a circumferential type.

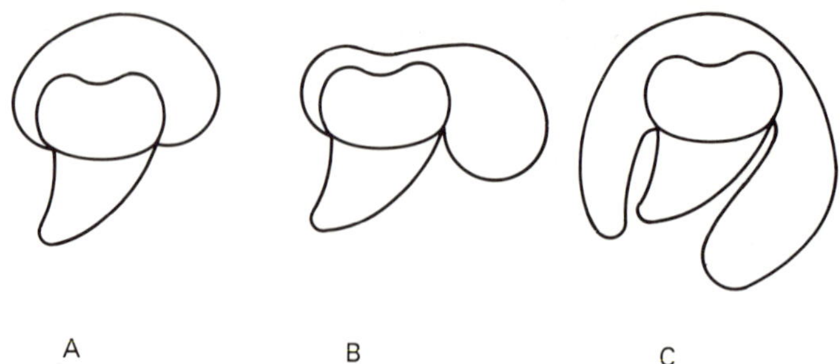

Figure 5.8. Diagram illustrating the manner in which the dental follicle may expand to produce the radiographic appearances of [A], central; [B], lateral; and [C], circumferential type dentigerous cysts.

Radicular cysts arising from deciduous teeth may mimic dentigerous cysts radiologically (Lustmann and Shear, 1985; Wood *et al.*, 1988).

Dentigerous cysts appear to have a greater tendency than other simple jaw cysts to produce some resorption of the roots of adjacent teeth (Struthers and Shear, 1976). In a radiographic study of root resorption produced by jaw cysts, Struthers and Shear (1976) observed root resorption in 11 of 20 dentigerous cysts (55 per cent) in which there was contiguity of cyst and root (**Figures 5.9** and **5.10**). By comparison, root resorption was detected in only six of 33 radicular cysts (18 per cent) and in none of their sample of 26 keratocysts. They suggested that the dentigerous cyst's potential for root resorption may be derived from its origin from dental follicle and the ability of the latter to resorb the roots of the deciduous predecessors of the teeth, the crowns of which they surround. They felt that variations in root resorptive potential could not be explained by differences in intracystic pressure as Toller (1948) had shown that dentigerous and radicular cysts have very similar intracystic pressures. The important role of dental follicle in the resorption of bone has been demonstrated experimentally by Cahill and Marks (1980).

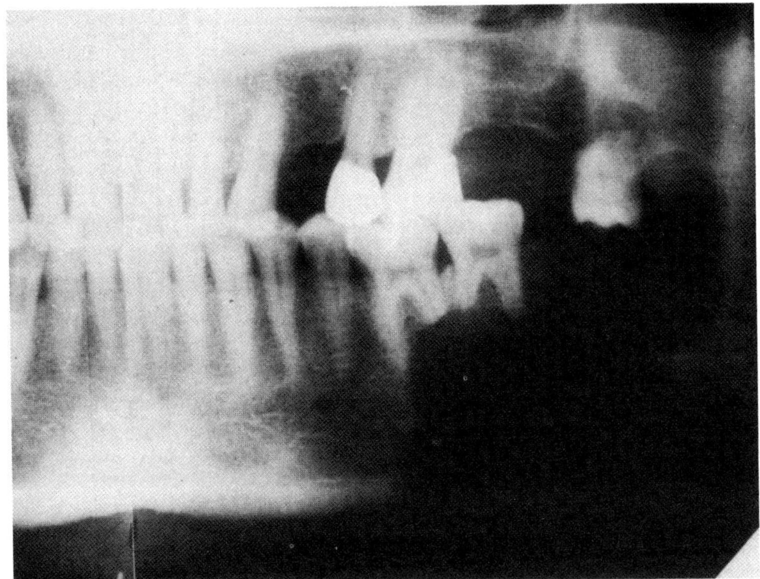

Figure 5.9. Dentigerous cyst which has displaced the mandibular third molar from which it has arisen and produced resorption of the roots of the adjacent molars.

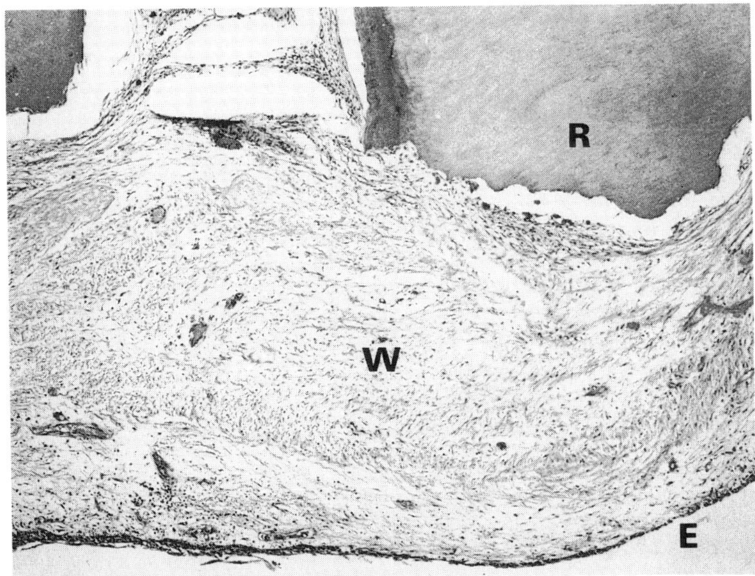

Figure 5.10. Dentigerous cyst wall with resorption of the adjacent tooth root. [E], epithelial cyst lining derived from reduced enamel epithelium; [W], cyst wall derived from dental follicle; [R], root of adjacent tooth. (H & E; × 85.)

There is evidence that vital cyst tissue in culture releases a potent bone-resorbing factor that is predominantly a mixture of prostaglandins E_2 and E_3 (Harris and Goldhaber, 1973; Harris *et al.*, 1973; Harris and Toller, 1975; Harris, 1978). The source of this resorbing factor was thought to be the capsule and its leucocyte content. Arendorf (1981) has suggested that prostaglandin E_2 may play a similar role in the resorption of cementum and dentine. Data reported by Harris (1978) indicated a lower level of prostaglandin-like material (measured as PGE_2) released by dentigerous cysts (12.2 ± 9.4 ng/mg) than by radicular (16.6 ± 13 ng/mg) or by keratocysts (20 ± 11 ng/mg). Of interest, however, is the fact that the four lesions with the highest activities regardless of group, including the ameloblastoma, with a mean of 59.25 ± 17.5 ng/mg, all resorbed the apices of adjacent teeth.

Matejka *et al.* (1985b) also found that PGE_2 was the predominant prostaglandin synthesized by radicular cysts but also found evidence of PGI_2 synthesis in a large number of radicular cysts. They believed that the surrounding granulation tissue with its associated inflammatory cells was the likely site of this synthesis and is thus one of the factors responsible for the osteolytic effects of radicular cysts. They suggested that these effects appear to be mediated at least in part by the synthesis of leucotrienes (with which prostaglandins share a common precursor, arachidonic acid), with a resultant increase in the production of PGI_2. The two dentigerous cysts that they investigated were the only two in their sample of 12 in which they found $PGF_{2\alpha}$. Further evidence that PGI_2- generation in human radicular cysts is stimulated by leucotrienes C_4 and D_4 in chronic inflammatory processes, was reported by Matejka *et al.* (1985a).

Meghji, Harvey and Harris (1989) investigated the possibility that interleukin 1 may be produced by odontogenic cysts and may account for the raised levels of prostaglandin and collagenase synthesis by the cyst capsules. They referred to previous work which had shown that interleukin 1 and tumour necrosis factor accounted for much of the bone resorbing activity attributed to osteoclast activating factor produced by mononuclear leucocytes. These cytokines are particularly associated with chronic inflammatory lesions. Using radicular and dentigerous cysts, they demonstrated synthesis *in vitro* of a macromolecular factor with osteolytic activity which has the characteristics of interleukin 1. The stimulation of fibroblast collagenase and prostaglandin E_2 synthesis in their cyst wall culture media as well as stimulation of fibroblast and osteoblast proliferation, also suggested interleukin 1 activity to the authors. They believed that the source of the interleukin could be the monocyte/macrophage infiltrate, the stromal fibroblasts and the epithelial cyst linings; and that the interleukin 1 released by the cysts could lead to a number of osteolytic cell reactions: the stimulation of osteoclasts to resorb bone, and the connective tissue cells to produce prostaglandins which will be responsible for further osteoclast activation. It also stimulates connective tissue cells to produce collagenase which is involved in the destruction of bone matrix.

Pathogenesis

There can be little doubt that dentigerous cysts develop around the crown of unerupted teeth, whatever causes failure of eruption of the latter. In an analysis of the distribution of 761 unerupted teeth in 304 patients, Mourshed (1964a) showed that the vast majority were mandibular (378) or maxillary (328) third molars. Maxillary canines were next, a long way behind (15), followed by mandibular second premolars (11), maxillary second molars (eight), mandibular second molars (seven), mandibular canines (six) and maxillary second premolars (four). The mandibular and maxillary first premolars, a maxillary central incisor and a supernumerary tooth were each involved once. A similar study was done in our own department to determine the distribution of 1259 impacted teeth in a consecutive sample of radiographs taken in various departments of our hospital during the year 1981 (Brown *et al.*, 1982). The distribution and frequency of individual impacted teeth determined in this way is compared in **Table 5.4** with the anatomical distribution of 184 dentigerous cysts as illustrated in **Figure 5.4.** In the case of mandibular third molars, the frequency of impaction (48.1 per cent) is roughly the same as the frequency of cyst formation (45.7 per cent). The maxillary third molars, however, have a comparatively much higher frequency of impaction (29.6 per cent) than cyst involvement (5.4 per cent) suggesting that this tooth might have a relatively lower risk than its mandibular counterpart of developing a dentigerous cyst. By the same token, maxillary canines would appear to have a somewhat higher relative risk of developing dentigerous cysts than mandibular canines. The relative risks of the other teeth are shown in the extreme right-hand column of **Table 5.4**.

Table 5.4 Comparison of frequency of impacted teeth with frequency of dentigerous cyst formation in two independent Witwatersrand samples

Tooth	*Impacted (I)*		*Dentigerous cyst involvement (DC)*		*DC%/I%*
	(No.)	*(%)*	*(No.)*	*(%)*	
Mandibular third molar	606	48.1	84	45.7	0.95
Maxillary third molar	372	29.6	10	5.4	0.18
Maxillary canine	150	11.9	36	19.6	1.65
Mandibular canine	44	3.5	7	3.8	1.09
Mandibular second premolar	41	3.3	14	7.6	2.30
Maxillary second premolar	27	2.2	7	3.8	1.73
Maxillary second molar	6	0.5	1	0.5	1.00
Mandibular first premolar	5	0.4	9	4.9	12.25
Maxillary central incisor	2	0.2	3	1.6	8.00
Mandibular second molar	1	0.1	2	1.1	11.00
Maxillary first premolar	1	0.1	1	0.5	5.00
Other teeth	4	0.3	9	4.9	16.33
Total	1259	100	184	100	

Mourshed (1964a) has calculated that the frequency of dentigerous cysts is 1.44 in every 100 unerupted teeth. Toller's estimate (1967) was that possibly one in 150 unerupted teeth might develop a dentigerous cyst, and the risk seems to be greater in individuals over 30 years than in those who are younger. The anatomical environment of an unerupted tooth is proobably of some significance in determining the development of a cyst. As I have mentioned before, however, the differences in sex and race incidence do suggest that there is some other factor, as yet unidentified, but possibly innate, which may play some role in determining whether a cyst will develop.

It has been suggested that dentigerous cysts may be of either extrafollicular or intrafollicular origin and that those of intrafollicular origin may develop by accumulation of fluid either between the reduced enamel epithelium and the enamel, or within the enamel organ itself.

Atkinson (1972, 1976, 1977) described the formation of cysts derived from the enamel organ around the crowns of mouse molar teeth transplanted subcutaneously into an inbred strain (C57B1) of mice. In his 1976 paper, Atkinson showed that after initial degeneration, the enamel organ took the form of a squamous epithelium in which after 5–6 days squamous hyperplasia took place. Cystic degeneration within the hyperplastic epithelium produced cavities lined with a thick parakeratotic stratified squamous epithelium but as the cysts enlarged the lining changed to a thin non-keratinized stratified squamous epithelium.

Riviere and Sabet (1973) transplanted unerupted molar tooth germs from 7-day-old mice to the mammary fat pads of adult mice of the same inbred line. Cysts with a dentigerous relationship to the crown of the tooth developed in every instance that the graft retained its viability and they developed at about the same rate in all animals over a 3-week period.

Al-Talabani and Smith (1980) studied the cysts which formed adjacent to the developing crowns of tooth germ isografts in hamster cheek pouch. In isografts from 5-day-old animals, cysts frequently formed as a result of enamel organ degeneration soon after transplantation. Enamel hypoplasia was often a feature of the related teeth. They then examined 86 teeth associated with human dentigerous cysts and 43 of these showed areas of enamel hypoplasia on their occlusal surfaces or incisal edges. In tooth germ transplants from 2-day-old hamsters, cysts formed in about half of the specimens only after completion of enamel formation, 6 weeks after transplantation. In this group, the cysts developed by separation between the cells of the reduced enamel epithelium and enamel hypoplasia was not a conspicuous feature. The authors considered that there was a strong possibility of a direct relationship between the development of cysts and the occurrence of enamel hypoplasia in the involved teeth. They suggested the possibility that there may be two types of dentigerous cyst, with different causes and arising at different stages of tooth development. One would arise by degeneration of the stellate reticulum at an early stage of development and is likely to be associated with enamel hypoplasia. The other would develop after completion of the crown by accumulation of fluid between the layers of the reduced enamel epithelium. Enamel hypoplasia would not be a significant feature of this variety. This concurrence of dentigerous cyst with enamel hypoplasia of the contained tooth is an interesting one as the relationship occurs too frequently to be fortuitous. Another explanation for the association, not suggested by Al-Talabani and Smith (1980), may be that the presence of foci of enamel hypoplasia diminishes the adherence of reduced enamel epithelium to crown and provides the starting point for the development of the cyst.

I am inclined to reject the extrafollicular theory of origin of dentigerous cysts as those which have been reported as arising in this manner appear to be envelopmental or follicular keratocysts. The case reported by Gillette and Weinmann (1958), and which is frequently quoted in support of extrafollicular origin, is clearly an envelopmental keratocyst (see **Figure 2.10**, p. 24). Occasional dentigerous cyst linings show projections which resemble Tomes' processes of the ameloblasts protruding into the lumen from the superficial layer of epithelial cells. This suggests that in these instances the superficial cells were derived from the ameloblasts and provides evidence that in these cases, dentigerous cysts arose by accumulation of fluid between the reduced enamel epithelium and the enamel, and not in the stellate reticulum. Furthermore, it must be unusual to be able to demonstrate an intact cyst lining around the crown of the unerupted tooth. In my experience, the epithelial lining of the dentigerous cyst invariably terminates at the neck of the involved tooth. Therefore, while not excluding the possibility that some dentigerous cysts develop within the enamel organ, and this certainly seems to happen in the tooth germ transplant experiments, I believe that in humans these cysts form between the reduced enamel epithelium and the enamel.

Another theory of origin which has been proposed is that the crown of a permanent tooth may erupt into a radicular cyst of its deciduous predecessor. This phenomenon probably does occur, but only exceptionally rarely, because radicular cysts involving the deciduous dentition are so uncommon (Lustmann and Shear, 1985). In such a case the erupting tooth may indent rather than penetrate the wall of the radicular cyst and this should be apparent histologically, if not macroscopically (**Figure 5.11**), (Gebhardt and Lenz, 1985; Wood *et al.*, 1988).

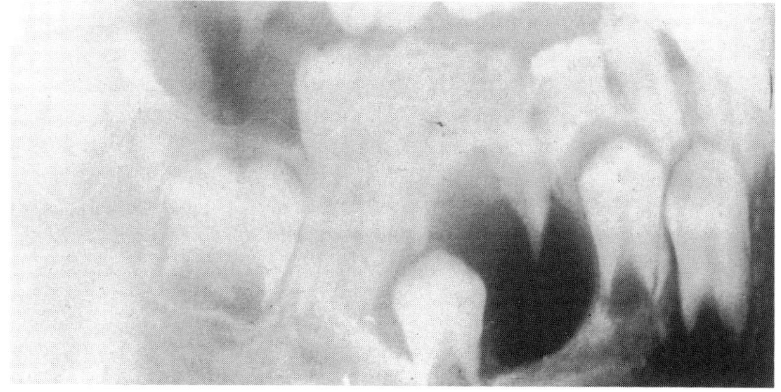

a

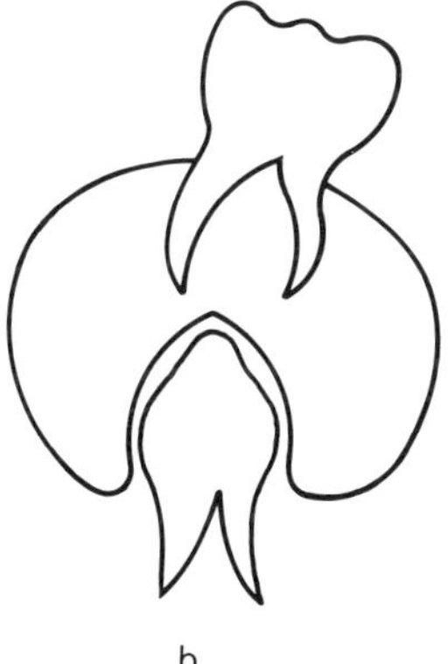

b

Figure 5.11. (a) Radicular cyst associated with a deciduous mandibular second molar tooth appears to be in a dentigerous relationship with the erupting premolar. (b) Diagrammatic representation of the probable relationship, where the erupting tooth has indented the radicular cyst wall. (Radiograph by courtesy of Dr. J. Lustmann.)

A variation of this concept is that inflammation at the apex of a deciduous tooth can lead to the development of an inflammatory follicular cyst (Shaw, Smith and Hill, 1980; Main, 1985; Benn, Ackermann and Altini, 1990; Benn, 1991). Benn's 1991 study included 15 patients ranging in age from 5 to 12 years. In 12 cases the inflammation arose from a non-vital deciduous predecessor, while two patients had

Garré's osteomyelitis. The mandible was involved in 10 cases and the maxilla in five. The premolar teeth were associated with the cysts in nine cases, the canines in three and the second molars in two cases, presumably in the patients with Garŕe's osteomyelitis. Macroscopically, all the cysts were attached to the necks of teeth showing virtually no root formation. Histologically, the most commonly occurring feature was the presence of non-keratinized stratified squamous epithelium of varying thickness with focal areas of arcading. All cases showed some degree of inflammation.

There would appear therefore to be some evidence of an inflammatory aetiology in the pathogenesis of some dentigerous cysts. Nevertheless, individual cases need to be assessed critically. Attachment of the cyst wall to the neck of the associated tooth is an essential feature; and microscopically, the cyst lining should demonstrate a readily identifiable component of reduced enamel epithelium before a diagnosis of dentigerous cyst is made. Most of the cases reported by Shaw, Smith and Hill (1980) were resolved after extraction of the involved primary tooth and curettage of the socket; and their brief description of the histological findings is consistent more with radicular than with dentigerous cyst linings. These are more likely to be rare examples of radicular cysts associated with deciduous teeth and which have been indented by the erupting permanent successors, as indicated in **Figure 5.11**.

Assuming then that the dentigerous cyst develops around an unerupted tooth by accumulation of fluid between the reduced enamel epithelium and the enamel, or between layers of reduced enamel epithelium, how does this happen? Main (1970b) suggested that the pressure exerted by a potentially-erupting tooth on an impacted follicle obstructs the venous outflow and thereby induces rapid transudation of serum across the capillary walls. The increased hydrostatic pressure of this pooling fluid separates the follicle from the crown, with or without reduced enamel epithelium. With time, capillary permeability is altered so as to permit the passage of greater quantities of protein above the low concentration of the pure transudate. Studies by Skaug (1973), Skaug and Hofstad (1973) and Browne (1975) on dentigerous cyst fluids have indicated total soluble protein levels, albumin/globulin ratios and immunoglobulin levels similar to those in serum. Browne (1975) suggested, therefore, that in dentigerous cysts the fluid arises as an exudate from the vessels in the capsule and is only slightly modified by any local immunoglobulin synthesis in the cyst wall. However, immunoglobulins and immunoglobulin-containing cells are present in the walls of odontogenic cysts, and in an immunohistochemical study of immunoglobulin-containing plasma cells in keratocysts, dentigerous and radicular cysts, Smith *et al.* (1987) showed that IgG-containing plasma cells were the predominant species in all three, with a much lower percentage of IgA- and few IgM-containing plasma cells. There was a significantly higher percentage contribution of IgG-containing plasma cells and a significantly lower percentage of IgA-containing plasma cells in dentigerous cysts than in keratocysts. There was also intense extracellular staining of IgG in the dentigerous cyst. The authors suggested that the Igs found in odontogenic cyst fluids may be derived from local synthesis in the cyst capsule as well as an inflammatory exudate.

Glycosaminoglycans, predominantly hyaluronic acid but also appreciable amounts of heparin and chondroitin-4-sulphate, are present in the fluids and walls of dentigerous cysts (Skaug and Hofstad, 1972; Smith, Smith and Browne, 1984, 1988a and b). Release of the glycosaminoglycans from the walls and their diffusion into the cyst fluid, is thought to play an important role in expansile cyst growth by increasing the osmolality of the cyst fluid and hence raising the internal hydrostatic pressure of the cyst. A more detailed account of the role of glycosaminoglycans in odontogenic cysts, is given in Chapter 2, p. 18.

Many dentigerous cysts show evidence of acute and chronic inflammation in their walls, and in these instances exudation must play some part in the expansion of the cyst. Moreover, the passage of desquamated epithelial cells and inflammatory cells into the cyst cavity must contribute to the increase in intracystic osmotic tension and thereby probably to further expansion of the cyst. Toller (1970b) has shown that the mean cyst fluid osmolality of seven dentigerous cysts was 10 mosmol higher than the mean serum osmolality but that this increase was not statistically significant. He believed (Toller, 1967) that the likely origin of dentigerous cysts is a breakdown of proliferating cells of the follicle following impeded eruption. Although he conceded that the factors favouring fluid accumulation which were postulated by Main may possibly play a role, he believed that raised osmolality of the cyst fluid makes an important contribution to cyst expansion. As the cyst expands, there may be some compensatory epithelial proliferation to cover the greater surface area of connective tissue, but this is slight, as demonstrated by the low mitotic rate in dentigerous cyst epithelium (Browne, 1975). Furthermore, Stenman *et al.* (1986) have shown that dentigerous cyst epithelium has little capacity for *in vitro* growth, compared with keratocyst epithelium.

The role of prostaglandins in resorption of bone and consequently the enlargement of dentigerous as well as of other cysts, has been dealt with earlier in this chapter.

Main (1970b) made the point that the pooling fluid separates the follicle from the crown, with or without reduced enamel epithelium, on the basis of the work of Stanley, Krogh and Pannuk (1965) who studied 70 non-cystic follicles from the third molars of patients ranging in age from 13 to 69 years. They concluded that follicles separated from enamel in patients below 22 years of age tend to leave the still-cuboidal reduced enamel epithelium attached to tooth, while above this age the progressively more squamous epithelium becomes increasingly more readily detached. The frequent occurrence of ‘epithelial discontinuities’ described by Toller (1966a) in about one-third of uninfected dentigerous cysts suggests that in some of these cysts the reduced enamel epithelium may separate in parts and adhere to the enamel in other parts.

Pathology

Sometimes the cyst is removed intact but more often the thin wall is torn during the surgical procedure. Pathologists should do a careful dissection of the gross specimen to determine that the cyst surrounding the crown of the tooth is indeed a dilated follicle and that it attaches at the amelocemental junction. Some keratocysts may appear, in the gross specimen, to be dentigerous cysts, but their extrafollicular location will be demonstrated on dissection except with examples of follicular keratocysts, the nature of which will only be revealed on histological examination (**Figure 2.11**, p. 25). In an inflamed dentigerous cyst the wall may be thickened.

I have seen a few cases of early adenomatoid odontogenic tumour which have appeared radiologically and in the gross specimen as dentigerous cysts. The clue to the presence of adenomatoid odontogenic tumour may be provided in the gross specimen by the observation of small white or yellow nodules on the luminal surface of the cyst wall. Similarly, the presence of the nodules of plexiform unicystic ameloblastoma referred to later in this chapter may be predicted by careful examination of the gross specimen. Histological sections should, of course, always be prepared from these areas of irregularity.

Histological examination usually shows a thin fibrous cyst wall which, being derived from dental follicle, consists of young fibroblasts widely separated by stroma and ground substance rich in acid mucopolysaccharide. The epithelial lining, which is in fact reduced enamel epithelium, consists of 2–4 cell layers of flat or cuboidal cells (**Figure 5.12**). Characteristically, the epithelial lining is not keratinized and most of those which have been described as keratinized have usually been adjacent keratocysts. Very rarely, a dentigerous cyst lining may apparently form keratin by metaplasia (**Figure 5.13**). Discontinuities in the epithelial lining may be seen in the presence of an intense inflammatory infiltrate in the adjacent capsule, or, as suggested by Toller (1966a) through partial adherence to enamel. Sometimes, the superficial layer of the epithelial lining is low columnar and retains the morphology of the ameloblast layer which, of course, it originally was.

In some cysts part of the epithelial lining may contain mucus-producing cells. Browne (1972) found them in 36 per cent of mandibular and in 53 per cent of maxillary dentigerous cysts in his series, and made the interesting observation that the frequency of such mucous cells increased in proportion to the age of the patients. Ciliated cells occur very rarely. The presence of these mucous and ciliated cells are thought to result from metaplasia. Another rare example of metaplasia in dentigerous cysts is provided by the occasional presence of sebaceous glands in their walls (Gorlin, 1957; Spouge, 1966). Hyaline bodies (Rushton, 1955) are sometimes seen.

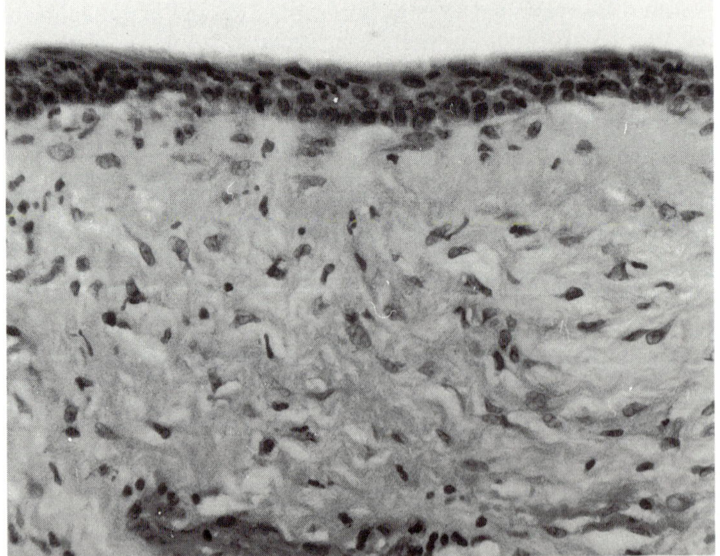

Figure 5.12. Wall of a dentigerous cyst lined by a thin epithelium of 2–4 layers of undifferentiated cells derived from the reduced enamel epithelium. (H & E; × 250.)

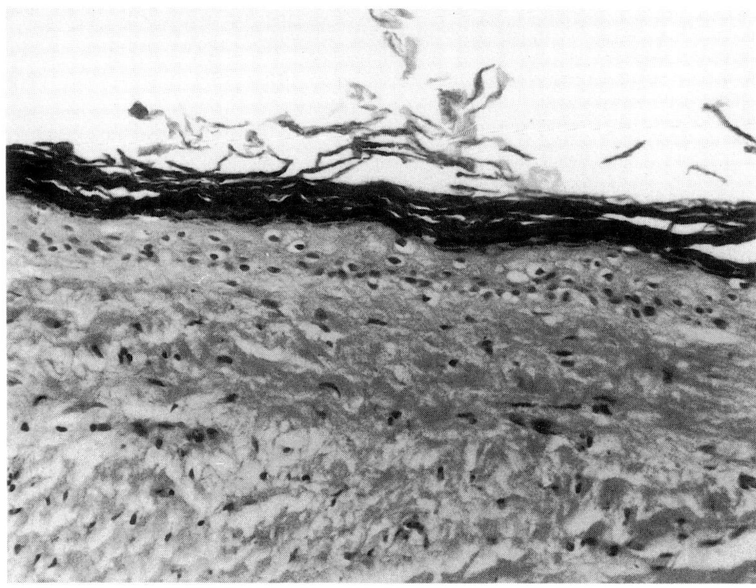

Figure 5.13. A rare example of keratinizing epithelium lining a dentigerous cyst. (H & E; × 220.)

Localized proliferation of the epithelial lining may occur in response to inflammation. Occasional bud-like thickenings of the epithelium may be seen in the absence of inflammation and sometimes there may be budding of the basal cells into the fibrous capsule. Nests, islands and strands of odontogenic epithelium are often seen in the capsule. Wright (1979b) reported the presence, in the capsules of a series of dentigerous cysts, of epithelial proliferations which resembled the squamous odontogenic tumour (Pullon *et al.*, 1975). None of the cases has recurred following conservative surgery. Undifferentiated epithelium lining dentigerous cysts, like reduced enamel epithelium of dental follicles, yielded consistently negative results for blood group antigens A and B in the hands of Wright (1979a). On the other hand, Vedtofte, Pindborg and Hakomori (1985) were able to demonstrate the A, B and H type 2 antigens in follicular, radicular and keratocysts. They ascribed the variation between their findings and those of Wright (1979a) to technical and sampling differences. Gardner and O'Neill (1988) also found that five of seven dentigerous cysts which they studied were markedly positive for blood group antigens A, B and H type 2. Two exhibited only a few positive cells.

Hormia *et al.* (1987) used immunohistochemical staining with monoclonal antibodies to study and compare the cytokeratin content of odontogenic cysts, normal gingival epithelium and ameloblastomas. Their results showed that keratocysts, radicular cysts and dentigerous cysts have distinct profiles of cytokeratin polypeptides and that with the exception of some dentigerous cysts they all lack large cytokeratins typical of keratinizing squamous epithelia. The entire epithelium of dentigerous cysts was stained intensely with PKK2 (which reacts with cytokeratin polypeptides 7, 17 and 19 and typical of basal epidermal cells); and KA1 (typical of squamous epithelium) antibodies. PKK1 (which reacts with cytokeratins 8, 18 and 19); K_M4.62 (which reacts with cytokeratin 19); and K_S8.12

(which reacts with cytokeratins 13 and 16) antibodies also reacted with the epithelium of these cysts but the labelling varied in intensity between samples, different areas of the same sample and between the cells. Two of the dentigerous cysts, unlike any other cysts, also contained a layer of cells expressing cytokeratin polypeptide No. 18 (K_S 18.18; PKK3). These cysts were negative for KA5 (indicating the absence of cytokeratins 1, 9, 10 and 11); and K_K 8.60 (indicating absence of cytokeratins 10 and 11) antibodies. Two other dentigerous cysts were negative for PKK3 and K_S 18.18 antibodies, but were strongly positive for KA5 and K_K 8.60 antibodies.

On the question of whether dentigerous cysts arise between the reduced enamel epithelium and the enamel, or by a split in the enamel organ itself, the authors proposed that their results suggested that two histogenetic entities could occur which could not be distinguished by routine histological examination. They also pointed out that their results indicated that dentigerous, but not other cyst types, may share with some cases of ameloblastoma, the expression of cytokeratin polypeptide No. 18. The cytokeratin 18-positive cells could have a specific histogenetic origin and could consequently have distinct functional characteristics. Another possibility, they suggested, is that the expression of cytokeratin polypeptide No. 18 in dentigerous cysts is a sign of oncofetal transformation in these lesions. Further studies are required to determine whether the presence of cytokeratin polypeptide No. 18 in dentigerous cyst epithelium might be associated with ameloblastomatous changes in the cyst.

Seven dentigerous cysts were included in the sample of 50 odontogenic cysts investigated by Matthews, Mason and Browne (1988) for the expression of keratins, epithelial membrane antigen (EMA), carcinoembryonic antigen (CEA) and rat liver antigen (RLA) by their epithelial linings. Using monospecific antibodies, keratins 7, 8 and 18 were poorly expressed with reactivity being detected only in isolated surface cells in some dentigerous cysts. Keratin 19 was detected in the epithelial linings of all cyst specimens and was normally expressed by the majority of epithelial cells irrespective of their level within the epithelium and/or differentiation. Keratin 10/11 was rarely expressed by dentigerous cyst linings although isolated positive cells or groups of cells were present in some specimens. The majority of dentigerous cysts were reactive with antibodies specific for keratin 13 and an epitope shared between keratins 13 and 16. CEA and EMA antigens were detected in the majority of epithelial cells lining dentigerous cysts, the reactivity of the latter being consistently greater. RLA was expressed by the majority of suprabasal cells in all cyst linings and occasionally by all layers. Like Matthews, Mason and Browne (1988), Morgan, Seddon and Lane (1988) demonstrated the expression of keratin 7, which is not normally present in stratified squamous epithelia, in the superficial cells of the epithelial linings of dentigerous cysts.

The dentigerous cyst as a potential ameloblastoma

A number of workers have claimed that many ameloblastomas arise in dentigerous cysts but I have seen no evidence to support such a contention. Indeed, the fact that dentigerous cysts are rarer in South African blacks, compared with whites, whereas ameloblastomas are very much more common in blacks (Meerkotter, 1969; Shear and Singh, 1978) provides contrary evidence. While ameloblastomas, being of odontogenic epithelial origin, may of course theoretically arise from dentigerous

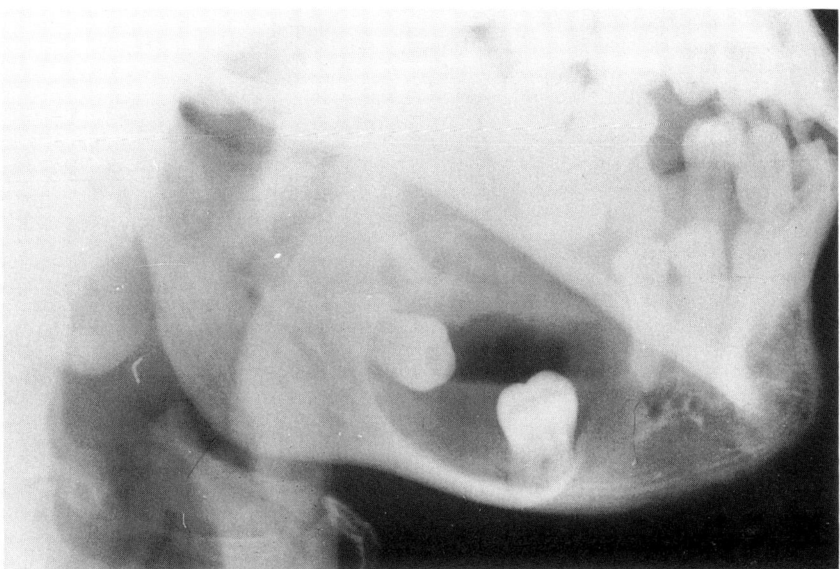

Figure 5.14. Ameloblastoma with the radiological appearance of a dentigerous cyst.

cyst lining as well as any other odontogenic epithelium, the belief that it commonly arises in this situation and that the dentigerous cyst should therefore be regarded as pre-ameloblastomatous, should be viewed with caution. Much of the confusion has, I believe, arisen for three reasons. First, an ameloblastoma, like a keratocyst, may involve an unerupted tooth, particularly a third molar at the angle of the mandible, and this may be incorrectly interpreted as a dentigerous cyst on radiographs (**Figure 5.14**). When subsequently the lesion is removed and diagnosed histologically as an ameloblastoma, the erroneous conclusion may be reached that the ameloblastoma developed from the dentigerous cyst.

The second possible reason for believing that many ameloblastomas develop from dentigerous cysts is that biopsies of ameloblastomas are often taken of an expanded locule lined apparently by a thin layer of epithelium. If the surgeon's provisional diagnosis is dentigerous cyst because of the radiological picture, the pathologist may well regard such histological features as consistent with the diagnosis. When the tumour is removed entirely and a diagnosis of ameloblastoma is made, once again this may be misinterpreted as having developed from a dentigerous cyst. Thirdly, as Lucas (1954) has pointed out, apparently isolated islets or follicles of epithelium are sometimes found in the cyst wall some distance from the epithelial lining. These have been interpreted as ameloblastoma although they bear only a superficial resemblance to the tumour.

Unicystic ameloblastoma

A number of workers have referred to the occurrence, in part of a dentigerous cyst lining, of a mural nodule of proliferating epithelium which closely resembles a plexiform ameloblastoma (Robinson and Martinez, 1977; Shteyer, Lustman and

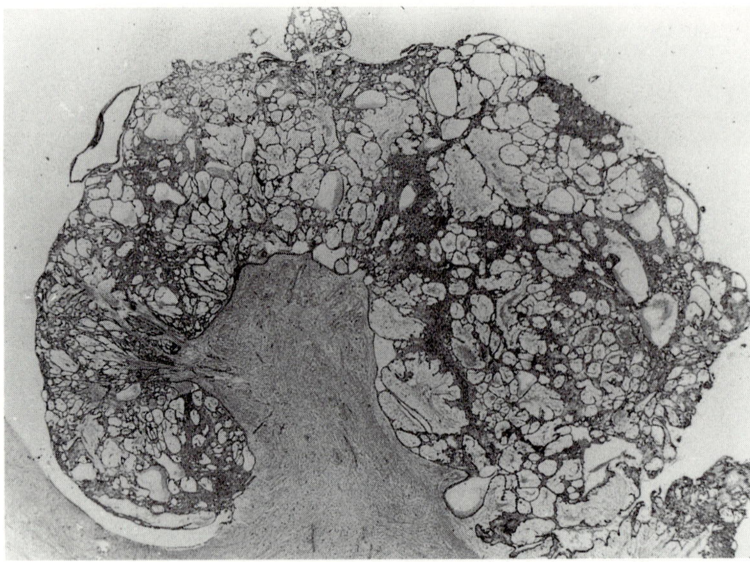

Figure 5.15. Group 2 unicystic ameloblastoma in a dentigerous relationship to the crown of an unerupted tooth. There is an intraluminal mural nodule consisting of tissue very similar to that of a plexiform ameloblastoma and there is no infiltration of the cyst wall. (H & E; × 8.)

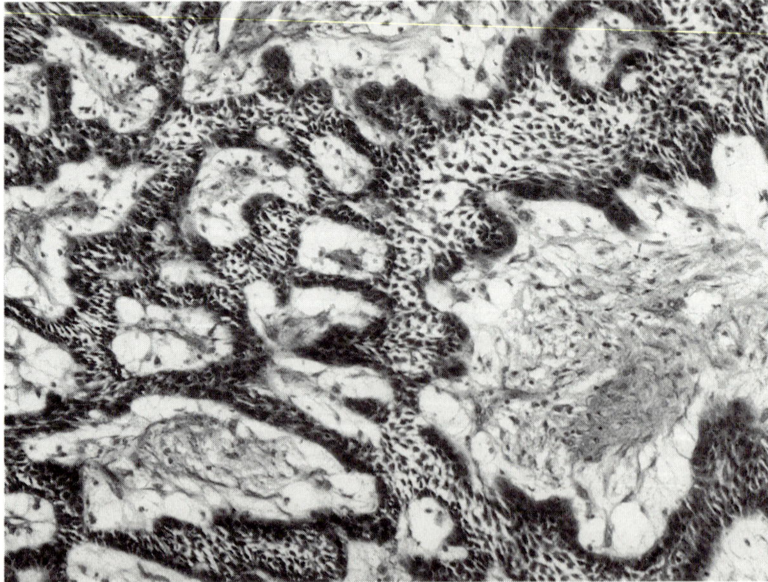

Figure 5.16. Higher magnification of another example of the phenomenon illustrated in Figure 5.15 showing the resemblance of the tissue to the plexiform ameloblastoma. (H & E; × 120.)

Lewis-Epstein, 1978; Gardner, 1981; Gardner and Corio, 1983, 1984). The nodule protrudes into the cyst cavity and varies in size but generally shows either no, or only limited, infiltration into the connective tissue capsule (**Figures 5.15**, **5.16**). Gardner (1981) regarded these lesions as ameloblastoma although he suggested that they require only conservative treatment, and proposed the term plexiform unicystic ameloblastoma. The use of this term has been regarded as unfortunate (Shafer, Hine and Levy, 1983) because of its similarity to the term 'plexiform ameloblastoma' and because the cysts do not exhibit epithelium typical of that described by Vickers and Gorlin (1970) as indicative of ameloblastoma. In the previous edition of this book, I was also critical of the reference to this lesion as an ameloblastoma, as it was not infiltrative, but cautioned that the pathologist should nevertheless examine numerous parts of such a cyst wall in order to exclude the possibility of infiltrating plexiform ameloblastoma elsewhere.

Gardner and Corio (1983, 1984) have countered this criticism by reporting cases of unicystic ameloblastoma that exhibit both patterns, namely, a plexiform nodule and plexiform ameloblastoma in the same lesion. In their 1984 study, they reported their findings in a series of 35 cases. Of 28 examples treated by enucleation or curettage, only three recurred (10.7 per cent), which is a much lower recurrence rate than that reported for typical solid or multicystic ameloblastomas. They cautioned that cases should nevertheless be followed for at least 10 years after treatment because of the small proportion that do recur. They believed that the plexiform unicystic ameloblastoma should be regarded as a histologic variant of unicystic ameloblastoma as its biological behaviour was no different from the others.

Another point of interest in the paper by Gardner and Corio (1984) is that they identified four cases of plexiform unicystic ameloblastoma which were not in a dentigerous relationship with a tooth.

We have undertaken a detailed study of the unicystic ameloblastomas in our department (Ackermann, Altini and Shear, 1988). In a series of 380 ameloblastomas recorded in the department during the 30-year period 1958–1987, 57 (15 per cent) were classified as unicystic. Males and females were affected approximately equally and most of the patients were black. The mean age of the patients at the time of diagnosis was 23.8 years (SD ±14.9) ranging from 6–77 years, with 48 per cent occurring in the second decade and 86 per cent in the second to fourth decades. The age distribution was significantly younger ($P < 0.001$) than that of patients with solid and multicystic ameloblastomas, an observation also made by previous workers in this field (Gardner, 1981; Robinson and Martinez, 1977).

The great majority of the lesions (92 per cent) occurred in the mandible. Some of the lesions were extensive, extending from angle to angle. Many affected the third molar region with extension up the ramus, while others involved the symphysis or body on one side only. Eleven of the lesions were associated with unerupted teeth (19 per cent) and of these only five (9 per cent) were related to the crown of a tooth in a true follicular manner.

Radiologically, the lesions were either well corticated unilocular radiolucencies or showed trabeculations which may lead to an erroneous diagnosis of multilocular cyst. Some were associated with unerupted teeth and could be mistakenly interpreted as dentigerous cysts, and the roots of adjacent teeth were frequently resorbed.

Microscopically, three distinct patterns could be identified, on the basis of which the sample was divided into three groups (**Figure 5.17**).

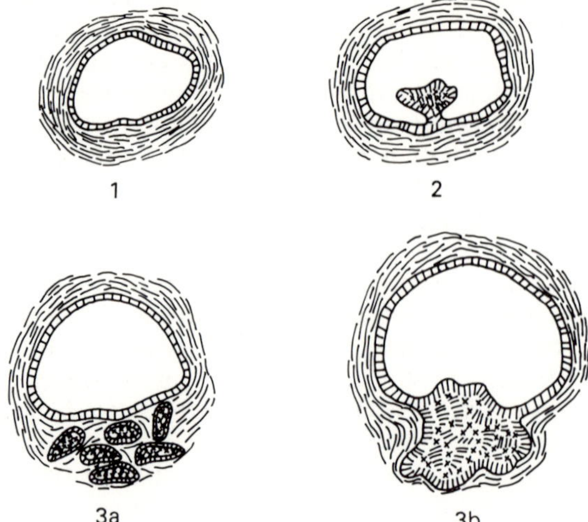

Figure 5.17. Classification of unicystic ameloblastoma into groups. *Group 1*, cyst lined by variable epithelium, sometimes showing criteria of ameloblastoma, often not, with no infiltration. *Group 2*, cyst with intraluminal plexiform epithelial proliferation with no infiltration. *Group 3*, cyst with infiltration of epithelium into cyst wall in either (a) a follicular or (b) a plexiform pattern. (Previously published (1988) in *J. Oral Pathol.* **17**, 541–546, and reproduced here by courtesy of the Editor.)

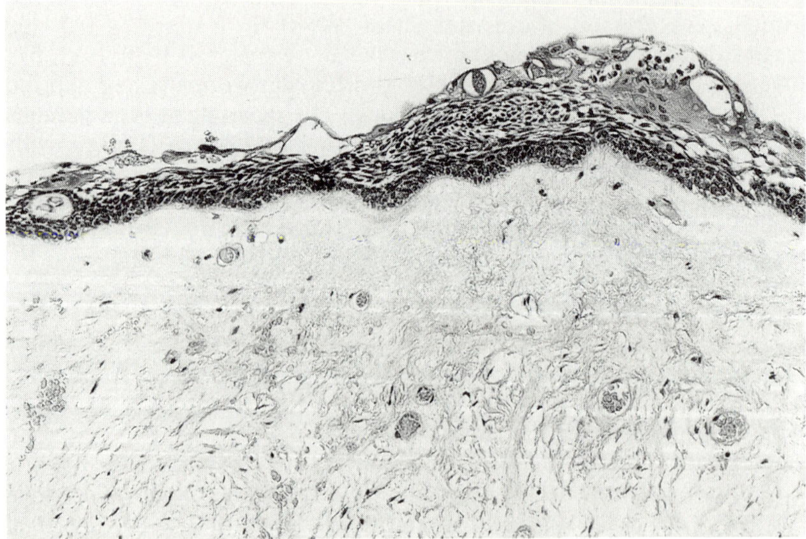

Figure 5.18. Lining of a unicystic ameloblastoma showing the features described by Vickers and Gorlin (1970). Subepithelial hyalinization is also a prominent feature. (H & E; × 125.) (Previously published (1988) in *J. Oral Pathol.* **17**, 541–546, and reproduced here by courtesy of the Editor.)

Group 1 comprises unilocular cystic lesions which are lined to a greater or lesser extent by epithelium which shows the criteria defined by Vickers and Gorlin (1970) for the diagnosis of ameloblastoma. These are columnar basal cells with hyperchromatic nuclei; nuclear palisading with polarization; and cytoplasmic vacuolation with intercellular spacing. Inactive odontogenic rests may be present within the fibrous cyst wall, but there is no evidence of infiltrating neoplastic epithelium. Subepithelial hyalinization is a very consistent feature of large ameloblastomatous cysts (**Figure 5.18**)

Group 2 comprises unilocular cystic lesions in which a mural nodule arises from the epithelial lining and projects into the lumen of the cyst. The nodule consists of odontogenic epithelium with a plexiform pattern which closely resembles that seen in the plexiform ameloblastoma (**Figures 5.15**, **5.16**). Part of the cyst lining may demonstrate the Vickers–Gorlin criteria, but there is no evidence of infiltration of the fibrous cyst wall by odontogenic epithelium (**Figure 5.19**).

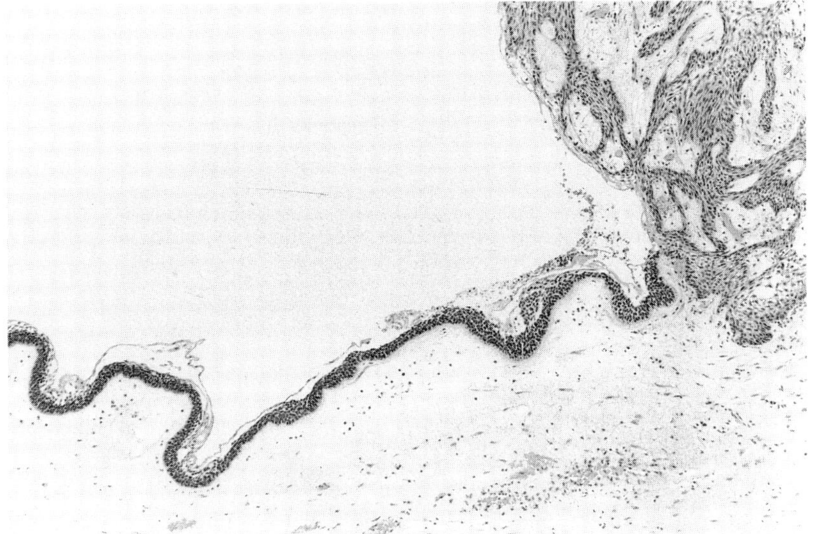

Figure 5.19. Part of of the lining of a Group 2 unicystic ameloblastoma showing the Vickers–Gorlin (1970) features. (H & E; × 80). (Previously published (1988) in *J. Oral Pathol.* **17**, 541–546, and reproduced here by courtesy of the Editor.)

Group 3 comprises unilocular cystic lesions in which invasive islands of ameloblastomatous epithelium of either the follicular or plexiform variety, which may or may not be connected to the cyst lining, are found in the fibrous wall of the cyst. Mural nodules of tumour tissue similar to those seen in Group 2, may also be present. The cyst lining may demonstrate the Vickers–Gorlin criteria in parts.

Substantial portions of the cyst lining in all three groups may lack the cytological features which are typical of ameloblastoma, and may instead be lined by a nondescript epithelium ranging from a thin epithelium of only 1–2 cell layers, to an acanthotic stratified squamous epithelium. Such cases will pose problems in histological diagnosis and cognizance must be taken of clinical and radiological details. It is also essential to sample multiple areas from the specimen before making a definitive diagnosis. Saku *et al.* (1991) reported that staining for the lectins *Ulex europaeus* agglutinin I (UEA-I) and *Bandeirea simplicifolia* agglutinin I (BSA-I) assisted in the differentiation between cystic ameloblastoma and odontogenic cysts. Using a substantial sample of ameloblastomas, keratocysts, dentigerous cysts and radicular cysts, they found that in the simple cysts, most of their specimens showed positive binding with UEA-I and BSA-I in the epithelial linings. No positive reactions were obtained for these two lectins in the epithelium of the ameloblastomas, except for limited UEA-I binding to keratinized cells in four cases.

With regard to the question of whether these lesions develop *de novo* or arise in existing odontogenic cysts, particularly dentigerous cysts, Ackermann, Altini and Shear (1988) pointed out that only a small number of their series were associated with the crowns of unerupted teeth in a true follicular relationship and there was no evidence at all that any other odontogenic cyst existed prior to the development of the lesions. As far as treatment is concerned, Ackermann *et al.* proposed that Groups 1 and 2 may be treated conservatively, while Group 3 must be treated aggressively in the same manner as solid and multicystic ameloblastomas.

Treatment

The treatment of dentigerous cysts is described in Chapter 18.

Chapter 6

Eruption cyst

An eruption cyst is in fact a dentigerous cyst occurring in the soft tissues. Whereas the dentigerous cyst develops around the crown of an unerupted tooth lying in the bone, the eruption cyst occurs when a tooth is impeded in its eruption within the soft tissues overlying the bone.

Clinical features

Frequency

Eruption cysts are not commonly seen in pathology departments and only 21 have been recorded in our archives in 32 years (0.8 per cent), (**Table 2.1**, p. 6). It is likely that they occur more frequently clinically and that as some burst spontaneously these are not excised and are therefore not submitted for histological examination.

Clinical presentation

The cysts are found in children of different ages, and occasionally in adults if there is delayed eruption. Deciduous and permanent teeth may be involved, most frequently anterior to the first permanent molar. The eruption cyst produces a smooth swelling over the erupting tooth which may be either the colour of normal gingiva, or blue (**Figure 6.1**). It is usually painless unless infected and is soft and fluctuant.

Sometimes more than one cyst may be present. There is often a brief history of about 3–4 weeks' duration during which they enlarge to approximately 1–1.5 cm. They are usually exposed to masticatory trauma. Transillumination is a useful diagnostic aid in distinguishing an eruption cyst from an eruption haematoma (Seward, 1973).

Radiological features

The cyst may throw a soft-tissue shadow, but there is usually no bone involvement except that the dilated and open crypt may be seen on the radiograph.

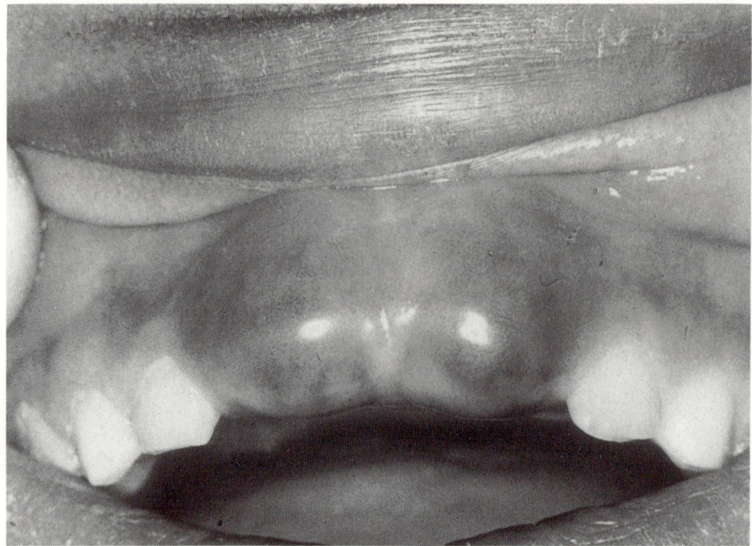

Figure 6.1. Eruption cysts involving the permanent maxillary central incisors.

Pathogenesis

The pathogenesis of the eruption cyst is probably very similar to that of the dentigerous cyst. The difference is that the tooth in the case of the eruption cyst is impeded in the soft tissues of the gingiva rather than in the bone. The factors which actually impede eruption in the soft tissues are not known, but the presence of particularly dense fibrous tissue could be responsible.

Pathology

As most eruption cysts are treated by marsupialization, the pathologist usually receives part of the cyst wall. The superficial aspect is covered by the keratinized stratified squamous epithelium of the overlying gingiva. This is separated from the cyst by a strip of dense connective tissue of varying thickness which usually shows a mild chronic inflammatory cell infiltrate. As the cysts are so frequently exposed to masticatory trauma the inflammatory infiltrate invariably increases in intensity towards the cyst lining, adjacent to which it is most intense. Sometimes it is possible to distinguish a line of demarcation between gingival and follicular connective tissues. The gingival connective tissue is relatively acellular and densely collagenous, and so has an eosinophilic hue. The follicular connective tissue is more densely cellular, less collagenous and has a more basophilic hue, presumably because of a higher content of acid mucopolysaccharide in the ground substance. Odontogenic epithelial cell nests may be present in the connective tissue.

In non-inflamed areas, the epithelial lining of the cyst is characteristically of reduced enamel epithelial origin, consisting in the main of 2–3 cell layers of squamous epithelium with a few foci where it may be a little thicker. Invariably, however, the epithelial lining is intensely inflamed. Acute inflammatory cells are found in the epithelium which proliferates in response to the inflammatory

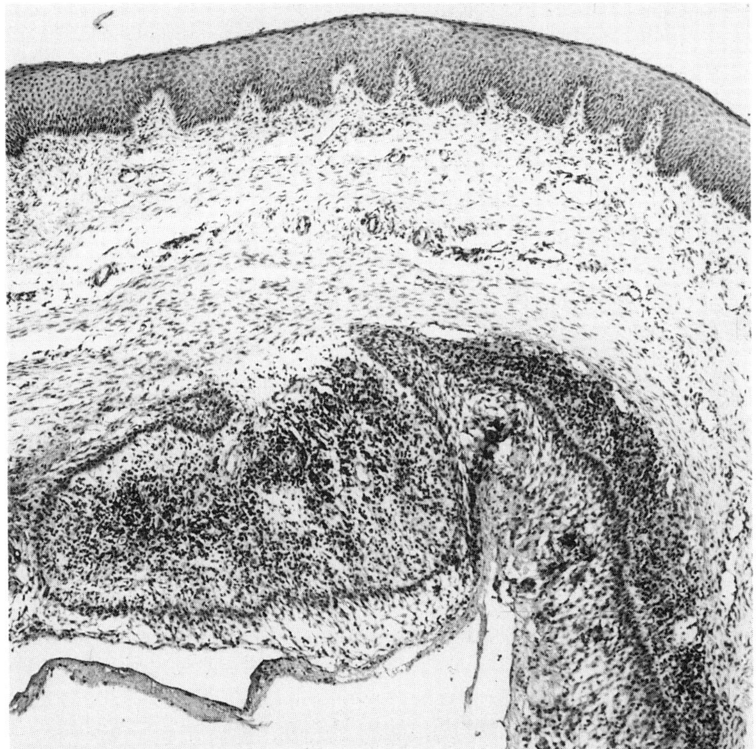

Figure 6.2. Eruption cyst. The surface epithelium is at the top and the cyst epithelium at the bottom of the photomicrograph. (H & E; × 70.)

stimulus, and may form characteristic arcades. Such epithelium is grossly spongiotic. The adjacent corium is hyperaemic and the seat of a chronic inflammatory cell infiltrate (**Figure 6.2**).

Treatment

Eruption cysts are treated by marsupialization. The dome of the cyst is excised, exposing the crown of the tooth which is allowed to erupt.

Chapter 7

Calcifying odontogenic cyst

The calcifying odontogenic cyst has many features of an odontogenic tumour and has in fact been classified as such in the World Health Organization's publication *Histological Typing of Odontogenic Tumours* (Kramer, Pindborg and Shear, 1992). The studies of Praetorius *et al.* (1981) have led them to conclude that what has previously been regarded as a calcifying odontogenic cyst actually comprises two entities, a cyst and a neoplasm.

The cyst itself is probably best classified as of developmental odontogenic epithelial origin. It was first described by Gorlin and associates (1962, 1964) who were impressed by its histological resemblance to the cutaneous calcifying epithelioma of Malherbe. Since then the lesion has been recognized in many pathology laboratories and a number of reports have appeared in the literature, amongst which have been papers by Abrams and Howell (1968), Ulmansky, Azaz and Sela (1969), Fejerskov and Krogh (1972), Freedman, Lumerman and Gee (1975), Altini and Farman (1975), Praetorius *et al.*,(1981), Nagao *et al.* (1983), Takeda, Suzuki and Yamamoto (1990), Buchner (1991) and Hong, Ellis and Hartman (1991).

Clinical features

Frequency

Despite the fact that the calcifying odontogenic cyst is now a well-recognized lesion, it is not very commonly encountered. We see only one or two cases a year in our department and regard the lesion as extremely rare. During the 32-year period 1958–89, 25 examples were recorded in our archives, representing 1 per cent of 2616 jaw cysts documented during that period (**Table 2.1**). Shamaskin, Svirsky and Kaugars (1989) reported 20 cases which had been recorded in their department over an 18-year period. Of these, 15 were central lesions and five peripheral. The age and sex distributions referred to below are derived mainly from a literature review combined with eight personally observed cases studied in the department by Altini and Farman (1975). To these data have been added 12 previously unreported cases presented by Praetorius *et al.* (1981) and another five examples documented in the department after the earlier survey (Rudick, 1981). Buchner (1991) pointed out that there are about five times as many central lesions reported in the literature as peripheral lesions.

Age

The age distribution of 87 cases is shown in **Figure 7.1**. The lesion occurs over a wide age range. The youngest recorded patient was 1 year old, the oldest 82 years, and there is a distinct peak in the second decade, a feature confirmed in the literature review of 215 lesions reported by Buchner (1991). Praetorius *et al.* (1981) have drawn attention to the bimodal age distribution seen in **Figure. 7.1** in support of their contention that two different entities may be involved.

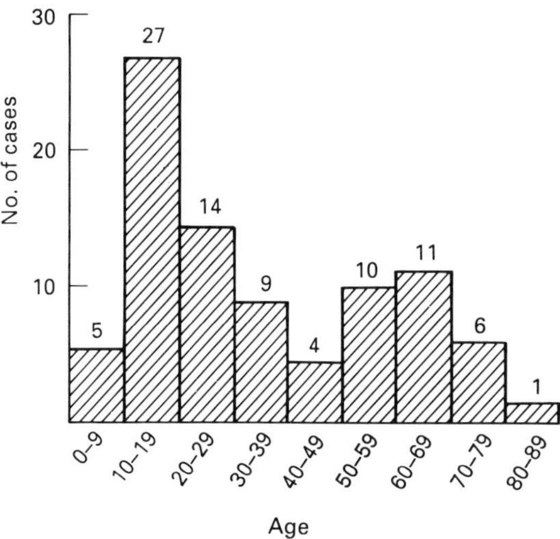

Figure 7.1. Age distribution of 87 patients with calcifying odontogenic cysts.

In a survey of 23 cases in the Japanese literature, Nagao *et al.* (1983) reported that with the exception of two patients, all were under 39 years with a peak in the second decade. Shamaskin, Svirsky and Kaugars (1989) found that of five extraosseous lesions, four were in patients over 50 years. In their literature review of 29 extraosseous cases, Kaugars, Kaugars and DeBiasi (1989) found that 16 patients were in their sixth decade or older. In their study of the peripheral calcifying odontogenic cyst, Buchner *et al.* (1991) observed a bimodal age distribution with peaks in the second and sixth decades.

Sex

There is an equal sex distribution, so that of 88 cases, 44 were male and 44 female. In Buchner's survey, 105 patients were males and 110 females. There is also an equal sex distribution in the series of extraosseous cases reported by Kaugars, Kaugars and DeBiasi (1989).

Race

No race predilection is apparent.

Site

The site distribution of 50 cases reported by Fejerskov and Krogh (1972) is illustrated in **Figure 7.2**. The mandible (23 cases) and maxilla (27 cases) were involved with almost equal frequency. The majority of cysts (36 cases) occurred in the jaw bones and 15 were found outside bone in the soft tissues related to the jaws. Of the series of 29 extraosseous cases documented by Kaugars, Kaugars and DeBiasi (1989), about one-half developed between the canines and none was posterior to the first molar. One case, recorded by Gorlin *et al.* (1964), was found in the parotid salivary gland. Freedman, Lumerman and Gee (1975) pointed out that 70 per cent of their sample occurring in patients before the age of 41 were in the maxilla whereas 80 per cent in patients older than 41 were in the mandible. In the Japanese study (Nagao *et al.*, 1983) the maxilla was involved in 17 cases and the mandible in six.

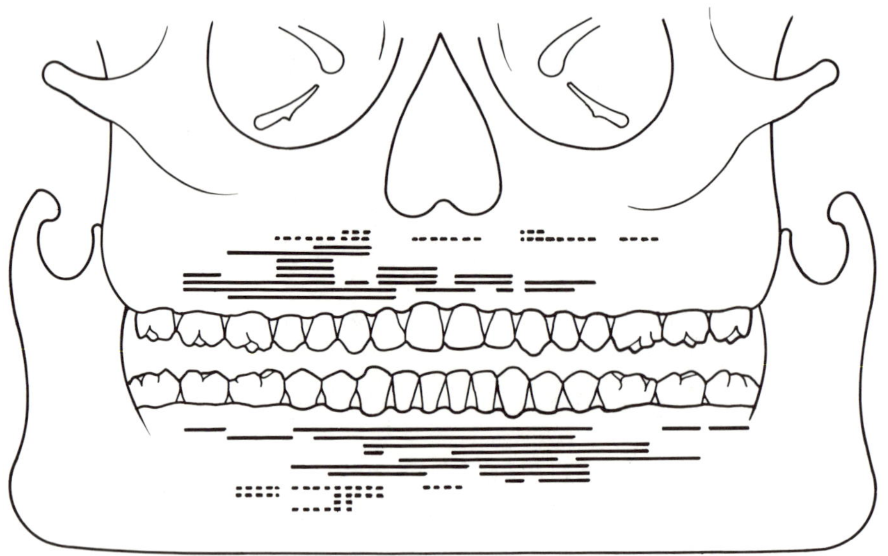

Figure 7.2. Anatomical distribution of 50 cases of calcifying odontogenic cyst. (By courtesy of Professor O. Fejerskov and the Editor, *Journal of Oral Pathology*. Previously published (1972) in *J. Oral Pathol.* **1**, 273–287.)

The most common site of occurrence has been the anterior part of the jaws. In the mandible, several cases have crossed the midline but this is less usual in the maxilla.

Most of the peripheral lesions were located in the maxillary or mandibular gingiva or alveolar mucosa anterior to the first molar (Buchner *et al.*, 1991).

Clinical presentation

Swelling is the most frequent complaint and has occurred in about one-half of the reported cases. Only rarely has there been pain. Intraosseous lesions may produce a hard bony expansion and may be fairly extensive. Lingual expansion may sometimes be observed. Occasionally the calcifying odontogenic cyst may perforate the cortical plate and extend into the soft tissues. In a few cases displacement of the teeth has been described. A remarkably large number of cases have been completely symptomless and have been discovered fortuitously during routine radiological examination.

Radiological features

The calcifying odontogenic cyst which occurs as an intraosseous lesion appears as an essentially radiolucent area. Some have a regular outline with well-demarcated margins. Others may be quite irregular and may have poorly defined margins. They are usually unilocular. Irregular calcified bodies of varying size and opacity may be seen in the radiolucent area (**Figure 7.3**) and in some cases the calcification may be

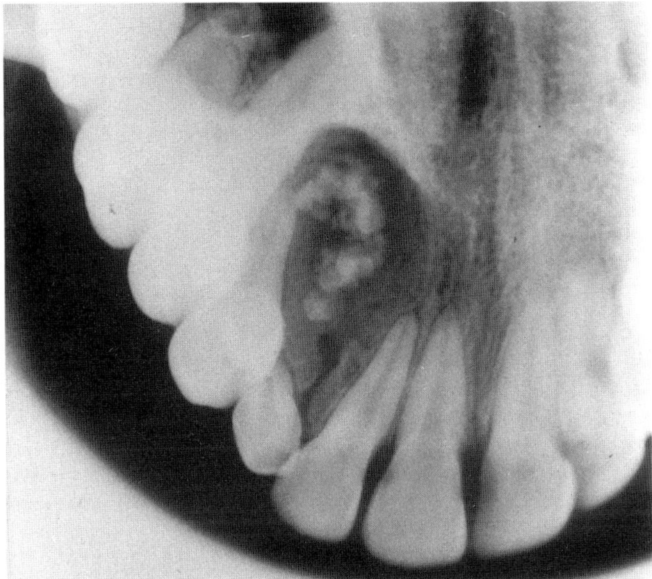

Figure 7.3. Radiograph of a calcifying odontogenic cyst. The features of a radiolucent area with irregular radio-opacities are not specific. (By courtesy of Professor J. E. Seeliger.)

substantial and occupy the greater part of the lesion. Dense opacities are likely to be present if the cyst is associated with a complex odontome, as it sometimes is. Some cases have been reported as being associated with an unerupted tooth. Displacement of teeth is often seen. Resorption of the roots of adjacent teeth is a frequent finding, and is regarded as an important radiological feature by Tanimoto *et al.* (1988). Local expansion sometimes occurs and perforation of the cortical plate, when present, may be radiologically demonstrable.

Pathogenesis and pathology

The histological features of a classic calcifying odontogenic cyst are characteristic and present few diagnostic problems. Elucidation of the pathogenesis is, however,

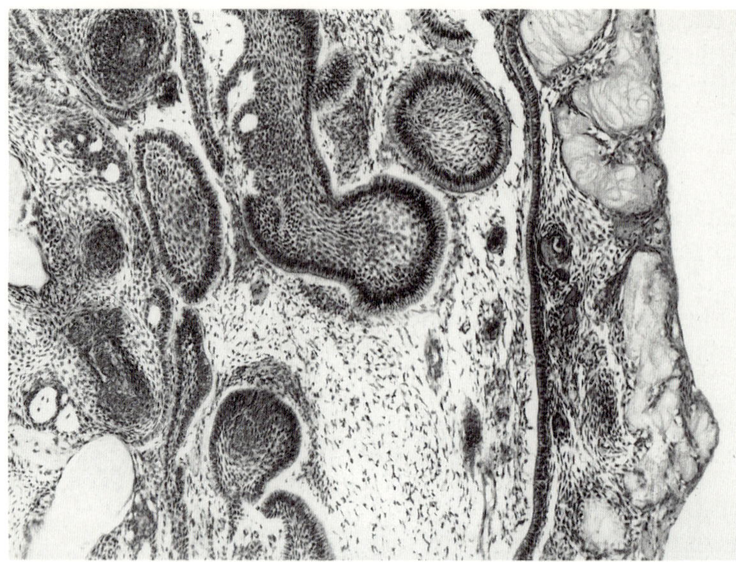

Figure 7.4. Calcifying odontogenic cyst associated with an ameloblastic fibroma. (H & E; × 85.)

considerably complicated by the fact that the epithelial lining of a calcifying odontogenic cyst appears to have the ability to induce the formation of dental tissues in the adjacent connective tissue wall; and that other odontogenic tumours such as the ameloblastoma, the odontoameloblastoma, the ameloblastic fibroma (**Figure 7.4**) and the ameloblastic fibro-odontome may sometimes be associated with it (Praetorius, 1975). Praetorius pointed out that the ghost cells which are so characteristic a feature of the calcifying odontogenic cyst also occur in other odontogenic cysts, the craniopharyngioma and the calcifying epithelioma of Malherbe, as well as in the other odontogenic tumours already mentioned. The mere presence of ghost cells in a lesion does not, therefore, justify the diagnosis of calcifying odontogenic cyst. In the first edition of this book I posed the question whether those calcifying odontogenic cysts which have other features of odontogenic tumours develop these secondarily, or whether they are themselves secondary phenomena in pre-existing odontogenic tumours. Takeda, Suzuki and Yamamoto (1990) were convinced that the cysts arise *de novo*, as were Praetorius *et al.* (1981) who concluded from their study that substantial evidence exists that the tumour develops from the wall of the cyst. They suggested that the calcifying odontogenic cyst is a unicystic process which develops from reduced enamel epithelium or remnants of odontogenic epithelium in the follicle, gingival tissue or bone. Dentinoid alone, or an odontome, may be found in the cyst wall, induced by the lining epithelium. Praetorius *et al.* (1981) classified these as Type 1, which may have three different patterns: *Type 1A* the simple unicystic type; *Type 1B* the odontome-producing type; and *Type 1C* the ameloblastomatous proliferating type. The neoplasm which possesses some of the histological features of the calcifying odontogenic cyst should, in the opinion of Praetorius *et al.*, be regarded as a separate entity, and they have classified it as *Type 2*. It occurs in older patients and consists of ameloblastomatous epithelium in which the development of cysts is a secondary feature. Areas of ghost cell formation and varying amounts of dentinoid are induced by the odontogenic epithelium. They have suggested the term 'dentinogenic ghost cell tumour' for this neoplasm. I have seen a case of this type in which enamel as well as dentine was found.

Hirshberg, Dayan and Horowitz (1987) reviewed the literature and identified six cases reported as calcifying odontogenic cysts which were solid masses with or without ameloblastomatous proliferation and without any association with other odontogenic tumours. In their review of 'odontogenic ghost cell tumours', Colmenero, Patron and Colmenero (1990) observed two different entities: one with infiltrating odontogenic epithelium and ghost cells which was locally aggressive like the ameloblastoma; and the other which was malignant with potential to metastasize. The latter entity is best described as an 'odontogenic ghost cell carcinoma' (Grodjest *et al.*, 1987). Scott and Wood (1989) reported a case with ameloblastomatous and basaloid features which behaved aggressively, and believed that as such a tumour has more in common with an ameloblastoma than a calcifying odontogenic cyst, its diagnostic designation should adequately reflect this. They proposed the term 'dentinogenic ghost-cell ameloblastoma'. I concur with this view and would suggest that the rare cases with enamel deposition as well as dentine, should be termed 'odontogenic ghost cell ameloblastoma' in keeping with the pattern used in the World Health Organization classification of odontogenic tumours (Kramer, Pindborg and Shear, 1992)

The calcifying odontogenic cyst is most frequently a unilocular lesion but multicystic lesions have been reported (Buchner, 1991; Hong, Ellis and Hartman, 1991). Satellite cysts may develop from odontogenic epithelial islands in the wall (Takeda, Susuki and Yamamoto, 1990). In the study of the peripheral lesions by Buchner *et al.* (1991), two-thirds were cystic and one-third were solid.

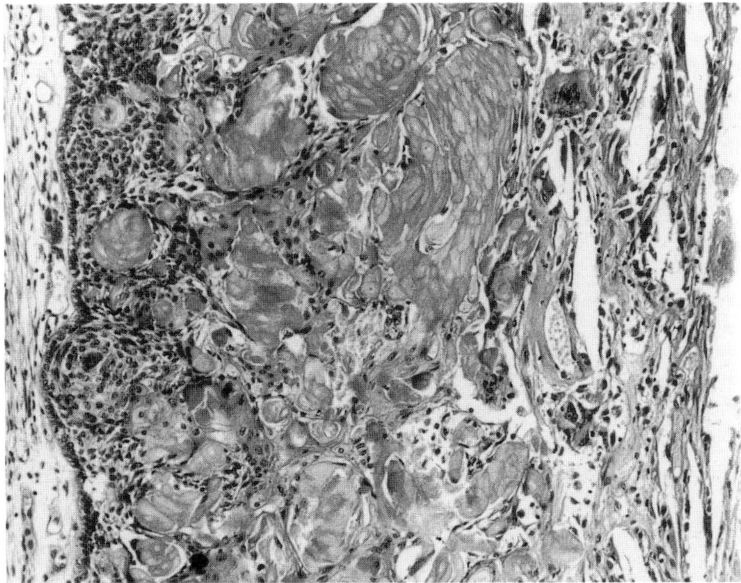

Figure 7.5. Lining of a calcifying odontogenic cyst containing 'ghost cells'. The basal cells of the epithelium are columnar and have their nuclei orientated away from the basement membrane. (H & E; × 95.)

The epithelial lining has characteristic odontogenic features with a prominent basal layer consisting of palisaded columnar or cuboidal cells and hyperchromatic nuclei which are polarized away from the basement membrane (**Figures 7.4, 7.5**). The epithelium may be a regular 6–8 cells thick over part of its length and be continuous with parts which may be very thin and others which are considerably thickened. Budding from the basal layer into the adjacent connective tissue and epithelial proliferations into the lumen are frequently seen.

The most remarkable feature of the calcifying odontogenic cyst is the presence of ghost cells which have been compared with those found in the calcifying epithelioma of Malherbe in the skin. These are found in groups, particularly in the thicker areas of the epithelial lining. The spinous cells in such situations may be widely separated by intercellular oedema and the epithelium around the ghost cells is often convoluted (**Figures 7.5, 7.6**).

The ghost cells consist of enlarged, ballooned, ovoid or elongated elliptoid epithelium. They are eosinophilic and although the cell outlines are usually well-defined, they may sometimes be blurred so that groups of them appear fused. A few ghost cells may contain nuclear remnants but these are in various stages of degeneration and in the majority all traces of chromatin have disappeared leaving only a faint outline of the original nucleus. The ghost cells represent an abnormal type of keratinization and have an affinity for calcification. They have the same histological reactions as keratin, giving a yellow fluorescence with rhodamine B (Praetorius, 1975). Hong, Ellis and Hartman (1991) showed that in formalin-fixed tissue the ghost cells expressed little or no cytokeratin reactivity and suggested that this, in association with their histological features, may represent the product of coagulative necrosis of odontogenic epithelium.

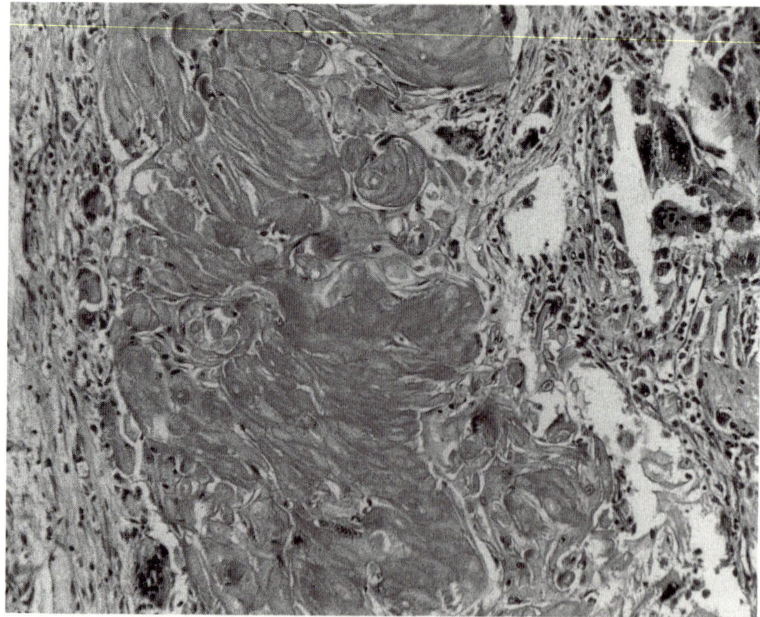

Figure 7.6. 'Ghost cells' have broken through the epithelium and evoked a foreign body giant cell reaction. (H & E; × 64.)

Ultrastructurally, they do not show the same features as keratin in epidermis and oral epithelia which are characterized by evenly distributed fine tonofilaments embedded in a matrix (Fejerskov and Krogh, 1972). The cytoplasm of some ghost cells in the study of Fejerskov and Krogh contained fine tonofilaments separated by small empty spaces. Most of the cells showed very thick electron-dense fibre bundles of relatively uniform size which were sharply defined against the large empty spaces in the cytoplasm. Endoplasmic reticulum, mitochondria, Golgi apparatus and ribosomes could not be identified. The cell membranes were intact with junctional complexes of various types.

Calcification may occur in some of the ghost cells, initially as fine powdery or coarse basophilic granules and later as small spherical bodies which ultrastructural studies have shown to represent dystrophic calcification (Sapp and Gardner, 1977).

The ghost cells may be in contact with the connective tissue wall of the cyst where they evoke a foreign-body reaction with the formation of multinucleate giant cells (**Figure 7.6**). In the fibrous wall there are usually strands and islands of odontogenic epithelium, either in direct contact with the epithelium or separately in the connective tissue. These vary from a few strands to extensive proliferations. Takeda, Suzuki and Yamamoto (1990) have done a histological study of satellite cysts and odontogenic epithelial islands in the connective tissue walls of these lesions. The satellite cysts could be grouped into the same three histological types described by Praetorius *et al.* (1981), but these did not always coincide with the typing of the mother cyst. An atubular dentinoid is usually found in the wall close to the epithelial lining and often in relation to the epithelial proliferations. It is frequently described as being found particularly in contact with masses of ghost cells (**Figure 7.7**). I have seen a number of examples of calcifying odontogenic cyst with complex odontomes in their walls.

Melanin deposits are sometimes present in the epithelial linings.

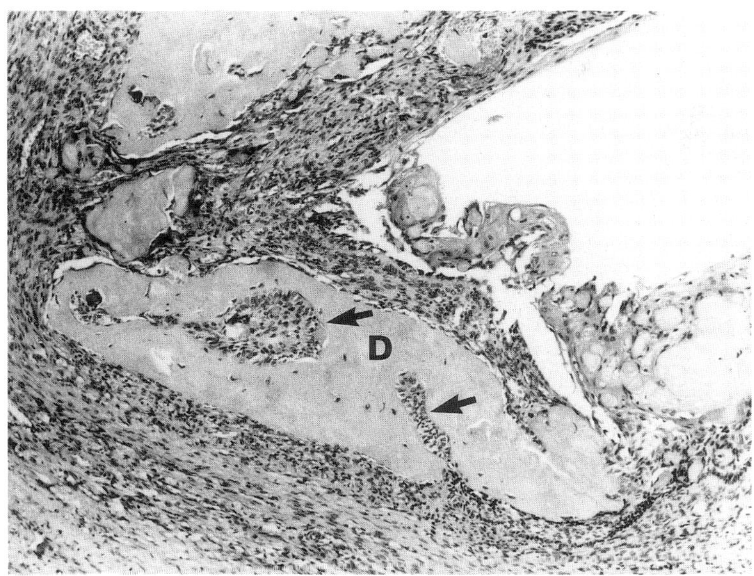

Figure 7.7. Induction of dentinoid [D] adjacent to epithelium (arrows) in a calcifying odontogenic cyst. (H & E; × 80.)

Treatment

The calcifying odontogenic cyst is treated by surgical enucleation unless it is associated with another odontogenic tumour such as an ameloblastic fibroma, in which case wider excision will be required. In the presence of a complex odontome, conservative removal will still be adequate. An ameloblastoma or one of its variants with foci of ghost cells must be treated radically. Although classic uncomplicated cases of calcifying odontogenic cyst may grow to a large size, reported recurrences are rare. For further details of the treatment, see the general consideration of the treatment of jaw cysts described in Chapter 18.

Chapter 8

Nasopalatine duct (incisive canal) cyst

The epithelial-lined cysts of non-odontogenic origin are thought to be derived from embryonic epithelial residues in the nasopalatine canal and, in the opinion of some workers, from epithelium included in lines of fusion of embryonic facial processes. The latter view is extremely controversial, as many embryologists and pathologists discount the possibility of such an origin, stating that the grooves between the processes are smoothed out by proliferation of the underlying mesenchymal growth centres, a process referred to as 'merging.' In only a few areas do developmental processes make ectoderm to ectoderm contact with subsequent ectodermal degeneration (Allard, Van der Kwast and Van der Waal, 1981a; Allard, 1982). An account of the embryology and anatomy of the anterior region of the palate will be found in the latter publications.

It is generally agreed that the nasopalatine duct cyst is an entity. It may occur within the nasopalatine canal or in the soft tissues of the palate, at the opening of the canal, where it is called the 'cyst of the palatine papilla'. The term 'nasopalatine duct cyst' is preferred to the synonymous 'incisive canal cyst'.

In recent years, doubt has been expressed as to whether the so-called 'median palatine cyst' is an entity or whether cysts in that region are merely posterior extensions of nasopalatine duct cysts. This point is discussed again later. Since 1968 we have therefore not made the diagnosis of median palatine cyst.

Clinical features

Frequency

The nasopalatine duct cyst is the most common of the non-odontogenic cysts and comprises, in our department, 287 of the 2616 jaw cysts registered in our department over a 32-year period (11.0 per cent) (**Table 2.1**). These include the cysts which were originally diagnosed as median palatine cysts and those which were predominantly in the soft tissues and were called cysts of the palatine papilla. Some indication of the frequency of nasopalatine duct cysts in the general population may be determined from studies on cadaver and dry skull material. Meyer (1931) examined 600 cadavers and observed a frequency of 1.5 per cent. This was similar to the frequency of 1.3 per cent reported by Chamda and Shear (1980) who found 13 cysts in 970 dry skulls in the Raymond Dart collection of the Department of Anatomy, University of the Witwatersrand. Killey, Kay and Seward (1977), however, reported detecting only two nasopalatine duct cysts in a series of 2394 dry skulls (0.08 per cent).

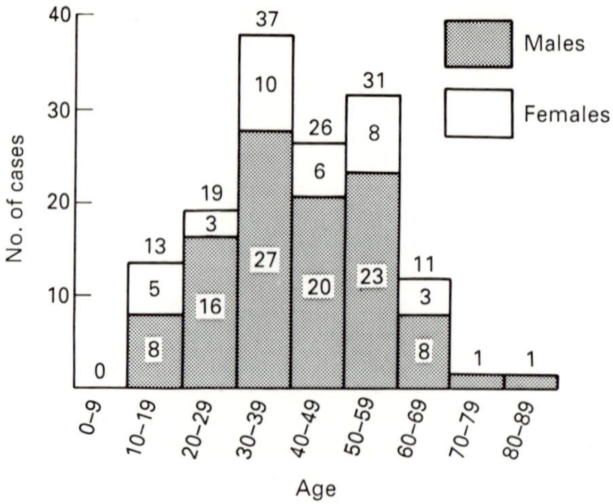

Figure 8.1. Age distribution of 139 patients with nasopalatine duct cysts.

Age

The age distribution of 139 of our cases is shown in **Figure 8.1**. There was no case in the first decade and the majority occurred in the fourth, fifth and sixth decades. When the age distributions of black and white patients are compared, the patterns are similar except that there are more black cases than white in the fifth decade and more white cases than black in the sixth decade (**Table 8.1**). The differences in age distribution between white and black patients are not statistically significant.

Table 8.1 Comparative age distributions of 68 black and 73 white patients with nasopalatine duct cysts

Age in years	*Black* (*No.*)	*Black* (*%*)	*White* (*No.*)	*White* (*%*)
0–9	0	0	0	0
10–19	6	8.8	8	11.0
20–29	9	13.2	9	12.3
30–39	19	27.9	18	24.7
40–49	18	26.5	10	13.7
50–59	9	13.2	23	31.5
60–69	6	8.8	4	5.5
70–79	1	1.5	0	0
80–89	0	0	1	1.4
	68	99.9	73	100.1

Sex

In our material there is a much higher frequency of nasopalatine duct cysts in males than females ($P < 0.002$) and this sex predilection appears to be more marked in blacks than in whites ($P < 0.025$). In a series of 157 patients, 119 were males (76 per cent) and 38 were females (24 per cent). This is a male:female ratio of 3.1:1. Of

Table 8.2 Sex distribution of black and white patients with nasopalatine duct cysts

	Male	*Female*	*Total*	*M:F ratio*
Black	69	13	82	5.3:1
White	50	25	75	2.0:1
Total	119 (76%)	38 (24%)	157	3.1:1
W:B ratio	1:1.4	1:0.5	1:1.1	

these, 69 were black males and 13 black females (5.3:1); 50 were white males and 25 white females (20:1) (**Table 8.2**). Killey, Kay and Seward (1977), Hedin, Klämfeldt and Persson (1978), Bodin, Isacsson and Julin (1986) and Swanson, Kaugars and Gunsolley (1991) also recorded a male preponderance, but in the series of Abrams, Howell and Bullock (1963), there was an equal sex frequency. In all, blacks and whites were equally involved.

Clinical presentation

The most common symptom is swelling, usually in the anterior region of the midline of palate (**Figures 8.2, 8.3**). Swelling also occurs in the midline on the labial aspect of the alveolar ridge (**Figure 8.4**) and in some cases 'through and through' fluctuation may be elicited between the labial and palatal swellings. The cyst may produce bulging of the floor of the nose. It is when midline swellings of the palate occur further posteriorly that diagnoses of median palatine cysts tend to be made.

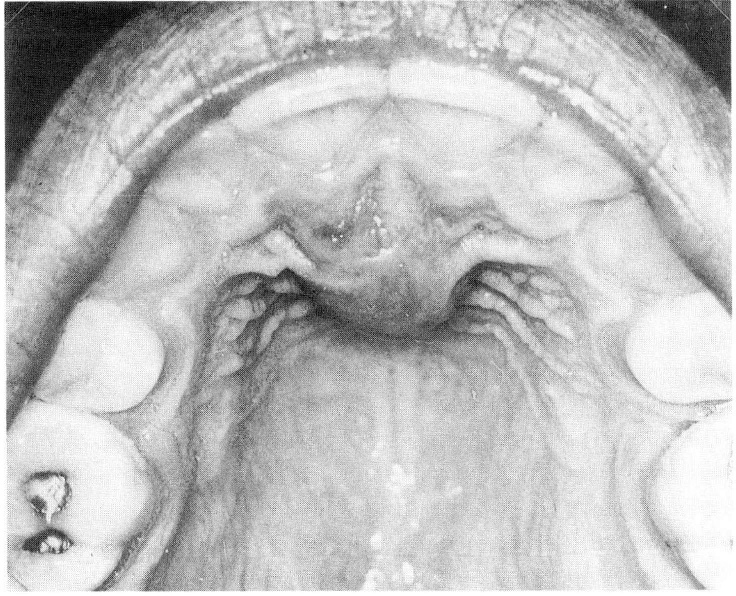

Figure 8.2. Small nasopalatine duct cyst. (By courtesy of Professor J. J. Pindborg.)

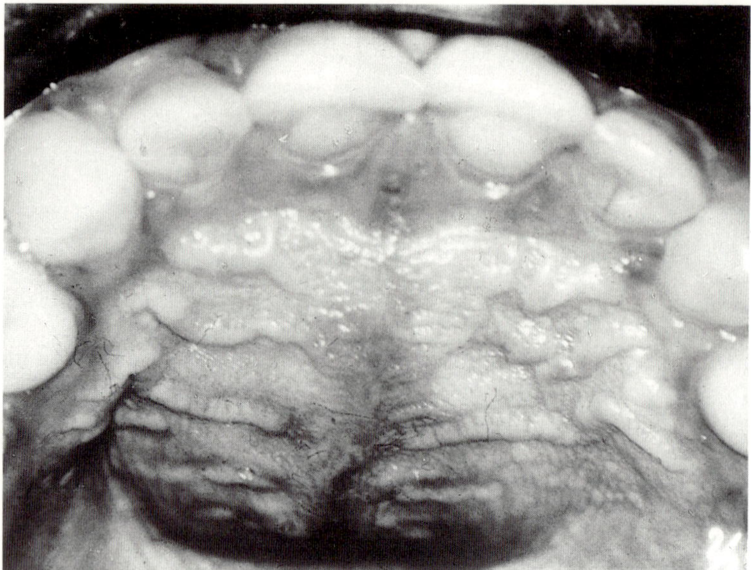

Figure 8.3. Large nasopalatine duct cyst extending posteriorly to involve much of the hard palate.

In a number of cases, the swelling is associated with pain by pressure on the nasopalatine nerves, and discharge, but sometimes discharge is the only complaint and in a few cases pain is the only symptom. Various combinations of swelling, discharge and pain may occur. The discharge may be mucoid, in which case the patients sometimes describe a salty taste, or it may be purulent and patients

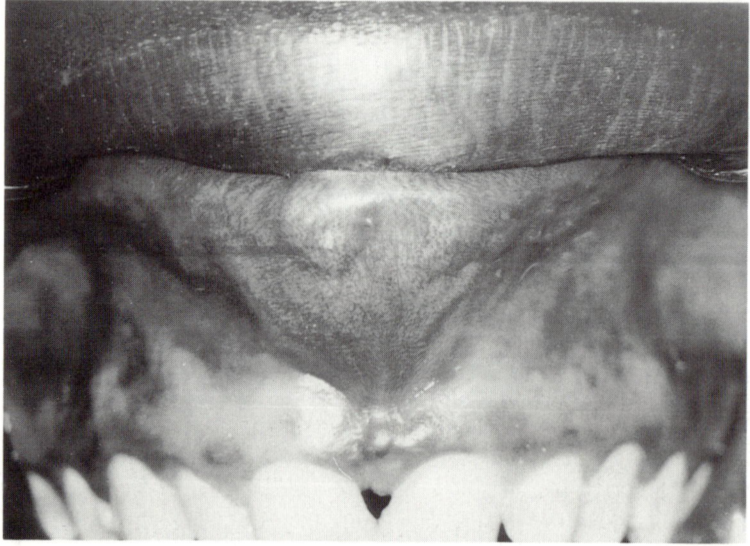

Figure 8.4. Nasopalatine duct cyst producing a midline swelling of the labial aspect of the alveolar ridge.

complain of a foul taste. In patients with cysts of the palatine papilla, there may be a history of recurrent swellings which periodically discharge and then 'go down'. Displacement of teeth is observed fairly often.

In general, symptoms are not severe and patients often disregard them for many years. They may also be completely symptomless and be discovered fortuitously by the dentist during routine radiological examination, and occasionally the presence of a cyst may become apparent after dentures are placed.

Nortjé and Farman (1978) and Hertzanu, Cohen and Mendelsohn (1985) have suggested that this lesion may produce more severe symptoms, and be more aggressive and larger in South African blacks. From a sample of 114 nasopalatine duct cysts, the latter authors selected all cases with a transverse diameter of greater than 30 mm. All of these occurred in blacks. They do point out, however, that late clinical presentation may be responsible for the large size at the time of diagnosis.

In establishing a diagnosis of nasopalatine duct cyst it is important to attempt to exclude the possibility of a periapical lesion by testing the pulp vitality of the incisor teeth.

Radiological features

The nasopalatine duct cyst occurs in the incisive canal and it may be difficult to decide whether a radiolucency in that area is a cyst or a large incisive fossa (**Figure 8.5**). In attempting to distinguish between the two, the study done by Roper-Hall (1938) is frequently quoted. In an investigation of 2162 skulls selected at random from a series of more than 6000, he found that the incisive fossae of 2154 were absent or small. Five were of medium size, one was enlarged but shallow and two were large and cystic. The shapes of the fossae were round, oval, diamond or

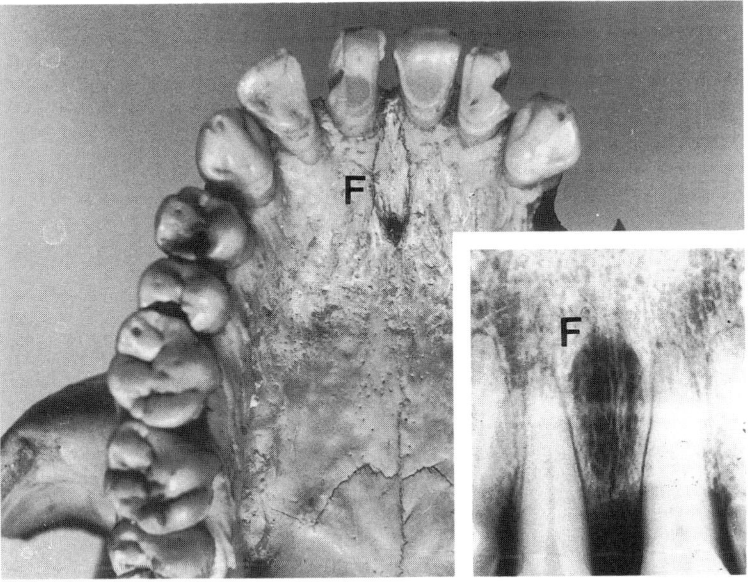

Figure 8.5. Incisive fossa [F] on a dry skull. Inset: Radiograph of an incisive fossa [F] on a different dry skull. (By courtesy of Dr R. Chamda.)

triangular and sometimes were funnel-shaped. Their anteroposterior measurement was usually greater than the width although the average measurements were 3 mm wide, 3 mm anteroposteriorly and 2–3 mm high. The largest fossa which was at all frequent was 5 mm wide and 7 mm anteroposteriorly. Of the seven which were larger than this, four were 6 mm wide and 8 mm anteroposteriorly, and one was 6 mm wide and 10 mm anteroposteriorly. The two cavities which were large and cystic were 7 mm × 15 mm and 7 mm × 14 mm respectively. Roper-Hall concluded that any radiograph of the fossa which shows a shadow less than 6 mm wide may be considered to be within normal limits, provided the patients have no other symptoms. Similar observations made by Killey, Kay and Seward (1977) on 2394 fossae confirmed Roper-Hall's views. In our own study, however, in which the dimensions of incisive fossae of 970 Negroid skulls were measured, the mean anteroposterior dimension and the width were both substantially greater than those in the previous reports (Chamda and Shear, 1980). The mean anteroposterior dimension and standard deviation in our sample was 10.19 ± 3.24 mm and the mean width 4.79 ± 1.33. Incisive fossa widths of greater than 6 mm were found in 148 specimens (15.3 per cent) of which 13 were associated with cysts. The greatest width in the non-cystic category was 8.05 mm. Anteroposterior dimensions of greater than 7 mm were found in 799 specimens (82.4 per cent) including the 13 cysts. The greatest anteroposterior dimension in the non-cystic category was 17.5 mm.

Radiographs, using a standardized technique, were taken of 164 of the skulls, selected at random. The mean anteroposterior dimension of the incisive fossae on these radiographs was 11.67 ± 3.27 mm and the mean width 4.50 ± 1.61 mm. The difference between these measurements and the actual measurements on the same 164 skulls was statistically significant. In some instances the ratio of skull:radiograph dimensions was more than unity and in others less than unity. Although the two sets of measurements correlated strongly with each other the range of variation around unity indicates that it is invalid to extrapolate skull dimensions from radiographic measurements even if a multiplication factor is used.

It would appear from this study that a radiographic shadow with anteroposterior dimensions of as much as 10 mm in the incisive fossa region may be within normal limits. In the absence of any other symptoms or signs, such patients should be observed and re-radiographed at intervals rather than be subjected to immediate surgery. Bodin, Isacsson and Julin (1986) proposed that if the width of the radiolucency exceeds 8 mm, is pronounced and has a thin cortical border on the periphery, exploratory operation should be considered especially if the lesion is asymmetrically bulging; and that radiolucencies exceeding 14 mm in diameter are always cysts.

Incisive canal cysts are found in the midline of the palate, above or between the roots of the central incisor teeth (**Figure 8.6**). In the latter case, the incisor roots may diverge. They are round or ovoid and some may appear heart-shaped either because they become notched by the nasal septum during their expansion, or because the nasal spine is superimposed on the radiolucent area, or if there are bilateral cysts. Cysts may develop bilaterally in both Stenson canals and in some instances the radiolucency may be seen laterally if a single cyst develops in one of the major lateral canals of Stenson (Stafne, 1969). Very large cysts extend posteriorly and superiorly and it is these which give rise to the diagnosis of median palatine cyst (**Figure 8.7**). Cysts close to the floor of the nose may be more clearly demonstrated on panoramic than on occlusal films (Nortjé and Farman, 1978). The

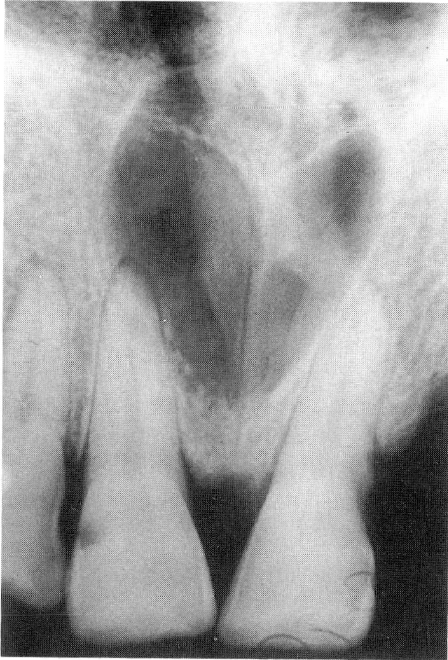

Figure 8.6. Radiograph of a nasopalatine duct cyst. The lamina dura of the tooth on the left is intact although the apex appears to be in the cyst.

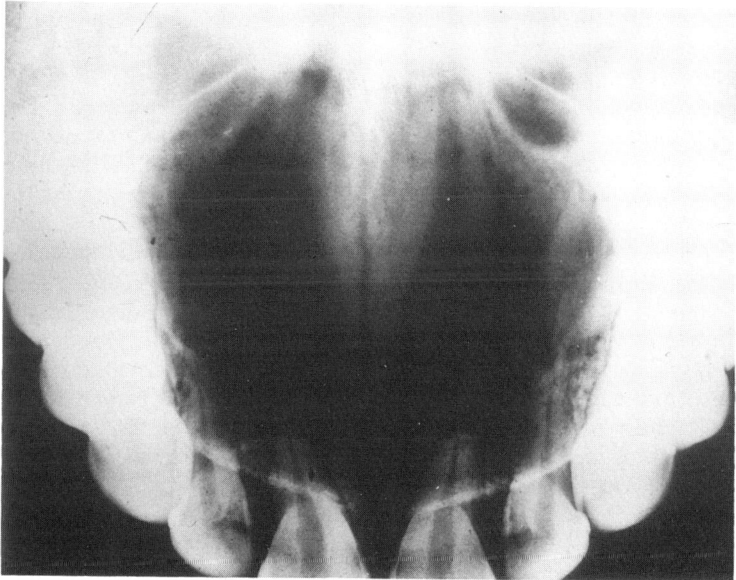

Figure 8.7. Radiograph of a large nasopalatine duct cyst which may give rise to a diagnosis of median palatine cyst.

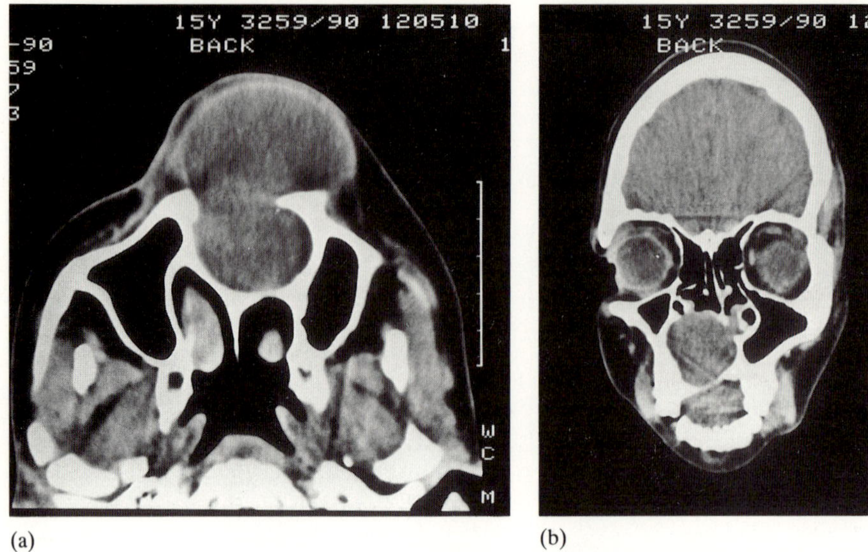

(a) (b)

Figure 8.8. (a) Nasopalatine duct cyst. Axial CT scan showing a well-defined mass extending through the alveolar ridge. (b) Nasopalatine duct cyst. Coronal CT scan showing bowing of the hard palate and extension of the mass into the nasal cavity. (By courtesy of Professor J. Lownie.)

margins of nasopalatine duct cysts are well-demarcated but exhibit varying degrees of cortication (Bodin, Isacsson and Julin, 1986; Nortjé and Wood, 1988). In the sample of 46 cases reported by the latter authors, the radiolucencies ranged from 9–52 mm in greatest diameter. Tooth displacement was common with their roots directed distally. Amorphous intraluminal calcifications were seen in a few cases. In the study of Bodin, Isacsson and Julin (1986), the great majority of radiolucent areas had lateral dimensions in the range 7–12 mm. In sample of 116 cases reported by Swanson, Kaugars and Gunsolly (1991), 6.4 per cent were 6 mm or less in diameter. Struthers and Shear (1976) observed some degree of root resorption with four of 11 nasopalatine duct cysts which were contiguous with tooth roots.

If the radiolucent area appears on a dental radiograph to be related to the apex of an incisor tooth, an occlusal view will usually demonstrate that the cyst and the apex are separated. In addition to the demonstration of pulp vitality, it may also be possible to see an intact lamina dura around the tooth apices (**Figure 8.6**).

The radiological investigation of nasopalatine duct cysts by tomography has been described by Lysell and Molin (1972). Hertzanu, Cohen and Mendelsohn (1985) suggested that CT appeared to be of value in the investigation of large lesions with destruction of bone and posterior and intranasal extension (**Figure 8.8**).

Woo *et al.* (1987) reported a case of a keratocyst which occurred in the anterior midline of the maxilla, simulating a nasopalatine cyst.

Pathogenesis

Nasopalatine duct cysts are thought to arise from the nasopalatine ducts in the incisive canal, but the aetiological factors associated with their formation and their pathogenesis are largely speculative.

In lower animals, the nasopalatine ducts are concerned in some way with the sense of smell. In man, vestigial remnants of this primitive organ of smell may be found in the incisive canals in the form of epithelial-lined ducts, epithelial cords, epithelial nests or combinations of these. Epithelial nests may show central degeneration. The frequency with which a continuous patent nasopalatine duct between the nasal and oral cavities occurs in man is uncertain as various authors have reported different findings. These are summarized by Abrams, Howell and Bullock (1963) who carried out similar studies on 24 fetuses. In none of these was there either a continuous patent duct or epithelial cords. In no instance did they find a patent oral opening of a nasopalatine duct, although nine patent nasal openings were identified. Sixteen fetuses had portions of nasopalatine duct with central lumina and three of these had an appearance suggestive of cystic degeneration. In their investigation the ducts were lined most frequently by squamous epithelium (82 per cent of cases) and most of these were in the oral and middle thirds of the incisive canals. A primitive or cuboidal lining was present in 41 per cent of cases, and these were predominantly in the nasal third. Although squamous epithelium lined some nasopalatine ducts in the nasal third of the canal, in no case was pseudostratified columnar epithelium found in the oral third.

The vomer-nasal organs of Jacobson are sometimes mentioned as a possible source of cysts in the incisive canal but this is most unlikely. They are bilateral structures which lie at the base of the nasal septum just above the nasal extremity of the incisive canals. They are believed to be associated with the nasopalatine ducts as olfactory organs in many animals, and have been demonstrated in human embryos (Abrams, Howell and Bullock, 1963).

As far as aetiology is concerned, it has been suggested that trauma or bacterial infection could stimulate the nasopalatine duct remnants to proliferate. There is, however, very little evidence to support such hypotheses. On the contrary, a number of factors tend to preclude these possibilities. If trauma to the area during mastication is the cause, why are the cysts found so infrequently when such trauma is very common? Why are the cysts so much more frequent in males than females? Some nasopalatine duct cysts, particularly those higher up in the canal away from the mouth, are relatively free of inflammatory infiltrate. Nor does one see arcading of proliferating stratified squamous epithelium as in inflamed radicular cysts. These latter two points do not of course definitely exclude the possibility of an inflammatory origin, as the inflammatory process could have subsided before the cyst was removed. They do, however, suggest that more evidence is required to support such a theory of onset. The fact that there may be an intense inflammatory cell infiltrate in the walls of cysts of the palatine papilla is not really adequate evidence to support an inflammatory origin, as cysts of this region are more than likely to be traumatized and thereby show a secondary inflammatory reaction.

The fact that mucous glands develop in association with nasopalatine ducts and are sometimes seen in the walls of the cysts has led to the suggestion that the cysts might be caused by secretion of mucin from the glands into the duct lumina, particularly when the duct is blocked. Factors against such an origin are that only very infrequently have connections between the mucous glands and the duct lumina been demonstrated and that the secretory pressure that would exist is unlikely to be adequate to produce bone resorption and form an intraosseous cyst.

Main (1970a) has postulated that nasopalatine duct cysts, like keratocysts, develop spontaneously. Although there is no proof for such a hypothesis, the concept is in accord with some of the facts. First, there is the observation that small cystic dilatations of portions of the nasopalatine ducts are occasionally seen in fetal material. It would explain the absence of inflammatory cell infiltrations from so many cases and also the relative infrequency of the cysts in relation to the frequency of trauma in the nasopalatine area. Main (1970a) has shown that nasopalatine duct cysts show a lesser tendency than keratocysts for epithelial proliferation, which partly explains their slow growth and moderate size. Main (1970b) believed that fluid accumulation is likely to be responsible for the enlargement of nasopalatine duct cysts but what leads to the initial collection of fluid in the cyst cavity is uncertain. Osmotic attraction of serum through normal capillary walls may occur and in the absence of drainage of this fluid (Toller, 1966b) the hydrostatic pressure would increase. Osmotically active particles are supplied by the breakdown of cells shed into the cyst cavity.

The mechanism which might initially trigger the spontaneous development of nasopalatine duct cysts, if this is indeed what happens, has yet to be identified. It seems to me possible that the occurrence of these cysts, as with other jaw cysts, may have some genetic determinant.

Histological features (Figures 8.9, 8.10, 8.11 and Table 8.3)

The epithelial linings of nasopalatine duct cysts are extremely variable. Stratified squamous, pseudostratified columnar, cuboidal, columnar, or primitive flat epithelium may be seen, individually or in combination.

Goblet cells may be found in pseudostratified columnar epithelial linings and cilia, although most frequently seen on the surface of pseudostratified columnar epithelia, may also be present in association with columnar and, very rarely, with cuboidal epithelium.

Table 8.3 Histological features in 86 nasopalatine duct cysts

		Numbers	*Percentage*
Epithelium			
Stratified squamous		67	78
entirely	33		
partly pseudostratified ciliated columnar	22		
partly cuboidal	10		
partly columnar	2		
Pseudostratified ciliated columnar		39	45
entirely	7		
partly squamous	22		
partly cuboidal	8		
partly columnar	2		
Fibrous cyst wall			
Neurovascular bundle		39	45
Large muscular-walled vessels		62	72
Mucous glands		6	7
Cartilage		6	7
Inflammatory infiltrate			
absent		21	24
mild		39	45
moderate		17	20
severe		9	11

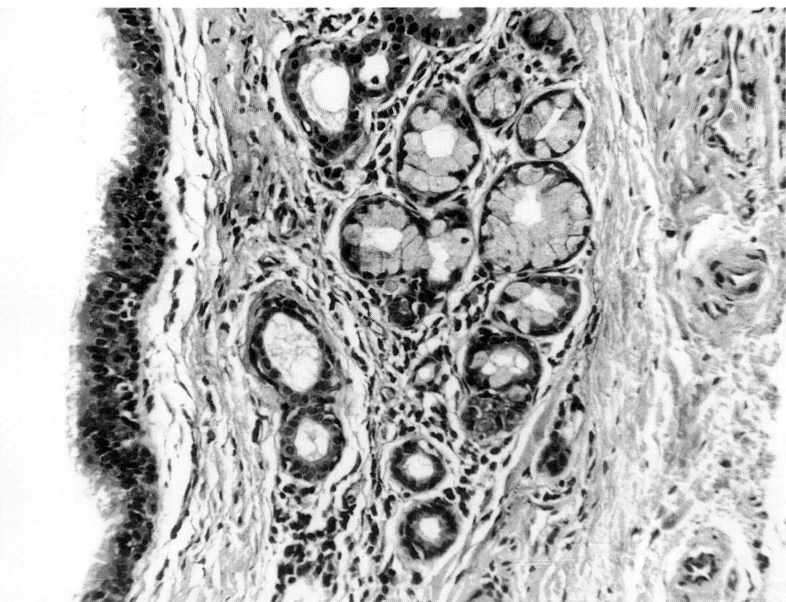

Figure 8.9. Nasopalatine duct cyst lined by pseudostratified ciliated columnar epithelium. Mucous glands are present in the wall. (H & E; × 200.)

Stratified squamous epithelium is found more frequently than any other, followed by pseudostratified columnar. In a series of 86 of our own cases which have been analysed histologically (**Table 8.3**), 67 (78 per cent) were lined by stratified squamous epithelium; 33 entirely, whereas 22 were lined in part by pseudostratified ciliated columnar epithelium. Thirty-nine cysts (45 per cent) contained pseudostratified ciliated columnar epithelium in part of their linings, but only seven were lined entirely in this way. Four cysts were lined in part by simple columnar and 18 by simple cuboidal epithelium. One was lined entirely by cuboidal epithelium. These distributions are very similar to those of Abrams, Howell and Bullock (1963). Similar histological analyses have been done by Allard, van der Kwast and van der Waal (1981a) and Bodin, Isacsson and Julin (1986). Although it has been stated that cysts lined by respiratory epithelium originate from nasopalatine duct adjacent to the nasal cavity, whereas those lined by stratified squamous epithelium develop from the lower portion of the duct, this should not be regarded as a rule. For one thing, cysts of the palatine papilla may be lined by pseudostratified ciliated columnar epithelium, and for another, it is rare to find a nasopalatine duct cyst lined entirely by one variety of epithelium. Furthermore, except for cysts of the palatine papilla, it is rare for a surgeon to state in his biopsy request what the anatomical level of any particular nasopalatine duct cyst was, so that it is not really possible to correlate position with histology. The fact that the majority of cyst linings have a combination of epithelial varieties is suggestive of their origin from pluripotential epithelium but the possibility that metaplasia occurs must also be considered.

A valuable diagnostic feature of nasopalatine duct cysts is the presence of nerves and blood vessels in the fibrous capsule (**Figure 8.11**). Abrams, Howell and Bullock

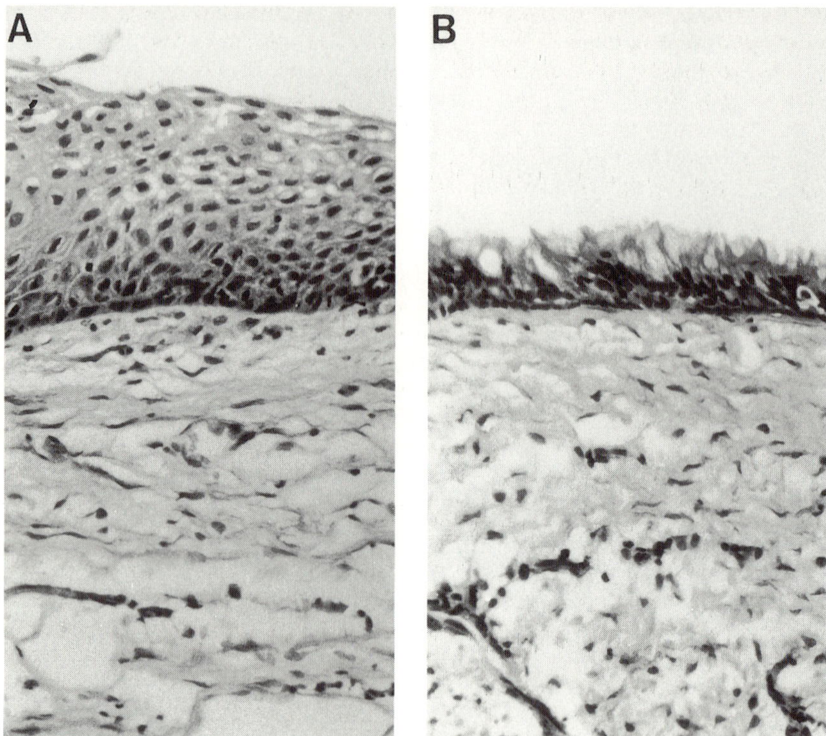

Figure 8.10. Different areas in the nasopalatine duct cyst illustrated in Figure 8.8. Part is lined by stratified squamous epithelium [A] and part by pseudostratified ciliated columnar epithelium [B]. (H & E; × 250.)

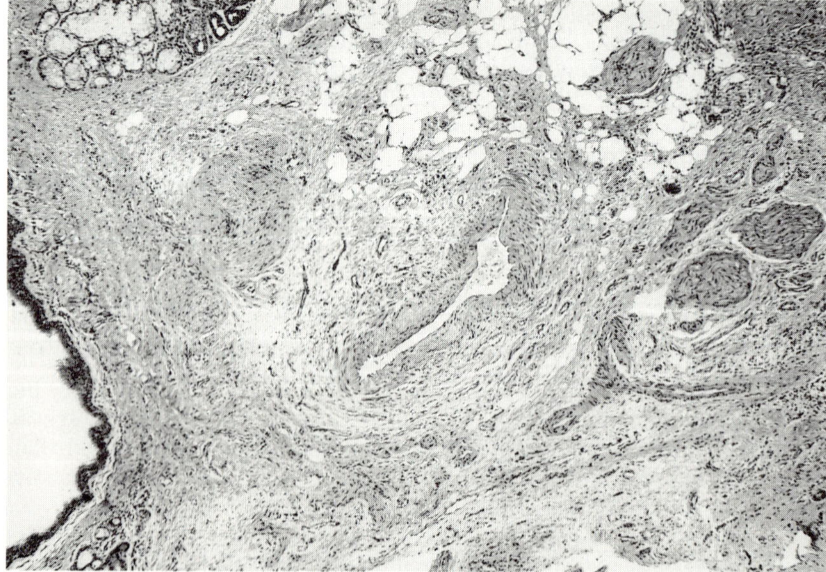

Figure 8.11. Neurovascular bundle in the wall of a nasopalatine duct cyst. (H & E; × 45.)

(1963) showed that moderate-sized nerves were present in 88 per cent of their series and in the remaining 12 per cent nerves were present, although few and small. In 87 per cent of their cases, muscular arteries and numerous small veins were present. Our own observations support the frequency with which these features are found. In our series, prominent neurovascular bundles were found in 45 per cent of cases and large muscular arteries in 72 per cent. The explanation for this phenomenon is that the long sphenopalatine nerve and vessels which pass through the incisive canal are either included in the cyst wall or are removed with the cyst in the course of surgical enucleation.

Small foci of mucous glands (**Figure 8.9**) were found in the fibrous capsules of approximately one-third of cases in the series of Abrams, Howell and Bullock (1963), and of Allard, van der Kwast and van der Waal (1981a) but in only 7 per cent of our own. As the foci are small, it is probable that their frequency would be higher if biopsy material were more extensively sampled. It has been suggested that the presence of mucous glands in a cyst wall is strong evidence in favour of the diagnosis of nasopalatine duct cyst, but I have seen them in an undoubted nasolabial cyst (see **Figure 10.5**, p. 134).

One patient in our series had bilateral cysts and in 19 cases (22 per cent) nasopalatine ducts or their remnants were present in the main cyst wall. In the study of Abrams, Howell and Bullock (1963), epithelial cell nests were found in the walls of 22 of 61 cysts (36 per cent).

As far as evidence of inflammation is concerned, we found that 21 of our cases (24 per cent) were relatively free of inflammatory cell infiltrate. In 39 (45 per cent) there was a mild chronic inflammatory cell infiltrate. In 17 (20 per cent) the chronic inflammatory process was graded as moderate and in nine (11 per cent) as severe. In two cases there was a superimposed acute inflammatory cell infiltrate.

Small islands of hyaline cartilage may very rarely be seen in the cyst walls. They were present in six of our cases (7 per cent) and Abrams, Howell and Bullock (1963) found cartilage in all four of their palatine papilla cysts. These authors pointed out that, unlike the incisive canal and surrounding palatal bone, the palatine papilla normally possessed a small accumulation of cartilage in its anterior aspect.

Redman (1974) and Stam, van der Waal and van der Kwast (1979) have reported the occasional occurrence in nasopalatine duct cysts of an epithelial lining containing granules of pigment which was identified histochemically as melanin and possibly also lipofuscin. These workers were impressed by the resemblance of this lining to olfactory epithelium where olfactory neurons and goblet cells are sparse. Redman suggested origin from nasopalatine duct which had differentiated into olfactory epithelium whereas Stam *et al.* considered that the epithelium developed from remnants of Jacobson's organ. El-Bardaie, Nikai and Takata (1989) reported two cases of pigmented nasopalatine duct cysts in which they were able to demonstrate dendritic melanocytes in the basal layer of the epithelium, thereby identifying the pigment as melanin.

Treatment

Nasopalatine duct cysts are treated by surgical enucleation. Details of the procedure are described in Chapter 18.

Chapter 9

The so-called median palatine, median alveolar, median mandibular and globulomaxillary cysts

Median palatine and median alveolar cysts

In recent years, the existence of separate entities of median palatine and median alveolar cyst has been questioned and they have been excluded from the World Health Organization Classification (Kramer, Pindborg and Shear, 1992). Previously it was thought that these cysts developed from epithelium entrapped in the process of fusion of embryonic processes. It is now felt that they represent posterior extension of an incisive canal cyst in the case of median palatine cyst, and anterior extension in the case of median alveolar cyst. The so-called median alveolar cyst may also, in a number of instances, be a keratocyst derived from dental lamina in the midline of the maxilla.

Reference has been made elsewhere (Chapter 3) to the presence of cysts along the midpalatal raphe which arise from epithelial inclusions at the line of fusion of the palatal folds and the nasal processes. After birth the epithelial inclusions usually atrophy and become resorbed, but some may produce keratin-containing microcysts (see **Figure 3.4**) which extend to the surface and rupture during the first few months after birth. These are not, however, what are usually referred to as median palatine or median posterior palatine cysts, which are described as intrabony cysts in the midline of the palate. If a median posterior palatine cyst indeed exists it would be necessary to postulate its origin as being by enlargement of a midpalatine raphe cyst, or from epithelial inclusions in the region (Courage, North and Hansen, 1974). The contingency of this occurring must be remote. The midpalatine raphe cysts and the epithelial inclusions lie close to the palatal epithelium. It seems unlikely that a median palatine cyst could develop in this site and produce extensive bone resorption without forming a large palatal swelling at a very much earlier stage of its natural history.

I have re-examined the histological sections of 15 cases which were diagnosed as median palatine cysts in our department until 1968 when we stopped making this diagnosis. Six of these were lined exclusively by stratified squamous epithelium while the remaining nine were lined in part by pseudostratified ciliated columnar, cuboidal or columnar epithelium. Of the six lined exclusively by stratified squamous epithelium, three contained neurovascular bundles in the wall and another two contained large muscular blood vessels. Two of this group also showed remnants of nasopalatine ducts in their walls. There was no evidence of mucous glands in the walls of any of the 15 cases. These histological features would be consistent with a diagnosis of a nasopalatine duct cyst.

As far as the median alveolar cyst of the maxilla is concerned, Sicher (1962) was convinced that there is no embryological basis for assuming that it develops from epithelium enclaved at the site of fusion between the right and left globular processes. 'Such a fusion', said Sicher, 'simply does not occur.'

Median mandibular cyst

A cyst occasionally occurs in the midline of the mandible. It produces a well-defined round or ovoid or irregular radiolucent area and may separate the roots of the lower incisor teeth (**Figure 9.1**). In some of the reported cases, the associated teeth have given non-vital pulp responses (Olech, 1957: Case 2; Albers, 1973; Kniha and Gokel, 1985) and in others they have all been vital (Olech, 1957: Case 1; Meyer, 1957; Lucchesi and Topazian, 1961; Blair and Wadsworth, 1968; Buchner and Ramon, 1974; White, Lucas and Miller, 1975: Case 1; Killey, Kay and Seward, 1977; Soskolne and Shteyer, 1977; Nanavati and Gandhi, 1979).

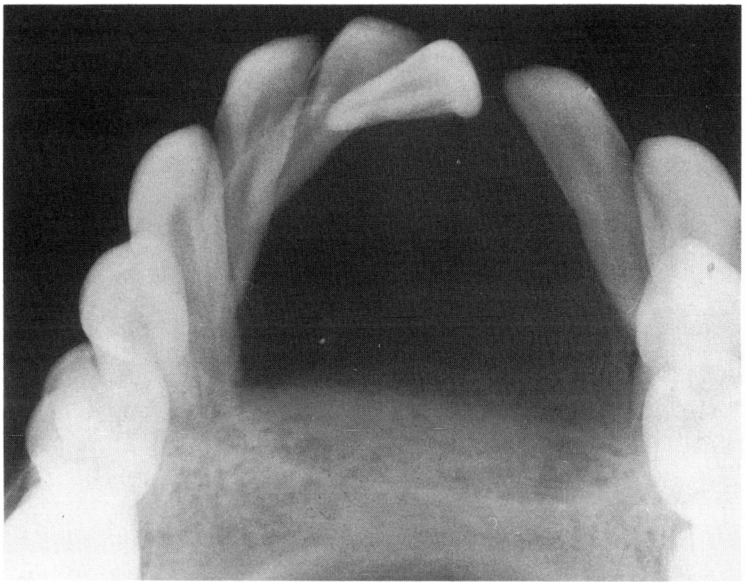

Figure 9.1. A so-called median mandibular cyst which proved to be a keratocyst on histological examination.

The presence of a cyst in the midline of the mandible associated with vital teeth tempted some workers to propose its origin from epithelial inclusions trapped in the area during embryonic development. This concept is, however, not tenable as the mandible forms in the mandibular process which develops as a single unit. As no fusion takes place between ectodermal processes it is not possible to postulate that epithelial entrapment occurs. There are still those, however, who argue otherwise. Allard (1982) has cited Patten (1961) who stated that if, during the process of merging, the mesenchyme inferior to the dividing groove becomes relatively inactive and the mesenchyme in the protruding eminences continues to grow at a normal or accelerated rate, the ectodermal surfaces could come into contact and form a source of fissural epithelium. Allard added however, that the rebuilding of the midline portion of the mandible about Meckel's cartilage, reduces the chances of survival of any enclaved epithelial nests.

Those cysts associated with teeth which have non-vital pulps are very likely to be radicular, and when these are lined by ciliated pseudostratified columnar epithelium it may very possibly be the result of secretory metaplasia. Olech's Case 1 and Meyer's case show histological features which resemble but are not identical to those of keratocysts. The two cases reported by Buchner and Ramon appear to be keratocysts. The published photomicrographs of the cases reported by Lucchesi and Topazian (1961) and by Blair and Wadsworth (1968) show a thin epithelial lining resembling reduced enamel epithelium and may possibly be lateral periodontal cysts, as is the case reported by Difiore and Hartwell (1987). The case of Killey, Kay and Seward (1977) was a solitary bone cyst, as was that of Zachariades, Papanikolaou and Koundouris (1982). Craig, Holland and Hindle (1980) have described an intraosseous dermoid cyst in the midline of the mandible and suggested that this possibility should be considered in the differential diagnosis of midline cystic lesions of the mandible. Tanimoto *et al.* (1983) analysed 12 cysts in the median mandibular region and believed that all could be either keratocysts, solitary, lateral periodontal or radicular cysts. Gardner (1988) surveyed 20 reported cases of median mandibular cyst and concluded that all could be odontogenic cysts. Allard (1982) has stated that in a series of about 8000 surgical specimens seen in the oral pathology department of his institution over a 10-year period, a diagnosis of median mandibular cyst could not be made with confidence in a single case. This would probably be the experience of most oral pathology departments.

There is little evidence, therefore, to indicate that the median mandibular cyst is an entity.

Globulomaxillary cyst

The globulomaxillary cyst has traditionally been described as a fissural cyst found within the bone between the maxillary lateral incisor and canine teeth. Radiologically it is a well-defined radiolucency which frequently causes the roots of the adjacent teeth to diverge (**Figure 9.2**). While there can be no doubt that cysts do occur in this region and that the pulps of the adjacent teeth may give positive vitality responses, there is now a considerable body of opinion against the idea that they are fissural cysts. The evidence against their being fissural cysts is in fact more substantial than the evidence in favour.

The first description of the globulomaxillary cyst has been ascribed to Thoma (1937), but I have not been able to verify this. It was believed for many years that they were fissural cysts arising from non-odontogenic epithelium included at the site of fusion of the globular process of the medial (frontonasal) process and the maxillary process. A variation of this concept was proposed by Ferenczy (1958) who considered that these cysts form at the junction of the premaxilla and maxilla, and that they should be called premaxillary-maxillary cysts. In 1962, Sicher seriously questioned the traditional theory of origin of globulomaxillary cysts, stating that on embryological grounds such an explanation was impossible. He believed that cysts in that region were probably keratocysts. Sicher's views were

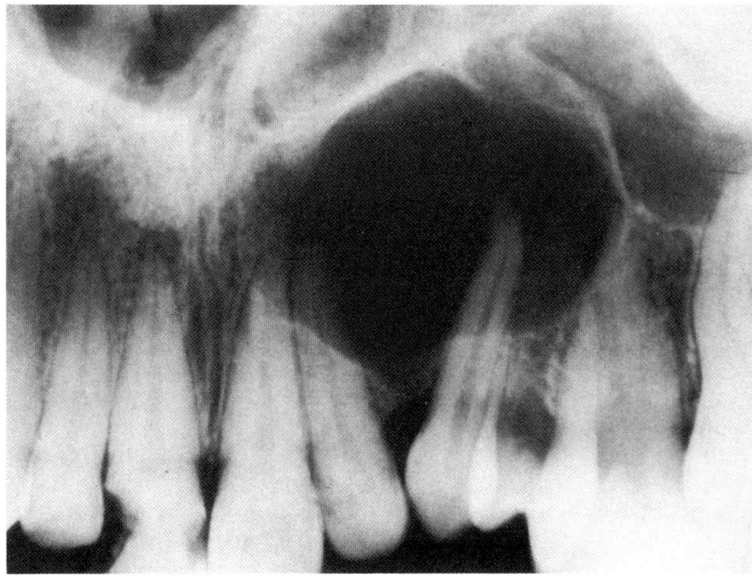

Figure 9.2. Status X-radiograph of a cyst in the 'globulomaxillary' region. Histologically this was a keratocyst.

strongly supported by Kitamura (1976) on the basis of his own extensive embryological studies.

Embryologists have pointed out (Arey, 1965) that the surface bulges seen in the nasomaxillary complex of the embryo and which are called 'facial processes' are not in fact prolongations with free ends which meet in the nasal region. Other than at the median palatal raphe there is no ectoderm-to-ectoderm contact which requires dissolution of the ectodermal surfaces prior to fusion and there is therefore no possibility of enclavement of ectodermal residues. The facial processes are in fact merely elevations or ridges which correspond to centres of growth in the underlying mesenchyme. These are covered by a continuous sheet of folded epithelium. As these growth centres proliferate and develop, the surface furrows between them become more shallow and eventually smooth out (**Figure 9.3**).

A critical study of the whole question of globulomaxillary cysts was reported by Christ (1970). In a survey of the literature over the 50-year period 1920–69, he found very few cases which fulfilled the criteria for acceptance, namely, a radiograph of the lesion, positive vitality of adjacent teeth, and tissue sections or photomicrographs of the histological material. He pointed out that his literature review revealed that a wide variety of other lesions present clinically and radiologically as globulomaxillary cysts. These included adenomatoid odontogenic tumours, myxoma and haemorrhagic bone cyst. Many cases were reported in the literature as globulomaxillary cysts despite the fact that there were non-vital or absent lateral incisors or canines (**Figure 9.4**).

He also reviewed 27 cases from his own departmental records and found that only three satisfied the criteria for inclusion in his study. Histologically, two of these appeared to be keratocysts and the other was thought to be of odontogenic origin. He suggested, therefore, that the globulomaxillary cyst is in fact an

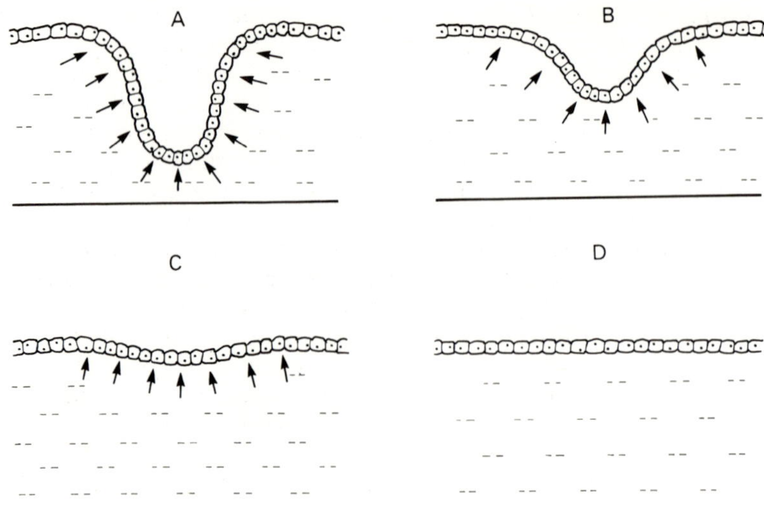

Figure 9.3. Diagram illustrating how proliferation of growth centres in mesenchyme obliterates the surface furrows between them. (After Kitamura, 1976.)

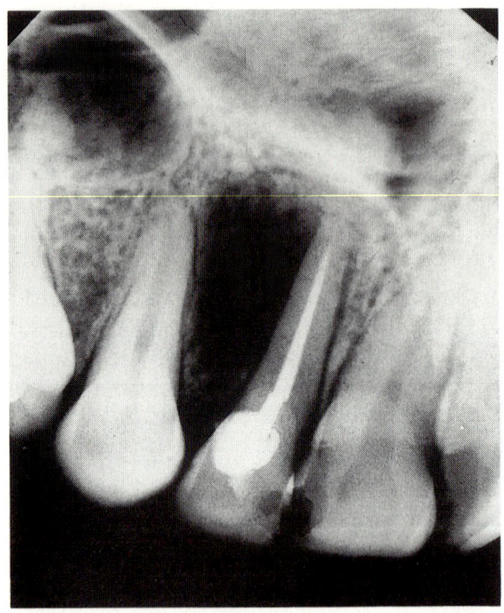

Figure 9.4. Radiograph of a lateral radicular cyst, arising from a non-vital maxillary lateral incisor, in the globulomaxillary area.

strongly supported by Kitamura (1976) on the basis of his own extensive embryological studies.

Embryologists have pointed out (Arey, 1965) that the surface bulges seen in the nasomaxillary complex of the embryo and which are called 'facial processes' are not in fact prolongations with free ends which meet in the nasal region. Other than at

A review in 1975 of 17 of our own cases accessioned as globulomaxillary cysts tended to support Christ's views. Only six of them showed any semblance of respiratory epithelium. Two of the cases had the classic histological features of keratocysts; four were associated with missing or root-treated teeth and fulfilled the criteria for diagnosis as radicular (**Figure 9.4**) or residual cysts; four had histological features very much like those seen in lateral periodontal cysts; and in five the clinical information was quite inadequate for a definitive diagnosis. There remained two possible cases, and even in these the clinical information was equivocal and the respiratory epithelium in the cyst linings could be explained on the basis of metaplasia. The 18 globulomaxillary cysts included in **Table 2.1** are relics of that earlier period. We no longer make this diagnosis in our department. Wysocki (1981) came to the same conclusion following his analysis of 37 cases which had been diagnosed clinically as globulomaxillary cysts. On histological examination 19 were radicular cysts, six periapical granulomas, four developmental lateral periodontal cysts, three keratocysts, three central giant cell granulomas, one calcifying odontogenic cyst and one odontogenic myxoma. Other lesions such as the adenomatoid odontogenic tumour, ameloblastoma and haemorrhagic bone cyst have also been reported in the globulomaxillary region and misdiagnosed as such on clinical and radiological grounds. Kuntz and Reichart (1986) have reported a case of an adenomatoid odontogenic tumour simulating a globulomaxillary cyst and Vedtofte and Holmstrup (1989) have described a series of inflammatory cysts in the globulomaxillary region which they considered to be paradental cysts.

A different point of view on the pathogenesis has, however, been put forward by Little and Jakobsen (1973). They quoted Patten (1961) in support of their belief that processes which join by merging may still entrap epithelium between them if mesenchymal growth is retarded below the groove that separates them. They believed, too, that the 'epithelial wall' which forms by fusion of the medial nasal process and the maxillary process at the inferior margin of the nasal pit is another potential source of epithelial remnants, despite the fact that these have not been found in studies of normal fetal tissues. Although agreeing that the globular process is not involved, they believed that a developmental cyst could arise from these epithelial residues. They suggested that cysts in this region of the maxilla may therefore be of either odontogenic or non-odontogenic epithelial origin.

While this is clearly an intriguing question most of the evidence presently available leads to the conclusion that the so-called globulomaxillary cyst is not an entity but that a variety of cysts and tumours can occur as well-demarcated radiolucent lesions in the lateral incisor-canine region of the maxilla.

Chapter 10

Nasolabial (nasoalveolar) cyst

The nasolabial cyst occurs outside the bone in the nasolabial folds below the alae nasi. It is traditionally regarded as a jaw cyst although strictly speaking it should be classified as a soft-tissue cyst. As the alveolus is not involved, the term nasolabial is preferred to nasoalveolar cyst.

Clinical features

Frequency

Nasolabial cysts are rare lesions and our own material consists of only 18 examples seen in 32 years (see **Table 2.1**, p. 6). Roed-Petersen (1969), in an extensive review of the literature, found information relating to 155 patients with nasolabial cysts and has done a statistical analysis of the combined data of 111 of these patients plus five of his own cases. A survey of cases reported subsequent to Roed-Petersen's review has been reported from our department (van Bruggen *et al.*, 1985). This identified another 45 examples of which 25 had sufficient documentation for analysis (Brons and Jongebreur, 1967; Crawford, Korchin and Greskovitch 1968; Harada *et al.*, 1968; Fanibunda, 1970; Santora, Ballantyne and Hinds, 1970; Stoelinga, 1971b; Karmody and Gallagher, 1972; Brandao, Ebling and Faria e Souza, 1974; Campbell and Burkes, 1975). The data presented below are based on Roed-Petersen's 116 cases, the 25 examples just referred to, and 10 from our own files: a total of 151 cases. Another review of the literature is that by Wesley, Scannell and Nathan (1984).

Age

There is a wide age distribution ranging from 12 to 75 years, with a peak frequency in the fourth and fifth decades (**Figure 10.1**).

Sex

There is a considerable preponderance of females with nasolabial cysts. In the sample of van Bruggen *et al.* (1985) 119 patients were females (79 per cent) and 32 males (21 per cent), a female: male ratio of 3.7:1. This difference is statistically significant ($P < 0.001$). All of our own patients have been women. The series reported by Kuriloff (1987) included 19 women and seven men.

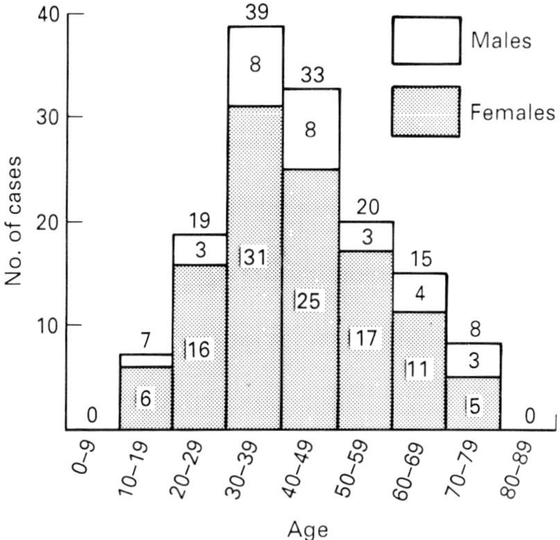

Figure 10.1. Age distribution of 141 patients with nasolabial cysts.

Clinical presentation

The duration of symptoms in recorded cases has varied from less than one month to as many as 40 years. The most frequent symptom is swelling and very often this is the only complaint. Sometimes the patients complain of pain and difficulty in nasal breathing. In some cases, difficulty with an upper denture has drawn attention to the problem, and occasionally the cysts are diagnosed fortuitously during routine examination. Cohen and Hertzanu (1985) reported a case which reached a huge

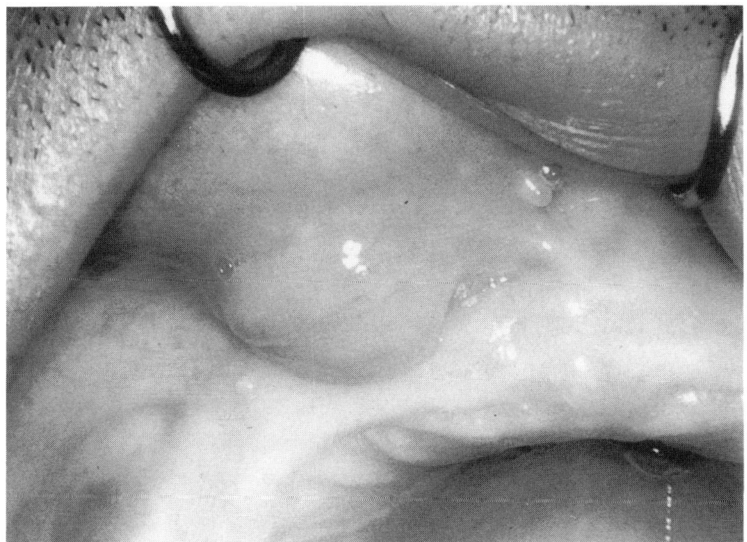

Figure 10.2. Intraoral swelling produced by a nasolabial cyst.

size, causing severe facial deformity. In most cases the cysts are unilateral, but in the study of van Bruggen *et al.* 16 patients had bilateral lesions (10.6 per cent).

The cysts grow slowly, producing a swelling of the lip. They fill out the nasolabial fold and may lift the ala nasi, distort the nostril and produce a swelling of the floor of the nose. Intraorally they form a bulge in the labial sulcus (**Figure 10.2**). The cysts are fluctuant and, on bimanual palpation, fluctuation may be elicited between the swelling on the floor of the nose and that in the labial sulcus. Infected cysts may discharge into the nose.

Radiological features

A detailed description of the radiological features has been provided by Seward (1962a). He pointed out that there is a localized increased radiolucency of the alveolar process above the apices of the incisor teeth. This radiolucency results from a depression on the labial surface of the maxilla which may be detectable in a tangential view. When the depression extends to the lateral margin of the anterior bony aperture of the nose there is resorption of the lower part of the nasal notch. The inferior margin of the anterior bony aperture of the nose is distorted by the lesion. As a result, standard occlusal radiographs show a pronounced posterior convexity in one-half of the bracket-shaped radio-opaque line which forms the bony border of the nasal aperture, instead of the usual double curve (**Figure 10.3**).

The cyst may be aspirated and a radio-opaque liquid introduced, after which it may be viewed in tangential and postero-anterior views of the jaws or in vertex occlusal views (**Figure 10.4**). It is normally a spherical or kidney-shaped lesion lying against the inferior and lateral borders of the anterior bony aperture of the nose, extending from the midline to the canine fossa.

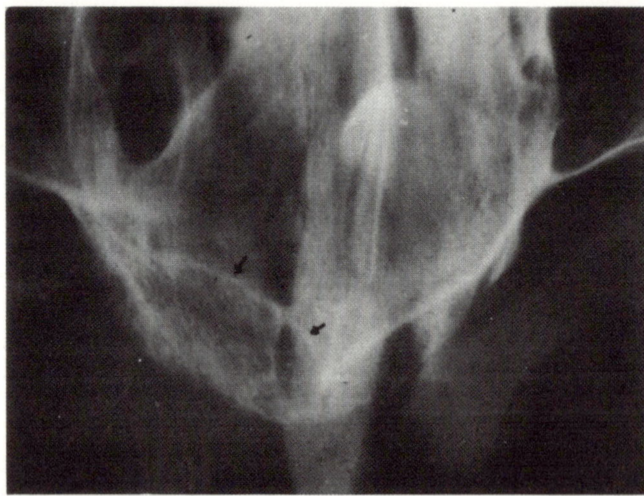

Figure 10.3. Standard occlusal view of a patient with a nasolabial cyst. There is posterior bulging of the right side of the bracket-shaped line, indicated by arrows. (By courtesy of Professor G. R. Seward and the Editor, *The Dental Practitioner*. Previously published (1962) *Dent. Pract.* **12**, 154–161.)

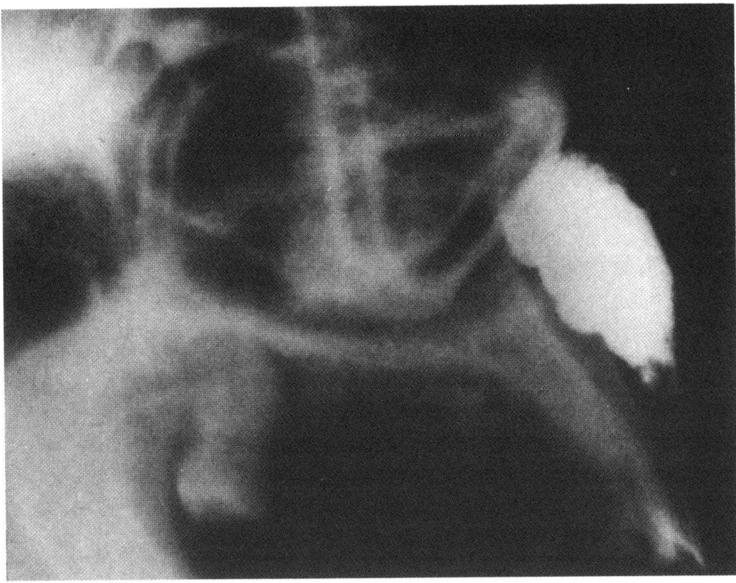

Figure 10.4. Nasolabial cyst demonstrated radiologically by aspiration of its fluid contents and injection of a radio-opaque fluid.

Pathogenesis

The pathogenesis of the nasolabial cyst is unresolved. The traditional concept, as described in many textbooks, was that the nasolabial cyst is the soft-tissue equivalent of the globulomaxillary cyst. It was therefore suggested that it arises from epithelium enclaved at the site of the globular, lateral nasal and maxillary processes. This concept, however, is not tenable as the embryological basis for it has been seriously disputed (see discussion in section on globulomaxillary cysts, Chapter 9). Flöe Möller and Philipsen (1958), Seward (1962a), Roed-Petersen (1969), Kitamura (1976), Allard (1982) and David and O'Connell (1986) have reviewed the various hypotheses proposed to explain the origin of nasolabial cysts, and there is considerable support for the proposal first put forward by Brüggemann (1920) that they develop from the lower anterior part of the nasolacrimal duct. When the margins of the lateral nasal and maxillary bulges coalesce, the ectoderm along the boundary between them gives rise to a solid cellular rod which at first develops as a linear surface elevation, the nasolacrimal ridge, and then sinks into the mesenchyme. Its caudal end proliferates to connect with the caudal part of the lateral nasal wall while its cranial extremity later connects with the developing conjunctival sac. This solid rod then becomes canalized to form the nasolacrimal duct (Warwick and Williams, 1973). The location of nasolabial cysts is such that they could conceivably develop from remnants of the embryonic nasolacrimal rod or duct, if not from the lower anterior portion of the mature duct. The mature nasolacrimal duct is lined by pseudostratified columnar epithelium and this is the type of epithelium usually found lining nasolabial cysts. Further embryological studies on the nasolacrimal duct could be of value in solving this problem.

There is general agreement that nasolabial cysts are of developmental origin, and this is reinforced by the finding of a 10.6 per cent frequency of bilateral cysts in the review done by van Bruggen *et al.* (1985). Roed-Petersen's survey referred to a report of nasolabial cysts occurring in father and daughter. Another remarkable feature is the high frequency in women, the only cyst of the oral regions other than the aneurysmal bone cyst to show a female preponderance. The reason for this is unknown.

Histological features

A histological analysis of nine examples in our collection done a few years ago, showed that all were lined by non-ciliated pseudostratified columnar epithelium (**Figure 10.5**). Goblet cells, varying in number from very few to very many, were seen in seven of them. In two cases there were small, localized areas of squamous metaplasia. In seven cases part of the epithelial lining consisted of either cuboidal epithelium or one to two layers of flat squamous cells. In some specimens the entire epithelial thickness was eroded leaving discontinuities.

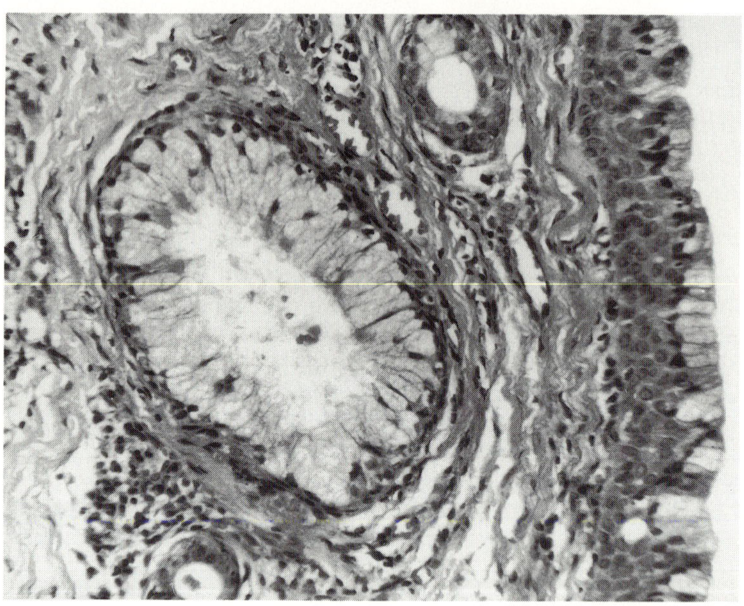

Figure 10.5. Nasolabial cyst. It is lined by pseudostratified columnar epithelium containing many goblet cells. In the example illustrated here, mucous glands are present in the wall. (H & E; × 190.)

The fibrous cysts walls were relatively acellular and either loosely or densely collagenous. Seven of the walls which consisted of loose connective tissue were very haemorrhagic. One cyst wall was fairly intensely infiltrated with chronic inflammatory cells while the others were relatively uninflamed. Mucous glands lay close to the epithelial cyst lining in three instances.

In Roed-Petersen's review, 64 cases which had been evaluated histologically were summarized. Pseudostratified columnar epithelium was the only type of lining in 26 cases (41 per cent). In nine, pseudostratified columnar epithelium was present in association with stratified squamous epithelium, and in 15 with cuboidal epithelium. Seven cases contained stratified squamous and cuboidal epithelium, four contained only cuboidal epithelium and three were lined by pseudostratified columnar, stratified squamous and cuboidal epithelium. In all, 53 of the cases (83 per cent) were lined wholly or in part by pseudostratified columnar epithelium. Goblet cells were present in 33 cysts and ciliated cells in 22.

Treatment

The treatment of nasolabial cysts is described in Chapter 18.

Chapter 11

Radicular cyst, residual cyst, paradental cyst and mandibular infected buccal cyst

A radicular cyst is one which arises from the epithelial residues in the periodontal ligament as a result of inflammation. The inflammation usually follows the death of the dental pulp and cysts arising in this way are found most commonly at the apices of the involved teeth. They may, however, also be found on the lateral aspects of the roots in relation to lateral accessory root canals. Rarely, inflammatory cysts may occur towards the cervical margin of the lateral aspect of a root as a consequence of an inflammatory process in a periodontal pocket. The latter lesion is perhaps best referred to as an inflammatory periodontal cyst or *inflammatory collateral cyst* (Main, 1970a, b). Quite often a radicular cyst remains behind in the jaws after removal of the offending tooth and this is referred to as a *residual cyst*. Cysts of inflammatory origin occurring on the lateral aspects of the roots of partially erupted mandibular third molars with an associated history of pericoronitis, have been described by Craig (1976) and termed the *paradental cyst*. A similar lesion, usually occurring on the buccal surfaces of the mandibular molars in young children, has been described by Stoneman and Worth (1983) and named the *mandibular infected buccal cyst*. These different inflammatory cysts of the jaws will be considered together in this chapter.

Radicular and residual cyst

Clinical features

Frequency

Radicular and residual cysts are by far the most common cystic lesions in the jaws, comprising 1368 (52.3 per cent) of 2616 jaw cysts in our series (see **Table 2.1**). This is a somewhat lower frequency than the figure of 68 per cent in the series of Killey, Kay and Seward (1977).

Age

The age distribution of 558 patients in our series is shown in **Figure 11.1**. Very few cases are seen in the first decade, after which there is a fairly steep rise, with a peak frequency in the third decade. There are large numbers of cases in the fourth and fifth decades, after which there is a gradual decline. A very similar age distribution was reported by Donath (1985). The low frequency in the first decade has been

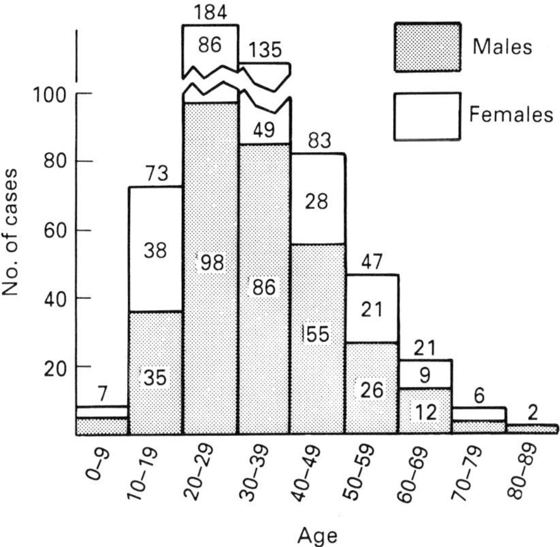

Figure 11.1. Age distribution of 558 South African patients with radicular cysts.

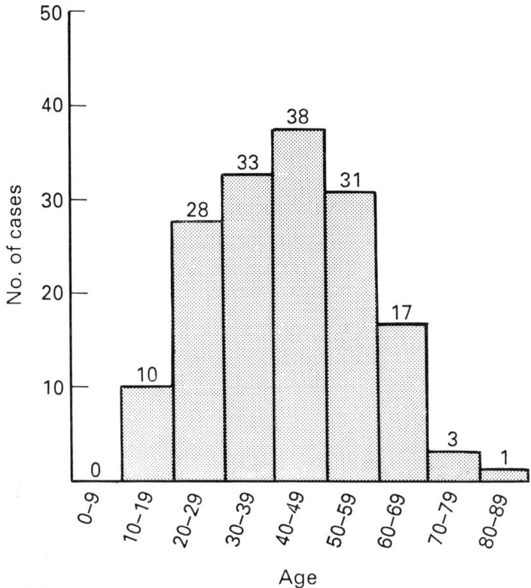

Figure 11.2. Age distribution of 161 English patients with radicular cysts.

shown in a number of studies and indicates that although dental caries is very common in children during the first decade, radicular cysts are not often found associated with deciduous teeth.

Interestingly, an age distribution analysis which I did some years ago of a group of English patients with radicular cysts (**Figure 11.2**) suggested that these cysts tend to be found at a somewhat older age in the English than the South African group.

Statistically, the difference is highly significant ($P < 0.001$ per cent) and may mean that the South African group is exposed to the relevant aetiological factor, mainly dental caries, at an earlier age than the English group.

Sex

Of 664 cases in our series, 388 (58 per cent) were in males and 276 (42 per cent) in females, a statistically significant difference ($P < 0.001$). The male preponderance occurred essentially in the fourth and fifth decades. The lower frequency in females, which has also been reported by other workers, may be because they are less likely to neglect their teeth, particularly the maxillary anterior incisors, in which area most radicular cysts occur. Males moreover are more likely to sustain trauma to their maxillary anterior teeth.

Race

In our sample white patients were involved with a frequency of about twice that of black patients.

Site

The anatomical distribution of 789 cysts from a pooled sample of South African and English patients is shown in **Figure 11.3**. They occur in all tooth-bearing areas of the jaws although about 60 per cent are found in the maxilla and 40 per cent in the mandible. There is a particularly high frequency in the maxillary anterior region (37 per cent) and there are a number of possible reasons for this. In addition to the hazard posed by dental caries, maxillary incisors have in the past, perhaps more frequently than other teeth, had silicate restorations placed in them, with

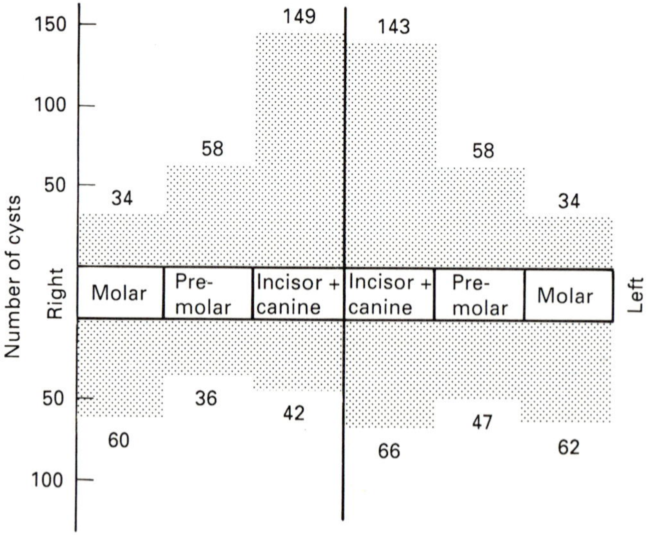

Figure 11.3. Anatomical distribution of 789 radicular cysts.

consequent high risk to their pulps. Then there is the high prevalence of palatal invaginations in the maxillary lateral incisors and the frequency with which pulp death supervenes in these teeth; and thirdly, maxillary anterior teeth are probably more prone than others to traumatic injuries which lead to pulp death.

Clinical presentation

Many radicular cysts are symptomless and are discovered when periapical radiographs are taken of teeth with non-vital pulps. Slowly enlarging swellings are often complained of. At first the enlargement is bony hard but as the cyst increases in size, the covering bone becomes very thin despite subperiosteal bone deposition and the swelling then exhibits 'springiness'. Only when the cyst has completely eroded the bone will there be fluctuation. In the maxilla there may be buccal or palatal enlargement whereas in the mandible it is usually labial or buccal and only rarely lingual. Pain and infection are other clinical features of some radicular cysts. It is often said that radicular cysts are painless unless infected. Some patients with these lesions, however, complain of pain although no evidence of infection is found clinically and no evidence of acute inflammation is seen histologically after the cyst has been removed. Likewise, some patients have clinically infected and histologically inflamed cysts which are not painful (Shear, 1961a).

A *sine qua non* for the diagnosis of a radicular cyst is the related presence of a tooth with a non-vital pulp. Occasionally, a sinus may lead from the cyst cavity to the oral mucosa.

Quite often, more than one radicular cyst may be found in a patient (Shear, 1961a; Stoelinga, 1973) and this has led a number of authors to believe that there are cyst-prone individuals who show a particular susceptibility to develop radicular cysts (Oehlers, 1970). This view is supported by the fact that radicular cysts are relatively rare in relation to the vast numbers of grossly carious teeth with dead pulps. It is possible that an immune mechanism may inhibit cyst formation in most individuals and that cyst-prone subjects have a defective immunological surveillance and suppression mechanism (Toller, 1970a). It is also possible that some individuals have a genetic tendency to develop radicular cysts.

Radicular cysts arising from deciduous teeth appear to be very rare. In a survey of the documents of 1300 radicular cysts recorded in our department over a 25-year period, only seven were associated with deciduous teeth (0.5 per cent). In an extensive review of the literature from 1898 (Lustmann and Shear, 1985), only 28 cases were found. The incidence is probably higher than these figures would suggest. Radicular radiolucencies related to deciduous teeth tend to be neglected and probably resolve after removal of the offending teeth. Nevertheless, the frequency is substantially lower than that of those associated with permanent teeth and one may speculate on the reasons for this. Pulpal and periapical infections in deciduous teeth tend to drain more readily than those of permanent teeth and the antigenic stimuli which evoke the changes leading to the formation of radicular cysts may be different. Periapical granulomas associated with deciduous teeth have not been subjected to the same extensive investigations that have been carried out on periapical granulomas of permanent teeth, which are discussed later in this chapter, in the section on pathogenesis.

Grundy, Adkins and Savage (1984) reported a series of cases of radicular cysts associated with deciduous teeth which had been treated endodontically with materials containing formocresol which, in combination with tissue proteins, is antigenic and has been shown to elicit a humoral and cell-mediated response. Some of the cysts in their series showed rapid buccal expansion and non-refractile eosinophilic material was observed in the epithelial linings.

In the study of Lustmann and Shear (1985), 23 personally-observed cases were reported. The patients' ages ranged from 4 to 12 years with one exceptional case aged 19 years. The male:female ratio was 1.6:1. The mandible was affected more frequently than the maxilla and the deciduous molars were the teeth most often involved. In nine cases buccal expansion was noticed and in eight cases the permanent buds were displaced. Caries was the most common aetiological factor.

Residual radicular cysts are those which are retained after removal of the offending non-vital tooth. There have been relatively few publications on the subject although it has been estimated that they represent approximately 10 per cent of all odontogenic cysts (Main, 1970a; Killey, Kay and Seward, 1977). High and Hirschmann (1986, 1988) have reported studies on series of asymptomatic and symptomatic residual cysts. They were interested in the factors which decide whether a radicular cyst will resolve or persist after tooth removal and the natural history and behaviour of these cysts once established. With regard to the asymptomatic cysts, they showed that there was a decrease in size with increasing age (r = 0.5; $P < 0.005$). There was an unexpectedly large number in the mandibular premolar region and there was a direct relationship between the age of the cyst and the radiological and histological evidence of mineralization ($P < 0.001$). There was an overall reduction in epithelial thickness with cyst age and all cysts showed minimal chronic inflammatory changes. They concluded that the vast majority of residual cysts are slowly resolving lesions. Nevertheless, they do persist and the authors did not provide evidence of complete resolution.

In their second paper, on their series of symptomatic cysts which produced pain or swelling or both, High and Hirschmann (1988) showed that the mean cyst size was larger than that of the asymptomatic sample, and that the negative correlation of size with cyst age was not as strong as with the asymptomatic sample ($r = 0.39$; $P < 0.05$). Cyst ages varied from 1 month to 20 years (figure corrected in reprint sent to me) and there was again a perplexingly high frequency in the mandibular premolar region. Acute and chronic inflammatory cell infiltration showed variable intensity and there was an inverse relationship between the percentage of polymorphonuclear leucocytes in the inflammatory infiltrate and cortication of the cyst wall radiographically ($P < 0.001$). There were no obvious causes for the inflammation in deeply positioned residual cysts. A chronic inflammatory process would certainly be present when the offending tooth is removed and the authors posed the question whether this could persist and gradually worsen as a result of lysosome or other irritant chemical release from dead or dying cells, and at some point trigger an acute inflammatory reaction.

Of significance, however, is that residual cysts persist and may, in due course, produce symptoms.

Radiological features

A number of studies have shown that it is difficult to differentiate radiologically between radicular cysts and apical granulomas. Mortensen, Winther and Birn (1970) examined histological material of 396 periapical lesions with a diameter of 5 mm or more, which had been classified preoperatively as cysts or granulomas on radiological evidence. A correct preliminary diagnosis had been made in 81 per cent of 232 granulomas but in only 48 per cent of 164 cysts. They also showed that the relative number of granulomas decreases with increasing size of the lesion whereas there is an increase in the relative number of cysts. Nevertheless it is interesting to note that of all the lesions measuring 10–14 mm in radiographic diameter, there were almost as many granulomas as cysts; and that in their group of lesions measuring 15 mm or more, approximately one-third were granulomas. Moreover, a little over one-third of their lesions measuring 5–9 mm were cysts on histological examination. Similar findings were reported by Stockdale and Chandler (1988).

These data certainly indicate that one cannot rely on the size of the lesion to establish a diagnosis except where the radiographic lesion is 2 cm in diameter or larger (Natkin, Oswald and Carnes, 1984). In addition, the large number of cysts which were incorrectly diagnosed as granulomas suggested to Mortensen, Winther and Birn (1970) that because of infection many cysts have a diffuse radiographic margin and therefore lack the circumscribed appearance usually ascribed to radicular cysts.

Biochemical procedures have been advocated to differentiate between periapical cysts and granulomas (Morse, Patnik and Schacterle, 1973; Morse, Wolfson and Schacterle, 1975; Morse, Schacterle and Wolfson, 1976). Aspirates of root canal fluids from patients with cysts showed an intense albumin pattern and definite patterns in the globulin zones, on polyacrylamide-gel electrophoresis. Fluids associated with periapical granulomas on the other hand showed only a faint to moderate pattern in the albumin zone.

The classic description of the radiological appearance of radicular cysts is that they are round or ovoid radiolucencies surrounded by a narrow radio-opaque margin which extends from the lamina dura of the involved tooth (**Figure 11.4**). In infected or rapidly enlarging cysts the radio-opaque margin may not be present. This can lead to diagnostic problems in the case of residual cysts. High and Hirschmann (1988) demonstrated a negative correlation between the loss of

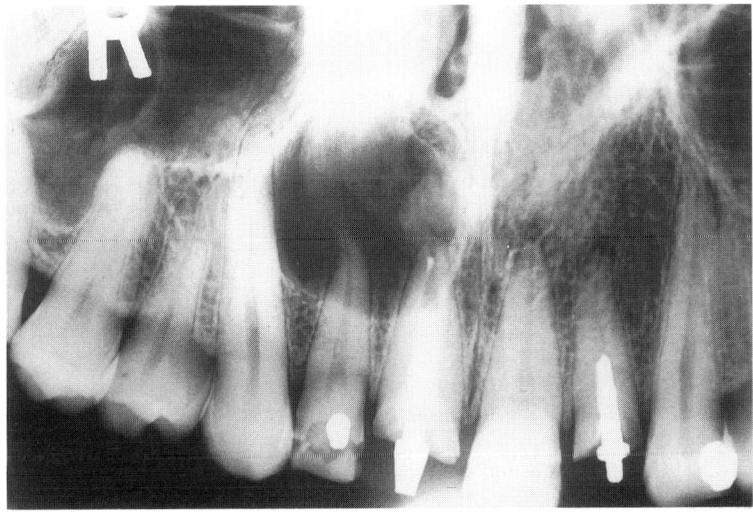

Figure 11.4. Radiograph of a radicular cyst.

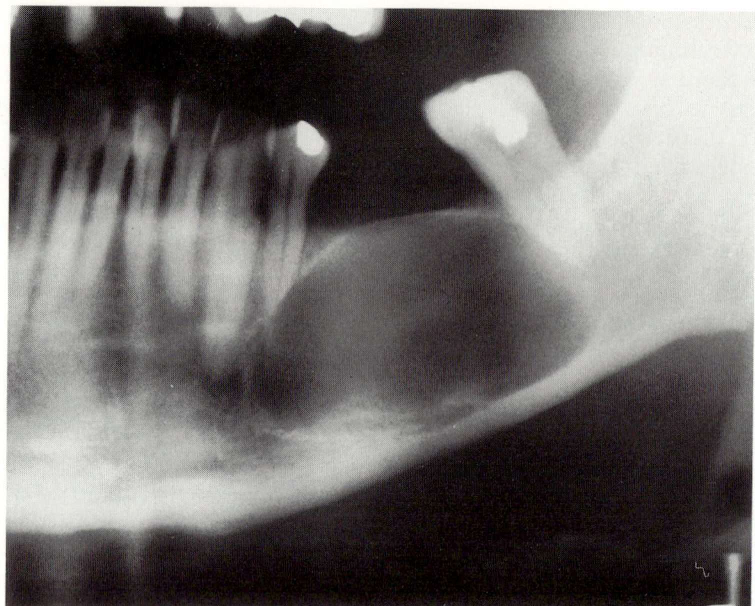

Figure 11.5. Radiograph of a residual cyst. This lesion must be differentiated from a keratocyst.

radiographic cortication and increasing intensity of acute inflammation ($r = 0.83$; $P < 0.001$). With a residual cyst, moreover, the differential diagnosis of keratocyst must be considered (**Figure 11.5**). A radicular cyst on the lateral margin of a root in association with an accessory root canal must be differentiated from a lateral periodontal cyst. Root resorption is rare, but may occur.

Pathogenesis

It is convenient to consider the pathogenesis of radicular cysts in three phases: the phase of initiation, the phase of cyst formation and the phase of enlargement. The mechanisms involved in all phases have been the subjects of extensive investigation and speculation and a great deal has been learnt over the past few years. It is generally agreed that the epithelial linings of these cysts are derived from the epithelial cell rests of Malassez in the periodontal ligament which come to lie in periapical granulomas associated with teeth with dead, often infected, pulps. There is also no doubt that these cell rests may proliferate, and when they do so, either *in vivo*, or in tissue culture experiments, there are consistent morphological and histochemical changes (Ten Cate, 1972). The proliferating cells show a decrease in nucleocytoplasmic ratio, they utilize glycogen, synthesize neutral lipid and ribonucleic acid, and show an increased glucose-6-phosphate dehydrogenase activity but depressed succinic dehydrogenase activity. The latter two chemical changes indicate that the activated epithelial cells preferentially use the hexose-monophosphate shunt.

Precisely how these epithelial cells are stimulated to proliferate is not clear. It would seem that some product of a dead pulp may initiate the process and that at the same time it evokes an inflammatory reaction, as there is evidence that proliferating odontogenic epithelium is associated with the presence of an acute inflammatory cell infiltration (Shear, 1963a). A feature of this infiltrate is that the polymorphonuclear leucocytes are found in the proliferating epithelium (Shear, 1964; Cohen, 1979; Johannessen, Nilsen and Skaug, 1983; Johannessen, 1986), and it may be that the substance which initiates the epithelial proliferation exerts a direct effect on the epithelium itself and is also chemotactic to polymorphonuclear leucocytes. Johannesen, Nilsen and Skaug (1983) demonstrated deposits of complement factor C3c and IgG in the basement membrane zone of the epithelium in periapical granulomas, and IgE within the epithelium, indicative of chemotactic factors which may be activated in this area. It has been shown that epithelial proliferation in periapical granulomas is more frequent with untreated than with treated root canals (Yanagisiwa, 1980).

There is also some evidence that local changes in the supporting connective tissue may be responsible for activating the cell nests (Grupe, Ten Cate and Zander, 1967) and that a decreased oxygen and increased carbon dioxide tension and a local reduction in pH produced in chronic inflammation may be the critical factors.

Immunological studies have made an important contribution in understanding the formation of periapical granulomas and radicular cysts, and both humoral and cell-mediated reactions have been implicated in the pathogenesis. Suggestions have also been made about the role of immune factors in the proliferation of epithelial cell nests. IgG is the predominant class of immunoglobulin demonstrated by immunofluorescence techniques in the immunoglobulin-containing cells of periapical granulomas. Stern *et al.* (1981) showed that 74 per cent of the antibody-producing lesional cells in periapical granulomas and cysts synthesized IgG, 20 per cent IgA, 4 per cent IgE and 2 per cent IgM. There were no significant differences between the solid and cystic periapical lesions. Smith *et al.* (1987) found 85 per cent IgG, 14 per cent IgA and 2 per cent IgM plasma cells, and intense extracellular IgG staining in their sample of radicular cysts. Complement C3 is demonstrable in the connective tissues. The antigens involved are presumed to be derived from bacteria. When these antigens gain entrance to the pulp or periapical tissues at certain concentrations, antigen–antibody complexes may form. These may coactivate complement, leading to increased vascular permeability and a leukotactic response (Pulver, Taubman and Smith, 1978). The presence of both IgE immunoglobulin-containing cells and mast cells, some of which undergo degranulation, suggest that anaphylactic hypersensitivity reactions may also play a role in periapical granulomas (Pulver, Taubman and Smith, 1978; Yanagisiwa, 1980; Torabinejad, Kettering and Bakland, 1981; Johannessen, Nilsen and Skaug, 1983; Perrini and Fonzi, 1985; Kontiainen, Ranta and Lautenschlager, 1986).

Infiltrates of T lymphocytes, indicating that cellular immune reactions are involved in their pathogenesis, were demonstrated by Stern *et al.* (1982) and by Skaug *et al.* (1984b) in human periapical granulomas; while the latter authors (Skaug *et al.*, 1984a) concluded that because of low complement component C3d receptor activity, B lymphocytes form only a minor component of the mononuclear cells in these lesions. However, the authors considered that further studies were necessary before conclusions could be made as to the significance of these findings. T helper cells (OKT4) were found by Nilsen *et al.* (1984) to be more numerous than suppressor/cytotoxic T (OKT8) cells and were considered to play an important role in the differentiation of B lymphocytes into Ig-producing plasma cells as well as in the activation of T lymphocytes (OKT3) into suppressor/cytotoxic T lymphocytes. By contrast, Kontiainen, Rauta and Lautenschlager (1986) and Babál *et al.* (1987)

showed that cells of the suppressor/cytotoxic phenotype (OKT8) dominated within T cells. Gao *et al.* (1988a) also found that suppressor/cytotoxic cells generally outnumbered T helper cells in the periapical granulomas, whereas the two cell types were of equal number, or the T helper cells predominated, in the cysts which they examined. The range of the cell ratios found by Gao *et al.* indicated to them the complex nature of the immune interactions in periapical lesions and that the ratio may be affected by many factors, including the stage of the lesion. This may also explain the discrepancy in the results reported by different workers. In a similar study on odontogenic cysts, including radicular cysts, Matthews and Browne (1987) found that although the helper T subset always predominated over the suppressor/cytotoxic T subset, the ratios varied between sites within individual specimens and inverse ratios were detected at some sites in several specimens.

The proportion of B lymphocytes in the study of Kontiainen *et al.* was approximately 20 per cent, and that of plasma cells was 2 per cent, lower than the 13 per cent plasma cells reported by Stern *et al.* (1982). B and T lymphocytes, predominantly the latter, were demonstrated in periapical granulomas by Torabinejad and Kettering (1985) and in granulomas and cysts by Gao et al (1988) who, like Nilsen *et al.* (1984), suggested that these lesions probably result from activation of both humoral and cell-mediated immunological reactions in response to egress of potential antigens from the root canal system into the periapical tissues.

Gao *et al.* (1988a) have contributed some ideas as to the reasons for the proliferation of the epithelium in periapical lesions, while acknowledging that these are not clear. In their study they observed that dense infiltrates of lymphocytes, HLA-Dr positive cells, and lysozyme- and α-1-antitrypsin-positive cells were always closely related to the proliferating epithelium in periapical granulomas and near the epithelial linings of the cysts. T helper lymphocytes were seen more frequently in the connective tissue around the epithelium and suppressor/cytotoxic lymphocytes within the epithelium. They speculated that activated T cells in periapical granulomas produce lymphokines that may act on the rests of Malassez causing proliferation and altered differentiation leading to cyst formation. The presence of α-1-antitrypsin in periapical granulomas and cysts has also been reported by Ylipaavalniemi (1977) and Wilk *et al.* (1983) who emphasized its protective effects, inhibiting autodigestion by proteolytic enzymes released by leucocytes and restricting the expansion of periapical lesions.

Matthews and Browne (1987) demonstrated intraepithelial HLA-Dr positive cells in most of their samples of odontogenic cysts and about one-third of their specimens showed extensive cytoplasmic HLA-Dr expression in their epithelial linings. Most specimens also showed a third population of intraepithelial cells which expressed a Langerhans cell phenotype although rarely having the classic dendritic morphology of these cells. The authors suggested that these might present antigens in the cyst fluid to the immune system. Their study indicated that the inflammatory cell populations, epithelial expression of HLA-Dr and occurrence of intraepithelial cells displaying a Langerhans cell phenotype are similar in all types of odontogenic cyst.

Contos *et al.* (1987) and Gao *et al.* (1988a) also demonstrated Langerhans cells in the epithelial linings of radicular cysts. In areas of intense inflammation, as evidenced by large numbers of lymphocytes, polymorphonuclear leucocytes and plasma cells, greater numbers of S-100- and HLA-Dr positive cells (Langerhans cells) were observed (Contos *et al.*, 1987). The finding of lymphocytes adjacent to stained Langerhans cells suggested increased antigen challenge and antigen-processing activity and that T lymphocytes may act as effector cells in the pathogenesis of the cyst, after receiving information from stimulated Langerhans cells.

In a subsequent study, Gao *et al.* (1988b) used immunohistochemical techniques with a panel of monoclonal antibodies to study patterns of keratin expression in quiescent cell rests of Malassez, in the proliferating epithelium of periapical granulomas, and in the epithelial linings of radicular cysts. Expression of keratin 19 was found throughout the entire range of epithelia examined while in the rests of Malassez they appeared to be paired with keratin 5. However, unlike the situation in normal oral epithelium where staining for keratin 19 is found in the basal region, in proliferating epithelium in the periapical granulomas, staining tended to be suprabasal, while in cyst linings staining was often restricted to the most superficial layers of the epithelium. With proliferation of the rests of Malassez, a more complex pattern of keratin expression was observed. As an early change, epithelia in periapical granulomas uniformly and strongly expressed keratin 14 and subsequently keratin 13 and some keratin 4. Further epithelial change to form a cyst lining was associated with a more clearly differentiated phenotype of non-keratinized stratified squamous epithelium. Although reactivities were not always strong, staining for keratins 8 and 18 (typical of the simple epithelial phenotype) was consistently observed in proliferating epithelium in granulomas and in cyst linings. Gao *et al.* suggested therefore, that proliferating odontogenic epithelium thus appears to have a phenotype different from normal epithelia but one which is perhaps similar to that of epidermis during embryogenesis. They suggested further, that during cyst formation the proliferation of the epithelial rests of Malassez, which is associated with an inflammatory reaction and local accumulation of various types of immune cells, may be stimulated by soluble mediators of inflammation to influence the epithelial phenotype.

Proliferating epithelium has a characteristic histological appearance. The epithelium, in section, forms arcades and rings, each encircling a core of vascular connective tissue. The reason for this appearance may be appreciated by considering the three-dimensional picture. When the epithelial cells proliferate, they do so in different planes, forming a mass rather than sheets or strands. Cores of vascular connective tissue extend into the epithelial mass from all directions and the resulting appearance in histological section is one of arcades and rings of epithelial cells surrounding these cores. This epithelial arcading is frequently seen in histological preparations of apical granulomas and radicular cysts (**Figure 11.6**).

The next phase in the pathogenesis of a radicular cyst is the process by which a cavity comes to be lined by the proliferating odontogenic epithelium. Two possibilities have been generally recognized, both of which are feasible and which may operate independently of one another. One concept proposes that the epithelium proliferates and covers the bare connective tissue surface of an abscess cavity or a cavity which may occur as a result of connective tissue breakdown by proteolytic enzyme activity (Summers, 1974). The other, and perhaps more widely supported theory, postulates that a cyst cavity forms within a proliferating epithelial mass in an apical granuloma by degeneration and death of cells in the centre.

There is histological evidence for the latter hypothesis. The proliferating epithelial masses show considerable intercellular oedema. These intercellular accumulations of fluid coalesce to form microcysts containing epithelial and inflammatory cells (**Figure 11.7**). The demonstration of high levels of acid

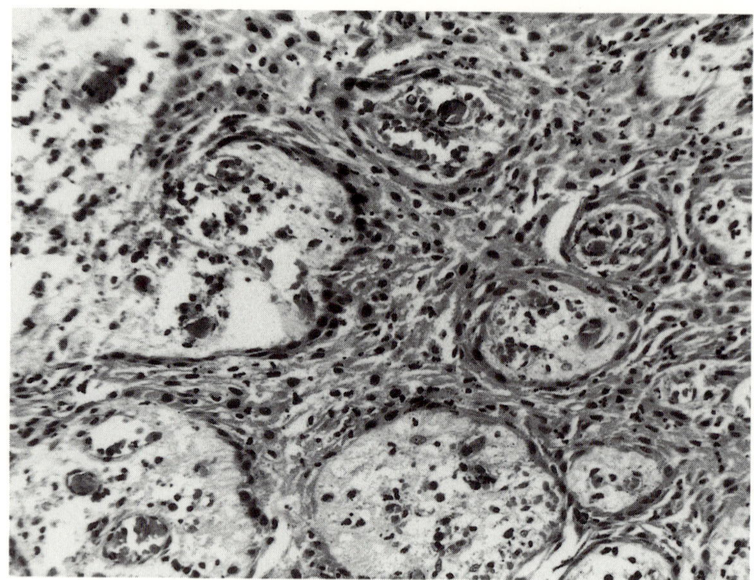

Figure 11.6. Arcades and rings of proliferating epithelium in an apical granuloma. (H & E; × 190.)

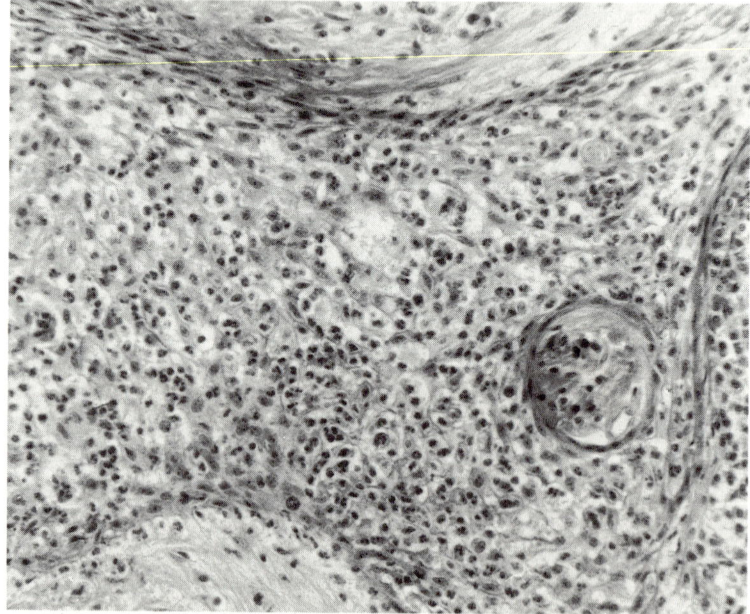

Figure 11.7. Degeneration of cells in the centre of a mass of proliferating epithelium in an apical granuloma. There is an intense infiltration of lymphocytes and polymorphonuclear leucocytes. Accumulations of intercellular fluid coalesce to form a microcyst. (H & E; × 175.)

phosphatase activity in the central cells of apical granulomas (Grupe, Ten Cate and Zander, 1967) and in the exfoliating epithelial cells of radicular cysts (Lutz, Cimasoni and Held, 1965), and the fact that Summers (1972, 1974) found that weak proteolytic activity was present centrally within the proliferating epithelium of apical granulomas, suggest that these cells are undergoing autolysis. Ultrastructurally, the epithelial cells in apical granulomas adhere to each other by fewer desmosomes than in normal squamous epithelium (Summers and Papadimitriou, 1975) and evidence of death of the central cells has been demonstrated in experimentally induced granulomas (Ten Cate, 1972). Microcysts may increase in size by coalescence with adjacent microcysts and, once established, the cyst increases in size by mechanisms which will be discussed later. Established radicular cyst fluid showed no spontaneous proteolytic activity (Ylipaavalniemi and Tuompo, 1977). Activation of proteolysis with 3 M sodium thiocyanate suggested, however, that a proenzyme might be present.

In his histological study of experimentally induced radicular cysts in monkeys, Valderhaug (1972) did not, however, see evidence of intraepithelial degeneration with formation of microcysts. He did observe quite frequently, though, that the degenerated central area of an apical granuloma became surrounded by proliferating epithelial cells.

In some periapical lesions, sheets of epithelial cells with distinct clefts are seen (Shear, 1963a) and in certain instances the cyst may be initiated in this way (**Figure 11.8**). Torabinejad (1983) has postulated, however, that it is not the lack of blood supply which accounts for the death of the central epithelial cells in an apical lesion, but that the development of the cavities in proliferating epithelium and the final destruction of these cells are mediated by immunological reactions. He suggested different ways in which activated epithelial cell nests can acquire antigenic

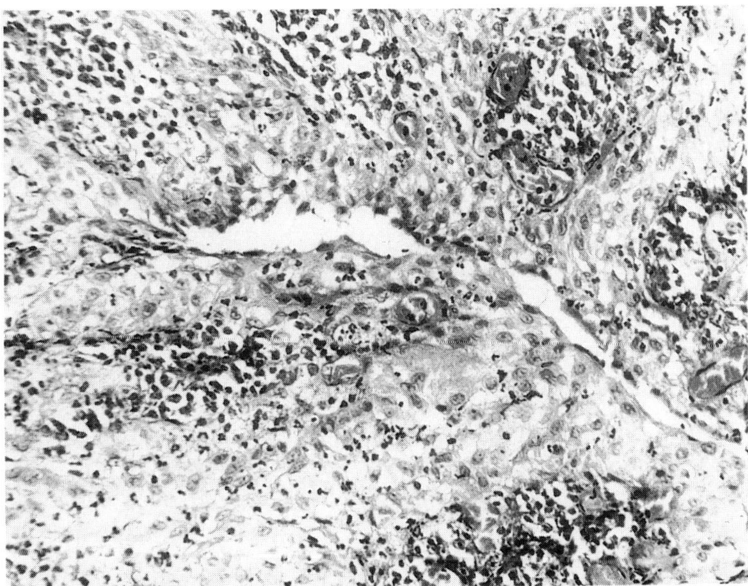

Figure 11.8. Sheet of epithelial cells in a periapical lesion. A distinct cleft has formed and this may initiate a radicular cyst. (H & E; × 215)

properties, but did not explain why the central and not the peripheral proliferating cells are targeted in this manner. Nevertheless, the participation of immunological processes in the breakdown of proliferating epithelium must be given serious consideration. However, despite the extensive immunological studies that have been done on the development of the periapical granuloma which have been described earlier in this chapter, relatively sparse attention has been given to the role of immune processes in the proliferation and central disintegration of the epithelium.

The third phase in the pathogenesis of the radicular cyst, its enlargement, has been the focus of considerable experimental work. Toller's studies provided evidence for the hypothesis that osmosis makes a contribution to the increase in the size of cysts. He showed (1970b) that the mean osmolality of the fluid from 21 apical and residual cysts was 290 ± 14.93 mosmol compared with a mean serum osmolality of 279 ± 4.68 mosmol. This difference is statistically significant ($P < 0.01$). Lytic products of the epithelial and inflammatory cells in the cyst cavity provide the greater numbers of smaller molecules which raise the osmotic pressure of the cyst fluid. Toller believed that the upper limit of permeability in most cysts is close to the molecular size of albumin, molecular weight 69 000, and that particles of larger size would find difficulty in diffusing across a cyst lining. Toller's *in vivo* dialysis experiments (1966b) using a radioactive crystalloid and a radioactive colloid showed that the diffusion rate of the crystalloid was fairly rapid in every case but that the colloid tended to be retained, whether subsequent histological examination revealed that the cyst wall was entirely lined by epithelium or not. This tended to confirm that cyst walls have the properties of a semipermeable membrane.

Electrophoretic studies (Toller, 1970a) demonstrated that radicular cyst fluids contain fewer, if any, of the larger protein molecules than the patients' own sera. Alpha-globulins were greatly diminished. Gamma-globulin varied greatly in quantity but in cysts which were not inflamed was present in small concentration. The small molecular sized albumin, and beta-1-globulin, were present in quantities comparable with serum but beta-2-globulin was usually absent. This suggested that these cyst fluids were simple dialysates from plasma through the cyst membranes which discriminate against the larger molecules. Skaug (1977) disagreed with this view. His studies on fluids from non-keratinizing cysts showed electrophoretic patterns which strongly indicated that serum-derived immunoglobulins were also present. Skaug did not, however, distinguish the radicular from the other non-keratinizing cysts. Koskimies, Ylipaavalniemi and Tuompo (1975) and Ylipaavalniemi, Tuompo and Koskimies (1976) have, nonetheless, shown that the protein patterns of radicular cyst fluids resemble those of serum. They were similar to those of dentigerous cysts, but keratocysts and residual cysts had considerably fewer protein zones than plasma.

Electrophoretic studies of the fluids of radicular and other non-keratinizing cysts have shown that more than half display levels of gamma-globulin much higher than the patient's own serum (Toller and Holborow, 1969; Toller, 1970a). In 19 cyst fluids in which levels of IgG, IgA and IgM were measured independently, all three were significantly raised in most of the non-keratinizing cysts. Immunofluorescent staining showed that lymphoid cell aggregates in the walls of radicular cysts often include numerous immunoglobulin-containing cells of the plasma cell series, many of them producing IgG, IgA or IgM, but IgA-staining cells were predominant. Pulver, Taubman and Smith (1978) have confirmed that there are larger numbers of IgA-containing cells in radicular cyst walls compared with periapical granulomas. While finding the potential role of IgA difficult to explain in this site, they pointed out that IgA-synthesizing plasma cells are the predominant Ig-containing cells in the lamina propria of the intestinal tract and bronchial and nasal mucosa where they presumably represent an immune response to multiple antigenic stimuli, chiefly microorganisms. These authors also found only traces of complement C3 in the cyst walls and suggested that this might have been consumed during the formation of antigen–antibody complexes.

The immunoglobulin-producing cells appear to be actively mobile and even capable of penetrating several layers of intact epithelial cells, thereby entering the cyst cavities. Sakuma (1973), Skaug (1974) and Ylipaavalniemi, Tuompo and Calonius (1976) supported the view that the gamma-globulins are of local origin and contribute to the protein levels of cyst fluids. Toller believed that this evidence suggests that there is an antigenic stimulus in the cyst wall and in the absence of demonstrable infection either the occult epithelium or its breakdown products are antigenic. This, he suggested, may be the mechanism whereby cysts undergo spontaneous regression. Those people who have a particular tendency to develop cysts may have an ineffective immunological surveillance and suppression mechanism. The question of regression of radicular cysts is discussed further in the chapter on their treatment.

Toller (1966b) also proposed the hypothesis that the contents of cyst cavities are subject to an osmotic imbalance with the surrounding tissues because of the absence of lymphatic drainage. He demonstrated this absence of lymphatic drainage by evacuating cyst cavities and refilling them with an aqueous solution of patent blue dye. At operation from 3 to 24 hours later, he was unable to detect any dye outside the cyst cavity. Neither the patients nor their urine were discoloured.

Main (1970b), however, felt that the retention of colloid in Toller's experiment may have resulted from a reduced internal hydrostatic pressure following aspiration of the fluid contents. He estimated the protein concentrations of cyst fluids by means of specific gravity and concluded that the radicular cyst fluid is essentially an inflammatory exudate. Skaug (1973, 1976a, 1977) confirmed that fluid from non-keratinizing jaw cysts contains high concentrations of protein but supported the view that accumulation of cyst fluid results essentially from inadequate lymphatic drainage of the cyst cavity. He suggested that plasma protein exudate and hyaluronic acid, as well as the products of cell breakdown, contribute to the high osmotic pressure of the cyst fluid. Ylipaavalniemi (1977) proposed that when the inflammation ceases a balance is probably established between the protein concentrations in cyst fluid and in serum.

Skaug (1974, 1977) has also commented on the question of permeability of cyst walls. He pointed out that the cyst capsule was not directly comparable with the biological membranes like capillary walls or cell membranes because of the many layers of cells of diverse function. These were the vascular endothelium, basement membranes, ground substance and cyst wall epithelium. The view that the cyst wall functions as a simple semipermeable membrane is therefore probably an oversimplification. It may nevertheless still be preferable to use the term permeability in connection with the passage of substances into or away from the cyst cavity.

Skaug found that the concentration of non-immunoglobulin plasma proteins in cyst fluids was proportional to their concentration in plasma and, as Toller did, that these were in inverse proportion to their molecular weights. The demonstration in cyst fluid of appreciable amounts of high molecular weight proteins suggested that the vascular permeability of cyst capsules was increased compared with the permeability of normal capillaries but there is nevertheless still a considerable restriction to free diffusion of plasma protein across the cyst capsule. Suzuki (1975) also demonstrated that there is an active transport mechanism for Na^+ and K^+ ions across the cyst wall and that there was a selective mechanism for the transfer of protein.

Toller (1948) showed that the internal hydrostatic pressures in 51 radicular cysts ranged from 56.6 to 95.0 cm H_2O with a mean of 70.0 cm. This figure is higher than that of capillary blood pressure and as the cyst expands there is resorption of the surrounding bone. Skaug (1976a) conducted similar experiments using a pressure transducer and either cannulation of the cyst cavity or cementing a two-way valve into a tooth which communicated through its root canal with a cyst. With a sample of 14 radicular cysts he found that the initial intracystic pressures ranged from 25 to 66 with a mean and SD of 47 ± 14.5 mmHg. In three cases in which pressure measurements were repeated 7–14 days after aspiration of cyst fluid, intracystic pressures in the same range as those originally recorded were found. This indicated that more fluid filters into the cyst cavity than is removed by the venous and lymphatic channels. The direction and the rate of fluid flow are determined by the balance of the differences in hydrostatic and osmotic pressures between cyst fluid and plasma (Skaug, 1976a).

Harris and Goldhaber (1973) have demonstrated that small fragments of vital cyst tissue produced resorption of mouse calvarium in tissue culture, whereas control tissue devitalized by rapid freezing and thawing failed to resorb bone. They postulated that intraosseous cyst expansion is facilitated by local enzyme or hormone-induced bone resorption and suggested that the active principle is a prostaglandin. In subsequent publications (Harris *et al.*, 1973; Harris, 1978) it was shown that cyst walls did release prostaglandin-like material in tissue culture. The synthesis of prostaglandins, their bone resorbing capacity and their possible role in the enlargement of jaw cysts is now well established in further experimental work (Matejka *et al.*, 1985a and b; Meghji, Harvey and Harris, 1989) and is described in Chapter 5 p. 84. In a detailed investigation of lipids in cyst walls and fluids, Suzuki (1984) suggested that jaw cyst enlargement is related to lipoperoxide and prostaglandin-like substances produced by lipid peroxidation of the cyst wall and fluid. In a study on the walls of radicular cysts, Matejka *et al.* (1986) showed by immunohistochemistry and radio thin layer chromatography, that PGE_2 is produced predominantly by plasma cells and histiocytic elements as well as endothelial cells and fibroblasts. Epithelial cells and granulocytes gave minimal positive staining, and lymphocytes gave a variable weak reaction to anti-PGE_2. On the other hand, 6-oxo-$PGF_{1\alpha}$ (the stable biologically inactive metabolite of PGI_2 – prostacyclin) was primarily found to be generated by endothelial cells and fibroblasts. The negative reaction of the cyst epithelium to both antibodies indicated that the granulation tissue and the inflammatory cells are the main source of prostaglandin synthesis in the walls of radicular cysts and may therefore be responsible for the resultant osteolytic activity. The authors cautioned however, that it is not yet certain whether the *in vitro* phenomena observed are also of biological relevance *in vivo*.

The possible role of local fibrinolysis in the growth of jaw cysts is not clear. In the radicular cyst, inflammatory episodes contribute to the activation of local fibrinolysis whereas with the ameloblastoma, the tumour tissue itself has the capacity to induce locally activated plasmin (Sugimura *et al.*, 1976). These facts do not, in themselves, indicate a role for fibrinolysis in cyst enlargement. Collagenolytic activity has been demonstrated in homogenates of radicular cyst walls and it has been suggested that this might influence their expansion (Uitto and Ylipaavalniemi, 1977).

Reference has been made in earlier chapters of this book to a series of papers on glycosaminoglycans which are present in the walls and fluids of odontogenic cysts (Smith, Smith and Browne, 1984, 1988a and b; Smith, Smith and Basu, 1989). These substances are derived from several sources in the cyst wall and diffuse into the cyst fluid where they probably contribute to the expansile growth of the cyst.

There do not appear to be data on the rate of radicular cyst growth although it has been estimated at approximately 5 mm in diameter annually (Livingston, 1927). They tend to expand progressively and if untreated may grow to a large size. The larger the cyst, however, the slower its relative increase in size.

Epithelial proliferation continues as long as there is an inflammatory stimulus, and Harris and Toller (1975) suggested that this contributes to enlargement of the cyst. When the stimulus to epithelial proliferation ceases, a situation which often occurs in a residual cyst, the epithelium is able to differentiate to a certain extent (**Figure 11.10**), although keratinization is very rare. Further increase in the capacity of the cyst cavity at this stage probably leads to thinning of the epithelial lining.

Studies in the experimental production of radicular cysts have been published by Valderhaug (1972, 1974) and Binnie and Rowe (1974). The latter authors studied 192 roots of immature pulpless teeth in eight young beagle dogs. The pulps had been filled with various materials. Epithelial cell nests were observed in 49 roots and proliferating epithelium in 14. Nine periapical cysts were found in four dogs. There was considerable variation between different dogs and this may reinforce the concept of individual susceptibility to the development of radicular cysts. In one dog, only one root showed epithelium, but in another there was epithelium associated with 19 of the 24 roots examined and four of these had formed cysts. All epithelial proliferations and cysts were associated with mild or severe periapical inflammation but their frequency was not related to the filling material used. An interesting feature of this study was the finding that epithelial remnants were present in only 37 per cent of specimens. If a similar situation obtains in humans, this alone may explain the existence of cyst-prone and non-cyst-prone individuals.

Valderhaug (1974) induced periapical inflammation in monkey primary teeth by removing the pulp tissue and leaving the root canals open to the oral cavity. About one-third of the experimental teeth developed periapical abscesses, granulomas and cysts without communication with the oral cavity. Proliferating epithelium was not observed in association with abscess formation. Many of the granulomas, however, contained islands and strands of proliferating epithelial cells. Small periapical cysts developed in some animals after long observation periods and these were lined by stratified squamous epithelium. ^{3}H thymidine was incorporated into the epithelial linings of the cysts and into the epithelium of the granulomas in inflamed areas. Uptake by epithelium could not be demonstrated at a certain distance from the inflammation nor on the control side.

Pathological features

The gross specimens may be spherical or ovoid intact cystic masses, but often they are irregular and collapsed. The walls vary from extremely thin to a thickness of about 5 mm. The inner surface may be smooth or corrugated. Yellow mural nodules of cholesterol may project into the cavity. The fluid contents are usually brown from the breakdown of blood and when cholesterol crystals are present they impart a shimmering gold or straw colour.

Almost all radicular cysts are lined wholly or in part by stratified squamous epithelium. These linings may be discontinuous in part and range in thickness from one to 50 cell layers. The majority are between six and 20 cell layers thick. The epithelial linings may be proliferating and show arcading with an intense associated inflammatory process (**Figure 11.9**) or be quiescent and fairly regular with a certain degree of differentiation (**Figure 11.10**). The inflammatory cell infiltrate in the proliferating epithelial linings consists predominantly of polymorphonuclear leucocytes whereas the adjacent fibrous capsule is infiltrated mainly by chronic inflammatory cells (Shear, 1963a; 1964; Cohen, 1979; Johannessen, Nilsen and Skaug, 1983; Johannessen, 1986). These proliferating epithelial linings show a considerable degree of spongiosis. When observed in the scanning electron microscope it is seen that the spongiotic spaces represent channels running between the epithelial cells and extend from the basal layer to the cyst lumen (Cohen, 1979). The polymorphonuclear leucocytes migrate along these channels and into the cyst cavity through interepithelial spaces on the luminal surface. Interepithelial spaces and channels in the cyst linings have also been demonstrated by means of transmission electron microscopy (Frithiof and Hägglund, 1966).

Orthokeratinized and parakeratinized linings are very rarely seen in radicular cysts. When they do occur, they are quite different morphologically from those seen in keratocysts (see **Figure 2.1**).

Secretory characteristics, in the form of mucous cells or ciliated cells, are frequently found in the epithelial linings (Shear, 1960b; Browne, 1972). Mucous cells occurred in as many as 40 per cent of Browne's series of radicular cysts. They

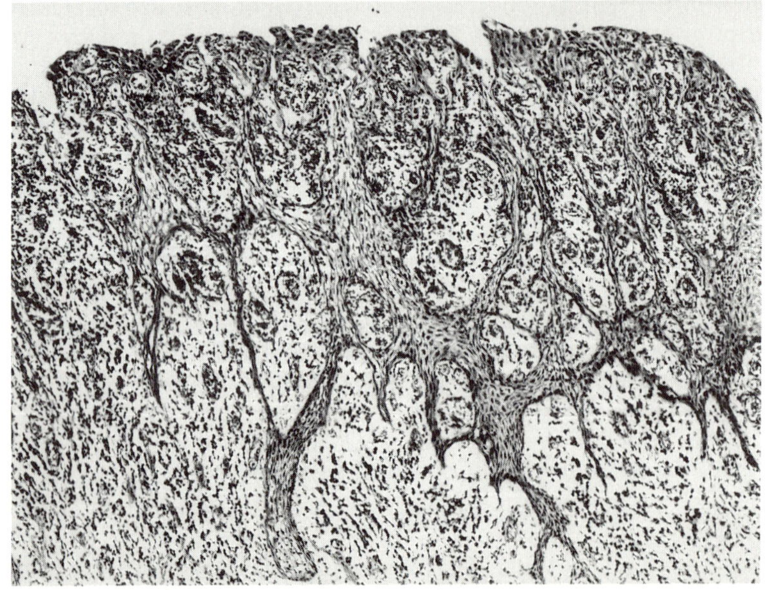

Figure 11.9. Proliferating epithelium lining a radicular cyst. (H & E; × 80.)

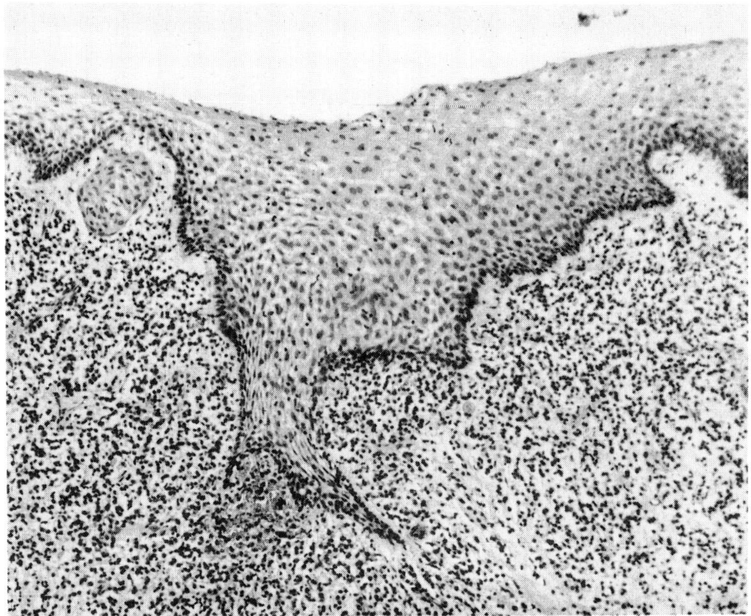

Figure 11.10. Quiescent epithelium lining a radicular cyst. (H & E; × 110.)

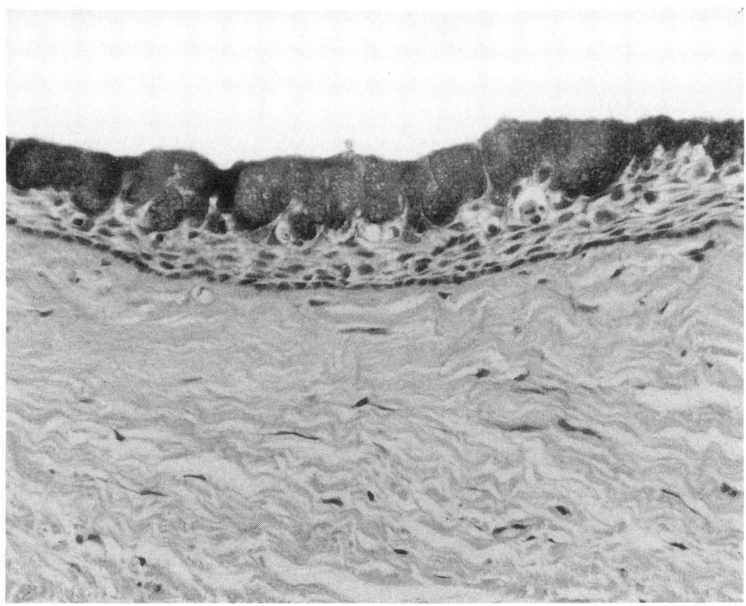

Figure 11.11. Mucous cells in the surface layer of the stratified squamous epithelial lining of a radicular cyst. (PAS-H; × 250.)

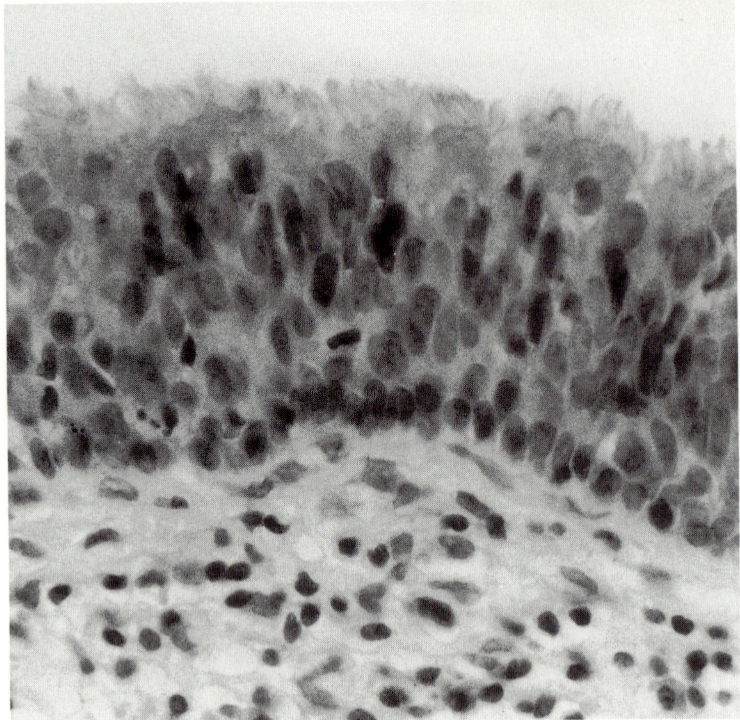

Figure 11.12. Ciliated epithelium in a radicular cyst. (H & E; × 640.)

may be present in the surface layer of a stratified squamous epithelial lining, either as a continuous row (**Figure 11.11**) or as scattered cells; and they may be found associated with ciliated epithelium (**Figure 11.12**). They are found in cysts occurring in all parts of the mandible and maxilla. Browne made the interesting observation that there is an increasing frequency of mucous cells with age, at the rate of 7 per cent per decade.

Most of the cases in which ciliated epithelium is found occur in the maxilla, but ciliated epithelium has been found in cysts in the anterior and posterior regions of the mandible. The presence of secretory epithelium in radicular cysts, particularly those in the mandible, is probably the result of metaplasia. Some cyst linings with these characteristics show features similar to those described by Fell (1957) in the process of metaplasia from stratified squamous to ciliated epithelium in explants of chick embryo skin grown under the influence of excess vitamin A.

Fujiwara and Watanabe (1988) reported an ultrastructural study of mucous cells and ciliated epithelium in a mandibular radicular cyst. These cells were indistinguishable from those found in the maxillary sinus or nasal cavity. In addition however, they commented on the presence of abnormal cilia belonging to the primary cilia group which have been documented in a variety of non-neoplastic and neoplastic tissues. The mechanism by which they are produced is obscure and the authors were unable to explain their significance in this radicular cyst.

In approximately 10 per cent of radicular cysts, hyaline bodies, first described by Dewey in 1918 and often referred to as Rushton's hyaline bodies, are found in the

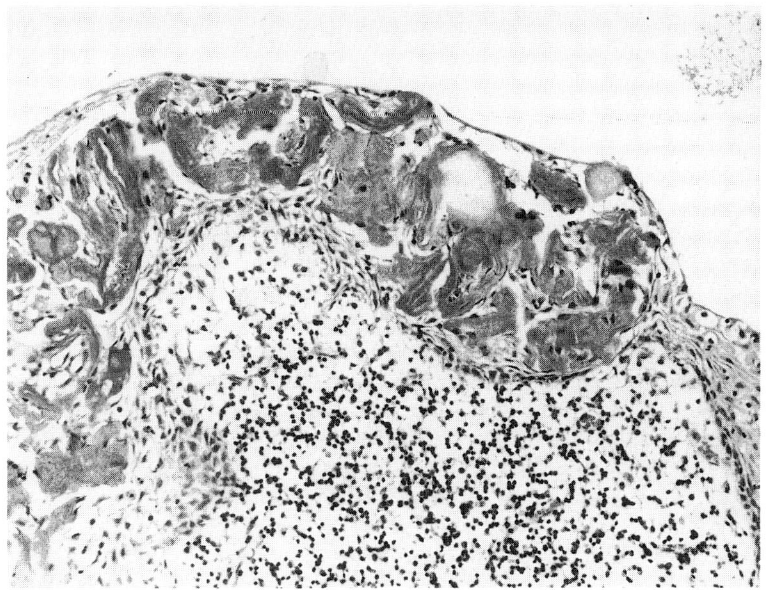

Figure 11.13. Hyaline and granular bodies in the epithelial lining of a radicular cyst. (H & E; × 140.)

epithelial linings (**Figure 11.13**). Only very rarely are they present in the fibrous capsule. The bodies measure up to about 0.1 mm and are linear, straight or curved or of hair-pin shape and sometimes they are concentrically laminated. They are brittle and frequently fracture. Circular or polycyclic bodies are also seen with a clear outer layer surrounding a central granular body.

Rushton (1955) believed that the hyaline bodies resembled, in appearance and the liability to fracture, the keratinized secondary enamel cuticle of Gottlieb. My own histochemical studies (Shear, 1961b) indicated that they contained cystine and I suggested that they were of odontogenic epithelial origin and probably a form of keratin. Wertheimer, Fullmer and Hansen (1962) and Wertheimer (1966) also found histochemical similarities to keratin but pointed out that the correspondence was not complete. They supported the view that the bodies were a secretory product of odontogenic epithelial cells formed in the same way as the secondary enamel cuticle, an opinion also held by Takeda (1985).

On the other hand Bouyssou and Guilhem (1965) and Sedano and Gorlin (1968) believed that hyaline bodies were of haematogenous origin; that they were derived from thrombi in venules of the connective tissue which have become varicose and strangled by epithelial cuffs which encircle them; and that they react histochemically as haemoglobin. They suggested that the thrombi shrink centrifugally and undergo splitting, or they may calcify. Dent and Wertheimer (1967) stated, however, that although hyaline bodies react to several haemoglobin and iron stains, the histochemical reactions for haemoglobin are not specific. I have found that hyaline bodies give a faint reaction with Pickworth's benzidine method for haemoglobin while a control of human erythrocytes stain intensely. Browne and Matthews (1985) stained cysts containing hyaline bodies for keratin, Factor VIII-related antigen, haemoglobin and fibrinogen, using immunoperoxidase methods. The hyaline bodies were negative for all these antigens but fibrinogen was detected in the cores of some circular and polycyclic forms. They concluded that their observations did not support the view that they are keratinous in nature, nor that they arise from erythrocytes or capillary endothelium, but they did tentatively propose that the presence of fibrinogen in the cores of some hyaline bodies could support the notion of a haematogenous origin of the granular bodies.

Although I agree that the circular or polycyclic forms are sometimes of a morphology which suggests that they are lying in a transversely sectioned blood vessel, there are some puzzling features about their distribution if they are of vascular and haematogenous origin. For one thing they are often seen in epithelium overlying connective tissue devoid of any blood vessels. For another, they are very rarely found in the fibrous capsules, and I have never seen them in this situation. Thirdly, if their pathogenesis is as described, it is most surprising that they occur so exceptionally rarely in other situations. As far as I am aware there is only one report of their occurrence in lesions other than jaw cysts. Takeda, Kikuchi and Suzuki (1985) have described their presence in a plexiform ameloblastoma. Furthermore, I have not seen them in nasopalatine duct cysts which are not of odontogenic origin.

Ultrastructural studies of the bodies (Allison, 1974; Jensen and Erickson, 1974; Morgan and Johnson, 1974) have been done on material recovered from paraffin blocks and from reserve tissue stored in formalin. The investigation of Morgan and Johnson failed to demonstrate any close relationships between the bodies and either red cells or blood vessels. They were also unable to demonstrate any cellular structures, or evidence of either cell stratification, desmosomes, or, except in one case, filamentous laminae. In this exceptional instance, they felt that there might be some similarity to the contents of poorly keratinizing epithelial cells. On the whole, however, they believed that their ultrastructural findings ruled out a keratinous origin. They were not able to exclude the possibility that the hyaline bodies represented a type of dental cuticle. Their conclusion was that the bodies are a secretory product of odontogenic epithelium deposited on the surface of particulate matter such as cell debris or cholesterol crystals in a manner analogous to the formation of dental cuticle on the unerupted portions of enamel surfaces. Later enzyme histochemical studies (Morgan and Heyden, 1975) lent support to this theory. Further studies by Allison (1977a, b), including microprobe and microradiographic analyses, also led him to the conclusion that hyaline bodies arise as an epithelial secretion. Additional support for the view that hyaline bodies are a product of the epithelium is provided by the immunohistochemical and scanning electron microscopic studies and X-ray microanalysis carried out by Rühl, Philippou and Mandelartz (1989) and Philippou, Rühl and Mandelartz (1990). By X-ray analysis, foreign material could be demonstrated in the cyst epithelium which could be macrophages, erythrocytes or degenerating epithelium. The authors suggested that this irritates the epithelial cells to produce a fine-grained matrix which encloses the coarse-grained foreign material and then undergoes different degrees of 'homogenization'. This they called the hyaline body Type II. The Type I hyaline body has no central granular component. Hyaline bodies Types I and II always consisted of a fine-grained substance which underwent 'homogenization' and consistently contained calcium and phosphate. Scanning electron microscopy showed that the hyaline bodies were more or less spherical structures consisting of concentrically laminated layers which on section resembled a cut onion. The surface of each layer had a fine-grained texture.

Jensen and Erickson (1974) ruled out the possibility that the bodies might be composed of keratin or the secondary enamel cuticle. Their observations were unable to support a haematogenous origin. El-Labban (1979) did her ultrastructural study of hyaline bodies on formalin-fixed and on one fresh osmium tetroxide-fixed specimen. Her findings provided no support for the hypothesis that the bodies are keratinous or that they form from epithelial secretory products. Her study indicated that the granular bodies are composed of amorphous material in which fragments of red blood cells could be seen. She concluded that the hyaline bodies were derived from degenerating red blood cells in which segregation of various components has occurred. She was not able to explain their almost exclusive occurrence in epithelium.

The presence of hyaline bodies may be suspected if, in examining the gross specimen, the pathologist sees small, smooth, white, dome-shaped swellings of the epithelial surface protruding into the cyst cavity.

Deposits of cholesterol crystals are found in many radicular cysts, but by no means in all (Shear, 1963b; Browne, 1971b; Trott and Esty, 1972). In my own series they were present in 28.5 per cent of cases, and in Trott and Esty's 30 per cent, whereas Browne reported a frequency of 43.5 per cent in his larger sample. It is likely, however, that if entire cyst linings were examined instead of random sections, the frequency would be higher. Browne has demonstrated a statistically significant correlation ($P < 0.01$) between the presence of cholesterol and haemosiderin. He postulated that the main source of cholesterol is that which is released from disintegrating red blood cells in a form which readily crystallizes in the tissues. Cholesterol from this source and also from serum accumulates in the tissues because of the relative inaccessibility of normal lymphatic drainage. Arwill and Heyden (1973) confirmed the origin from red blood cells. They showed that the crystals may form in congested capillaries in the inflamed areas as they appear to be enveloped by endothelial cells.

Trott, Chebib and Galindo (1973) supported the finding of a close correlation between the occurrence of cholesterol and haemosiderin-containing macrophages as well as free haemosiderin in the tissues. Their regression analysis showed, however, that only 35 per cent of the cholesterol may be formed from this association. They suggested that slow but considerable accumulation of cholesterol could occur through degeneration and disintegration of lymphocytes, plasma cells and macrophages taking part in the inflammatory process, with consequent release of cholesterol from their walls.

The possibility that circulating plasma lipids are a further source of cholesterol in cysts as they are in atherosclerosis must also be considered. A mechanism similar to that which is thought might occur in atheroma may operate (Shear, 1963b). Beta-lipoproteins in the plasma pass through the fragile thin-walled blood vessels in the inflamed portions of cyst wall in the same manner as the extravasating erythrocytes. There, the beta-lipoproteins split into cholesterol and its esters which are retained, and other lipid components such as phospholipids which are absorbed by the lymphatics. This view was supported by Skaug (1976b) who assayed cyst fluids for lipoproteins and cholesterol.

Once the cholesterol crystals have been deposited in the fibrous capsules of the cysts, they behave as foreign bodies and excite a foreign body giant-cell reaction (**Figure 11.14**). Arwill and Heyden (1973) suggested that these giant cells are derived from pericytes of the vessel wall. In histological sections the cholesterol crystals have been dissolved out and clefts are seen surrounded by dense

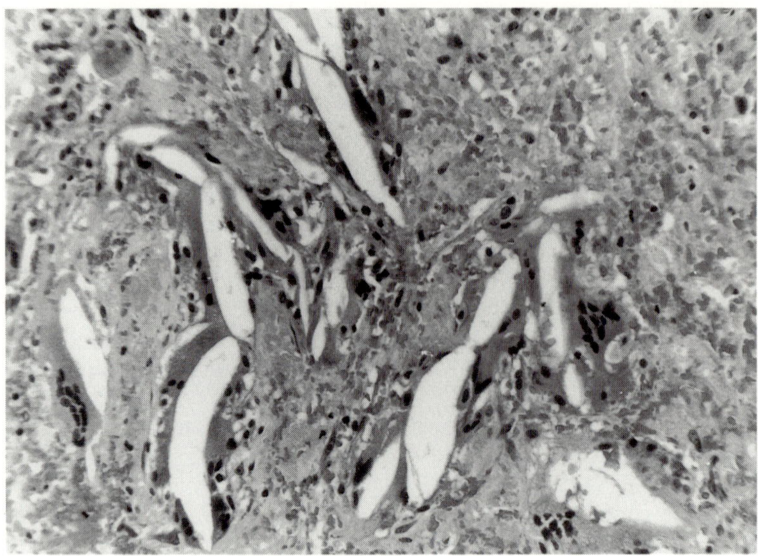

Figure 11.14. Multinucleate foreign body giant cells on the surface of cholesterol clefts in the wall of a radicular cyst. (H & E; × 200.)

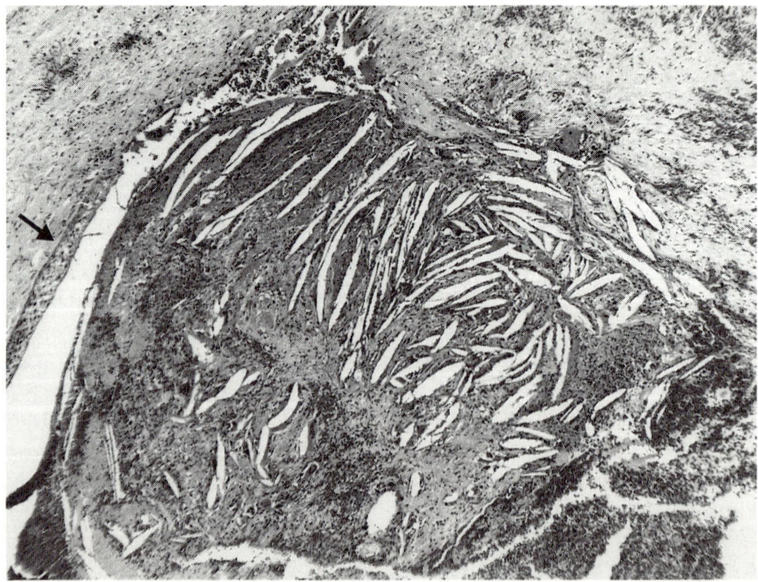

Figure 11.15. Mural nodule of cholesterol-containing granulation tissue fungating into the cavity of a radicular cyst. The epithelial lining of the cyst is indicated by an arrow. (H & E; × 40.)

aggregations of multinucleate giant cells. The cholesterol masses are extruded from the fibrous wall by the foreign body reaction. Invariably, the path of least resistance is into the cyst cavity as the external surface of the cyst may consist of dense fibrous tissue, bone and mucosa. When the reaction reaches the epithelial lining, this ulcerates. The granulation tissue containing the cholesterol fungates into the cyst cavity and appears macroscopically and microscopically as a 'mural nodule' (**Figure 11.15**). Once the entire mass has passed into the cavity the epithelial breach heals and the cholesterol crystals lie free in the cyst fluid (Shear, 1963b).

Buchner and David (1978) have demonstrated the presence of pigmented cells in the epithelial linings of a substantial proportion of radicular cysts. They identified these as macrophages containing the lipid pigment, ceroid. This, they thought, was derived in the same way as cholesterol, as part of the inflammatory process in the cyst wall.

In small periapical lesions a cavity may be present which is open to the root canal and is lined by epithelium. Simon (1980) has termed this a bay cyst.

A series of immunohistochemical investigations using monoclonal antibodies to study and compare the cytokeratin content and other antigens in the epithelial linings of odontogenic cysts, including radicular cysts, have recently been reported and are described in some detail in Chapters 2 and 5. Yamada *et al.* (1989) carried out an immunohistochemical investigation of the distribution of involucrin in radicular cysts. Involucrin is a 92 kD protein isolated from cultured human epidermal keratinocytes and synthesized in human squamous epithelial cells. It has been shown to be a useful histochemical marker for squamous cell differentiation. They showed that in proliferating epithelium lining radicular cysts, there was an irregular distribution of involucrin, whereas in the relatively well-differentiated epithelium in a quiescent cyst involucrin deposition was evenly distributed throughout the epithelium except for the basal layer.

The fibrous capsule of radicular cysts is composed mainly of condensed collagen peripherally and a loose connective tissue adjacent to the epithelial lining. A histochemical and immunohistochemical study using the Sirius red F3BA method and the avidin-biotin-peroxidase complex to detect Factor XIIIa in the fibrous cyst wall of radicular cysts was done by Toida *et al.* (1990). FXIIIa-containing interstitial cells increase in number in various human tissues associated with fibrosis. They demonstrated that the fibrous capsule of the radicular cyst was composed of three layers: an inner granulomatous layer, an outer fibrous connective tissue layer and an intermediate layer. FXIII was observed in certain connective tissue cells in all three layers. They were scanty in the inner layer where collagenous elements were also sparse but increased considerably in the moderately fibrous intermediate layer where they were dendritic or stellate-shaped. In the outer densely fibrous connective tissue layer, their numbers decreased slightly and were slender and spindle-shaped. These results suggested that FXIIIa-containing cells proliferate and differentiate prior to marked fibrosis and the authors proposed that these cells play an important part in the process of fibrosis in the radicular cyst wall.

Varying intensities of acute and chronic inflammatory cell infiltrate are present, particularly subepithelially. Acute inflammatory cells are seen particularly when the epithelium is proliferating. Usually, however, a chronic inflammatory cell infiltrate features in the fibrous capsule. Immunocytochemical studies on the walls of odontogenic cysts, including radicular cysts (Matthews and Browne, 1987), indicated that the cell populations are similar and consisted of HLA-Dr positive macrophage type cells and a mixture of T and B lymphocytes. An account, in greater detail, of the immunocytochemical work in this area is to be found in the earlier part of this chapter, in the section on the pathogenesis of the radicular cyst. Russell bodies are seen in about 50 per cent of cases.

Mast cells have been demonstrated (Mathiesen, 1973; Smith, Smith and Basu, 1989) in the epithelium and the connective tissue wall, particularly in the subepithelial zone. Reference has been made elsewhere in this book to their possible role in the pathogenesis of odontogenic cysts.

Remnants of odontogenic epithelium and occasional satellite microcysts may be found in the fibrous capsule and there have been reports of examples where epithelial proliferation is so extensive that it resembles squamous odontogenic tumour (Wright, 1979b; Simon and Jensen, 1985; Unal, Gomel and Gunel, 1987). The origin of this epithelium is almost certainly the cell rests of Malassez. When found in the wall of a dentigerous cyst, as has also been described (Wright, 1979b) or in the wall of a keratocyst (Hodgkinson *et al.*, 1978) the origin is likely to be cell rests of Serres. All writers on the subject are agreed that the treatment is that of the cyst of origin and that no subsequent therapy is required if this observation is made during histological examination of the cyst wall.

George, Gould and Behr (1984) described intraneural epithelial islands in the peripheral zone of the connective tissue capsule of a radicular cyst in the anterior maxilla.

Some cyst walls are markedly vascular. Haemorrhage is invariably present and haemosiderin deposits are seen in many specimens (Shear, 1963c).

Calcifications of various kinds are frequently present, and are a particular feature of residual radicular cysts which have been present for a long time (High and Hirschmann, 1986). Amorphous calcifications and trabeculae of woven bone occur most commonly and occasionally lamellar bone is found.

Frithiof and Hägglund (1966) examined 12 radicular cysts ultrastructurally. They found wide structural variations between specimens probably ascribable to differences in the degree of inflammation. In their ultrastructural study, Hansen and Kobayasi (1970a) found that the epithelium did not show the regular stratification usually seen in squamous epithelium. They described the presence of 'dark' and 'bright' cells. The dark cells they regarded as undergoing autolysis as they have a dense osmiophilic cytoplasm with indistinguishable organelles and they contain fat droplets, vacuoles and annular structures. Their nucleoplasm is dense and there are clumped chromatin masses. These cells also have poorly developed intercellular connections. The bright cells, on the other hand, have more distinct organelles, numerous mitochondria, ribosomes, granular endoplasmic reticulum and lysosomes, and are probably actively functioning cells.

Scanning electron microscopic observations on the inner surface of radicular cysts (Hurlen and Olsen, 1985) showed that sometimes the surface epithelium was fairly smooth with shallow foldings and ridges, and sometimes irregular and ruffled. Interepithelial spaces were seen in nearly all specimens. These were irregular in size and outline, and leucocytes could be seen penetrating them and lying on the surface of the epithelium, as were red blood cells in varying amounts. Four different types of crystal were seen, including cholesterol.

A microbiological study of the fluids of infected jaw cysts, predominantly radicular and residual, was reported by Iatrou *et al.*(1988), but the authors did not distinguish between cysts of different types in reporting their results. Gram-positive anaerobic cocci were the most frequent bacterial group, followed by Gram-negative anaerobic rods and Gram-positive aerobic cocci. Antibiotic sensitivity tests on the isolated organisms showed that the anaerobic cocci were most sensitive to chloramphenicol and minocycline, while all anaerobic rods tested were sensitive to metronidazole.

Carcinomatous change

A few well-documented cases have been reported which indicate that squamous carcinoma may occasionally arise from the epithelial lining of radicular and other odontogenic cysts. One such case, arising in a residual radicular cyst, was reported by Kay and Kramer (1962) while the case of Ward and Cohen (1963) appears from their published photomicrograph, to have originated in a keratocyst. Examples occurring in a radicular and in a dentigerous cyst were illustrated by Pindborg and Hjørting-Hansen (1974). Eversole, Sabes and Rovin (1975) reviewed series of cases of central epidermoid carcinoma and central mucoepidermoid carcinoma of the jaws. They found that 75 per cent of the former were associated with a cyst lining and 48 per cent of the latter were associated with either a cyst or an impacted tooth. An extensive review of the literature on the subject was published by Gardner (1969). He examined the evidence presented with each of 63 cases reported during the period 1889–1967 and concluded that 25 of these fulfilled the criteria for origin of squamous carcinoma from odontogenic cyst lining epithelium. Van der Waal *et al.* (1985) reported five cases of squamous carcinoma arising in odontogenic cysts: three residual, one keratocyst and one dentigerous cyst. Pearcey (1985) documented two cases treated with radiotherapy and suggested that such treatment might be an acceptable alternative to wide surgical resection.

Before the diagnosis of carcinoma arising from a cyst lining can be established, a number of alternative possibilities must be excluded (Kay and Kramer, 1962). It is possible that cyst and neoplasm may have developed independently adjacent to one another and ultimately fused in some parts. Careful questioning of the patient and clinical examination are necessary to exclude the possibility that the neoplasm arose primarily from the oral mucosa, or that it is a metastatic deposit in the jaw. A further possibility to be considered is that the lesion was initially an epithelial neoplasm which underwent secondary cystic change. Histological evidence of transition from a cyst lining through epithelial dysplasia to infiltrating squamous carcinoma provides acceptable proof (see **Figures 2.18**, **2.19**, **2.20** pp. 34, 35).

Despite the undoubted examples which occur from time to time, the frequency of neoplastic change is exceptionally rare in relation to the large numbers of cysts which are seen. Browne and Gough (1972) have suggested that keratin metaplasia in long-standing radicular and dentigerous cysts may precede carcinomatous transformation and examples of epithelial dysplasia are occasionally seen in jaw cysts without any evidence of carcinomatous transformation. There is no evidence however, that cyst epithelium is at particular risk and there is therefore no justification for regarding cysts as precancerous lesions.

Treatment

A detailed account of the treatment of radicular cysts is given in Chapter 18. I should like to give here, however, a pathologist's view on the question of the non-surgical treatment of these lesions

Oehlers (1970) believed that many periapical lesions left *in situ*, including cysts, are eliminated by the body once the causative agents are removed. This view was supported by Bhaskar (1972) who suggested that the vast majority of radicular cysts undergo resolution following conservative endodontic therapy. His hypothesis was based on endodontists' claims that 85–90 per cent of apical lesions disappear or become markedly reduced in size following conservative endodontic procedures. As available statistics indicate that 40–50 per cent of all apical lesions are radicular cysts and as it is difficult to distinguish between apical granulomas and radicular cysts on radiographs alone, Bhaskar concluded that the majority of radicular cysts can undergo resolution following root canal therapy and do not require surgical intervention. He suggested that during the endodontic procedure, instrumentation should be done slightly beyond the apical foramen. This produces a transitory acute inflammation which may destroy the epithelial linings of the radicular cysts and convert them into granulomas, thus leading to their resolution.

I have some difficulty in accepting Bhaskar's argument. First, it is difficult to obtain an accurate assessment of the relative proportions of periapical granulomas and cysts, and other workers have reported a lower frequency of cysts than did Bhaskar (Morse, Patnik and Schacterle, 1973). Many periapical granulomas are not submitted for histological examination and their frequency in pathology department archival material is no reflection of their incidence. Pathologists differ in the criteria which they use for the diagnosis of a cyst. Some require the presence of an epithelial lining whereas it has been clearly demonstrated that epithelial discontinuations occur to a greater or lesser extent in a substantial proportion of radicular cysts (Toller, 1966a). The contention that destruction of cyst lining epithelium will lead to resolution of the cyst is therefore untenable. Production of a transitory acute inflammation may, on the contrary, merely stimulate epithelial proliferation. What may happen to a cyst when endodontic instrumentation is done beyond the periapical foramen is that it becomes temporarily decompressed through the reduction of intracystic pressure. Bone deposition outside the cyst would show radiologically as an apparent reduction in size of the lesion.

While good evidence exists that periapical granulomas respond well to non-surgical endodontic treatment, the case for non-surgical treatment of radicular cysts has yet to be established. Morse, Patnik and Schacterle (1973), Morse, Wolfson and Schacterle (1975) and Morse, Schacterle and Wolfson (1976) have suggested that it is possible to differentiate between periapical cysts and granulomas by chemical analysis on aspirates of root canal fluids. Fluids from patients with cysts showed an intense albumin pattern and definite patterns in the globulin zones on polyacrylamide gel electrophoresis. Fluids associated with periapical granulomas on the other hand showed only a faint to moderate pattern in the albumin zone. These studies have not been followed up by clinical assessments of cases treated following this diagnostic procedure.

A useful critical analysis of published work on the non-surgical treatment of cysts and granulomas has been presented by Natkin, Oswald and Carnes (1984) who are sceptical of the potential for success of this approach to the treatment of radicular cysts.

Paradental cyst

Reference has been made elsewhere in this chapter to the development of inflammatory cysts on the lateral aspect of a root as a consequence of an inflammatory process in a periodontal pocket. Such a lesion has been referred to as an inflammatory periodontal cyst or inflammatory collateral cyst (Main, 1970a, b; 1985) to distinguish it from a radicular cyst associated with a lateral accessory root canal of a non-vital tooth; and from a developmental lateral periodontal cyst.

Such cysts probably arise by proliferation of cell rests of Malassez in the lateral periodontium. The sequence of events leading to their formation is likely to be similar to that which occurs when the cell rests of Malassez in the apical region of the periodontium are stimulated to proliferate as a result of an inflammatory stimulus from a non-vital pulp.

What is surprising, therefore, is that inflammatory collateral cysts are relatively so rare. We have recorded only 13 cysts under this heading over a 32-year period. In view of the high frequency of chronic periodontitis, the occurrence of inflammatory collateral cysts is very much lower than one might expect. The explanation for this may be that drainage occurs more readily from the lateral periodontium closely associated with the gingival crevice, than from the apical periodontium. The antigenic stimuli and the environment may therefore not be conducive to cyst formation.

Craig (1976) has written a detailed account of a cyst of inflammatory origin but with a different pathogenesis, which occurs on the lateral aspect of the roots of partially erupted mandibular third molars where there is an associated history of

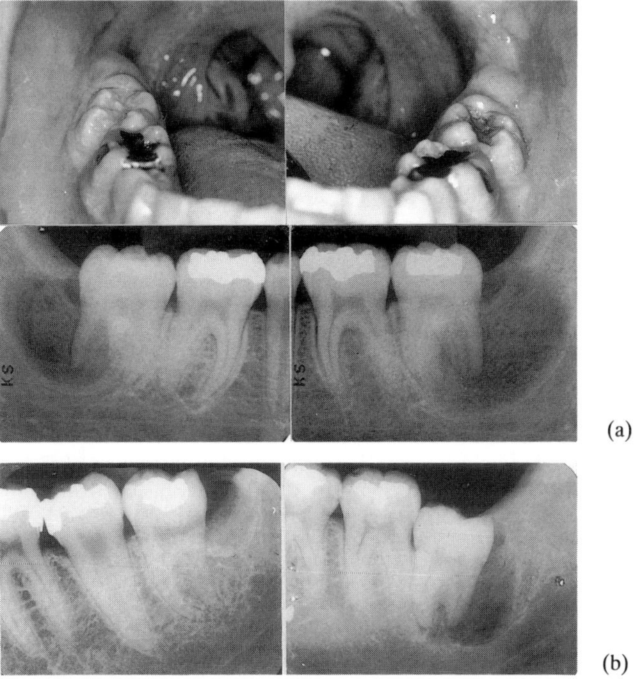

Figure 11.16 (a and b). Two cases of bilateral paradental cysts associated with erupting mandibular third molar teeth. The cysts are distal and buccal to the involved teeth. Note that the periodontal ligament space is not widened and that the distal part of the cyst is separate from the distinct distal follicular space. (By courtesy of Drs P. Vedtofte and F. Praetorius and C. V. Mosby Co. Previously published (1989) The inflammatory paradental cyst. *Oral Surg.* **68**, 182–188, Figs. 1 and 3.)

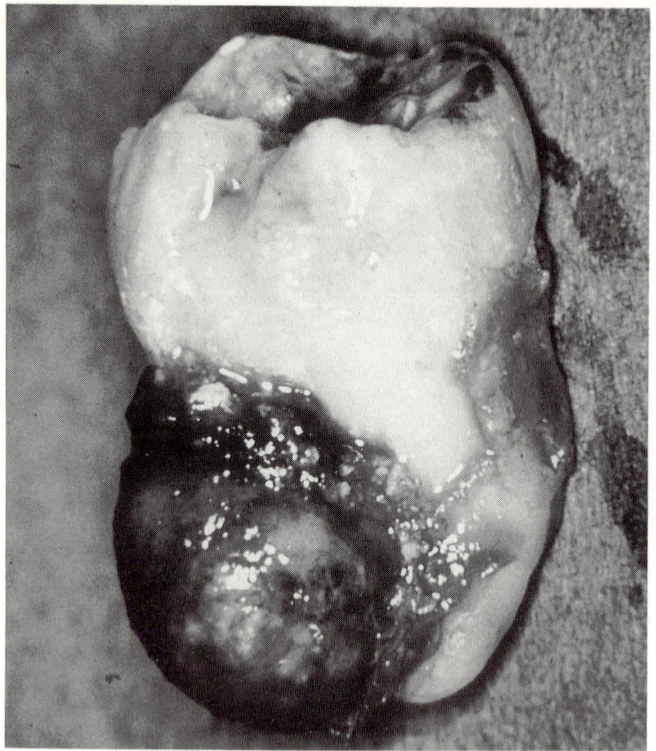

Figure 11.17. Gross specimen of a paradental cyst involving the distal and buccal surfaces of an impacted mandibular third molar tooth with pericoronitis.

pericoronitis (**Figures 11.16, 11.17**). He suggested that the term 'paradental cyst' was appropriate for this lesion.

His series consisted of 49 cases, which represented about 5 per cent of 1051 odontogenic cysts seen in his department over a 21-year period. Two-thirds of the cases occurred in patients in their third decade and there was a definite male preponderance (84 per cent). In all cases the involved tooth was associated with a history of pericoronitis. The teeth were vital. Radiologically a well-demarcated radiolucency occurred distal to the partially erupted tooth, but there was often buccal superimposition. The radiolucency sometimes extended apically but an intact periodontal ligament space provided the evidence that the lesion did not originate at the root apex (**Figure 11.16**).

Twenty-six cysts in Craig's series were located on the buccal aspect of the roots, 19 were distal and four were mesial. Craig was of the opinion, however, that there was some buccal involvement even in those cysts designated as of mesial or distal location. Macroscopically, the cysts on the buccal aspect of the roots covered the bifurcation and varied in size, some covering the entire buccal root surface (**Figure 11.17**). Of considerable interest is the fact that in 20 of 28 cases where the associated tooth was available for study, removal of the cyst from the buccal root surface revealed a developmental enamel projection extending from the amelocemental junction towards the root bifurcation.

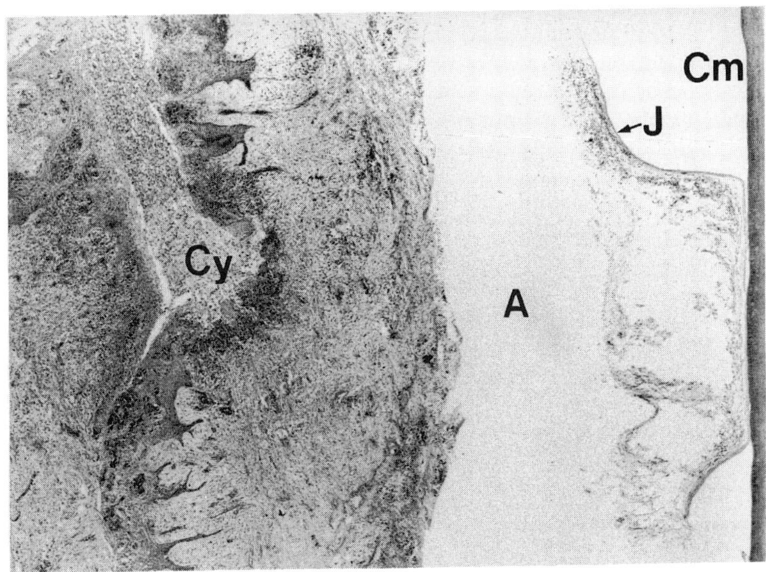

Figure 11.18. Paradental cyst [Cy] adjacent to the root of an impacted mandibular third molar. The cyst is lateral to the junctional epithelium [J] and hence does not appear to have arisen from reduced enamel epithelium. [A], separation artefact; [Cm], cementum. (H & E; × 35.)

Histologically, the cysts were lined by a hyperplastic, non-keratinized, stratified squamous epithelium. An intense inflammatory cell infiltrate is present associated with the hyperplastic epithelium and in the fibrous capsule adjacent to the epithelium (**Figure 11.18**)

It seems clear that the paradental cyst is of inflammatory origin and that it arises from odontogenic epithelium. Craig (1976) has suggested that either the cell rests of Malassez or the reduced enamel epithelium might provide the cells of origin. He favoured the latter source, arguing that in his study the rests of Malassez always appeared inactive and that if the Malassez rests were responsible the lesions should be equally distributed around the root surface. His serial sections indicated that the development of the paradental cyst may follow hyperplasia and cystic change in reduced enamel epithelium. He suggested that the presence of an extension of reduced enamel epithelium over the enamel projections might be the source, and could explain the frequent buccal location of the cyst.

Craig was of the opinion that the paradental cyst and the lesion described by Main (1970a, b) as an inflammatory collateral cyst are the same clinicopathological entity. In my opinion, however, even if rare, there appears to be a cyst which arises in the periodontium of an erupted tooth as a result of an inflammatory process in a periodontal pocket. Main's term 'inflammatory collateral cyst' is appropriate for such lesions.

Craig's paper on the paradental cyst was, for a number of years, the only detailed account of the entity. Recently, however, three substantial papers on the subject have appeared which corroborated Craig's observations (Ackermann, Cohen and Altini, 1987; Fowler and Brannon, 1989; Vedtofte and Praetorius, 1989). A lesion which is similar to the paradental cyst in many ways and may share the same aetiology and pathogenesis, has been described by Stoneman and Worth (1983) and named the mandibular infected buccal cyst. This lesion, however, affects predominantly the permanent first mandibular molar tooth in children and has sufficiently specific characteristics to warrant consideration as an entity. It will be given further attention later in this chapter.

Clinical features

Frequency

In the sample of 2616 jaw cysts in the archives of our department (**Table 2.1**), there were 65 paradental cysts classified over a 32-year period (2.5 per cent). The series of 50 cases of paradental cyst reported by Ackermann, Cohen and Altini (1987) represented 3 per cent of a sample of 1852 odontogenic cysts observed over a 20-year period. Vedtofte and Praetorius (1989) diagnosed 29 cases over a 5-year period.

Age

Virtually all the cases in the study by Ackermann, Cohen and Altini occurred between the ages of 10 and 39 with two-thirds of their sample in the third decade; the same as in Craig's material. Five of the six cases in the study of Fowler and Brannon affected patients in the third decade. Sixteen of 27 patients in the sample of Vedtofte and Praetorius occurred in patients in the first and second decades, but their material included 12 cases involving the first and second mandibular molars and represented their group of mandibular infected buccal cysts.

Sex

As in Craig's study, there was a considerable preponderance of males reported by Ackermann, Cohen and Altini and by Fowler and Brannon, whereas in the material of Vedtofte and Praetorius, there was an equal sex distribution.

Site

The cases of Ackermann, Cohen and Altini and Fowler and Brannon all involved the mandibular third molars and there was a history of pericoronitis in all of them. All the cases of Fowler and Brannon were attached to the buccal root surface and covered the bifurcation. In two of their cases there was an enamel spur at the bifurcation. Ackermann, Cohen and Altini found most of their cysts located distally and distobuccally and there were enamel spurs in two of eight teeth which were available for their retrospective study. All the papers emphasized that the involved teeth were vital. Bilateral examples occurred in a number of instances.

Radiological features

All authors reported a variable radiological picture but there are some features which appeared consistently and which seem to be useful in contributing to the diagnosis. These are that the periodontal ligament space was not widened and that the lesion was superimposed on the buccal root face. When there was a distal as well as a buccal radiolucency, the distal element was separate from the distinct distal follicular space. This is well illustrated in **Figure 11.16**.

Pathogenesis

There is not unanimity with regard to pathogenesis. Ackermann, Cohen and Altini, like Craig, favoured origin from reduced enamel epithelium but suggested that cyst formation occurs as a result of unilateral expansion of the dental follicle secondary to inflammatory destruction of periodontium and alveolar bone. This, they suggested, was different from the histogenesis of a dentigerous cyst where expansion of the follicle is the primary event with consequent bone destruction. In two of their cases they were able to demonstrate continuity of cyst lining with reduced enamel epithelium. While accepting that the paradental cyst was an entity, Fowler and Brannon suggested that it may be a variant of the dentigerous cyst or derived from an occluded periodontal pocket. Vedtofte and Praetorius were satisfied that the cyst was of inflammatory origin, initiated by a pericoronitis at the time of tooth eruption, and considered rests of Malassez and reduced enamel epithelium the most likely source of the cyst epithelium. It would seem as if there is some evidence to support origin from either rests of Malassez or reduced enamel epithelium. The case illustrated in **Figure 11.18** certainly seems to suggest that this particular cyst arose external to the junctional epithelium and is therefore unlikely to have originated in reduced enamel epithelium. Moreover, the histological resemblance of the paradental cyst to the radicular cyst argues in favour of origin from cell rests of Malassez. On the other hand, Ackermann, Cohen and Altini have demonstrated continuity of cyst lining with reduced enamel epithelium in two cases, and provided that they are not illustrating dentigerous cysts, such evidence must be taken seriously. What is required is a histological study of a substantial series of undoubted cases of paradental cysts sectioned in continuity with their teeth of origin.

Histological features

There is agreement that histologically, the paradental cyst is indistinguishable from the radicular cyst. It is lined by proliferating, non-keratinized, spongiotic stratified squamous epithelium of varying thickness. The fibrous capsule is the seat of an intense chronic or mixed inflammatory cell infiltrate (**Figure 11.18**).

Treatment

All authors agree that the lesion is treated by surgical enucleation and does not recur.

Mandibular infected buccal cyst

Reference has been made in the previous section to the lesion described by Stoneman and Worth (1983) as the 'mandibular infected buccal cyst'. This cyst has certain of the characteristics of the paradental cyst and is regarded by some workers to be a variety of it. However, it affects the permanent mandibular first and second molar teeth rather than the wisdom teeth, and a younger age group than the paradental cyst. Vedtofte and Praetorius (1989) who regarded the mandibular infected buccal cyst as a paradental cyst, argued that the age differences reflect the dates of eruption of the involved teeth. There is considerable evidence to support

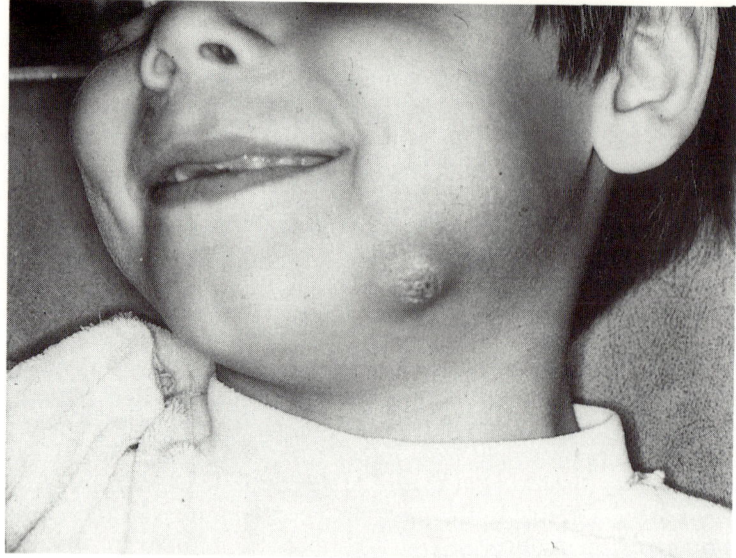

Figure 11.19. Young boy with mandibular infected buccal cyst involving newly erupted mandibular first permanent molar. Infection has extended through the bone and led to a facial abscess. (By courtesy of Dr D. W. Stoneman.)

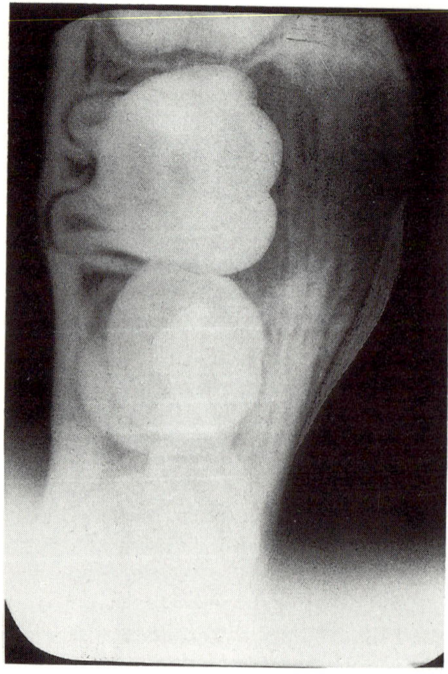

Figure 11.20. Occlusal view of mandibular infected buccal cyst. There is displacement and tilting of the right mandibular first molar tooth so that its apices lie close to the lingual margin. There is resorption of bone on the buccal aspect of the tooth and buccal expansion. Subperiosteal new bone has been deposited buccally, giving a laminated appearance. (By courtesy of Dr D. W. Stoneman and the Eastman Kodak Co. Previously published (1983) *Dent. Radiogr. Photogr.* **56**, 1–14, Fig. 12.)

the view that the two lesions represent different manifestations of the same disease process, both brought on by inflammation arising around the crowns of erupting teeth. However, the process in younger children, probably because of anatomical differences in the mandible, may be more extensive and present more severe clinical symptoms and signs (**Figure 11.19**), particularly when the first permanent molar is involved. For these reasons the lesion warrants its own designation, and is given separate consideration in this book.

Stoneman and Worth stated that the cyst may produce few or no clinical symptoms and minimal signs, but that there may be discomfort, pain, tenderness, painful occlusion and, rarely, suppuration (**Figure 11.19**). Swelling, particularly if inflamed, is the clinical feature most likely to induce the patient to seek advice. The diagnostic features are the young age of the patients, the mandibular molar site, the buccal periostitis, the usually vital pulp and the radiographic preservation of the continuity of the apical lamina dura. The cyst is always situated on the buccal surface of a mandibular molar, most frequently the first permanent molar, after partial or complete eruption. The associated tooth is usually tilted so that the apices are adjacent to the lingual cortex, a feature which is demonstrable in occlusal radiographs (**Figure 11.20**). The size of the cyst varies and may extend beyond the limits of the involved tooth and impinge upon and displace the crypt of the adjacent unerupted tooth.

The extension of the cyst in a buccal direction is variable, but frequently the outer bony cortex is lost. Facial swelling may follow and this may be inflamed. Rarely, an abscess forms and may point (**Figure 11.19**).

Radiological examination should include periapical, occlusal and panoramic views. With involvement of the periosteum new bone may be laid down, either as a single linear band or laminated if there are two or more layers (**Figure 11.20**).

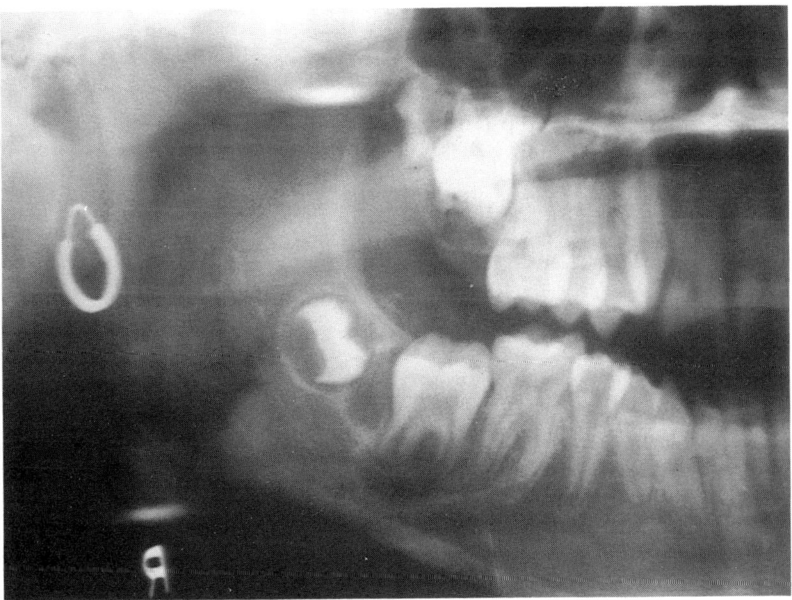

Figure 11.21. Mandibular infected buccal cyst involving erupting mandibular second permanent molar. (By courtesy of Dr D. W. Stoneman.)

Sometimes the new bone may be homogeneous. The cysts will be shown to lie on the buccal aspects of the affected molars. Usually there is involvement of the bone in the furcation and the entire interradicular bone may be lost. The inferior margin of the cyst is concave and rarely, the cyst may extend to the inferior border of the mandible but not leading to any external deformity (**Figure 11.21**).

Since the first report by Stoneman and Worth (1983), there have been a few publications, all of which confirm their original observations (Trask, Sheller and Morton, 1985; Camarda, Pham and Forest, 1989; Wolf and Hietanen, 1990; Packota *et al.*, 1990), although Packota *et al.* felt that these lesions were paradental cysts and that the use of the term mandibular infected buccal cyst should be discouraged. Neither the exclusively buccal location nor the selective involvement of the permanent mandibular molars have been adequately explained. As the affected teeth are not removed during treatment it has not been possible to establish whether the cysts were associated with enamel spurs at the bifurcation.

Treatment

It is generally agreed that enucleation of the cyst without removal of the associated tooth is the treatment of choice.

Chapter 12

Solitary bone cyst (traumatic, simple, haemorrhagic bone cyst)

The solitary bone cyst, which occurs in the mandible and very seldom in the maxilla, closely resembles and is probably identical to the solitary or unicameral bone cyst which is most frequently located in the metaphyses at the upper end of the humerus and the femur in children and adolescents.

Clinical features

Frequency

The solitary bone cyst is not a common lesion. We have had only 26 specimens in our departmental records during the 32-year period under review (1 per cent of jaw cysts), although other cases have been treated in the clinical departments of our hospital without any contents having been found for histological examination. There were 19 cases in the series of 3353 jaw cysts reported by Hoffmeister and Härle (1985), a frequency of 0.6 per cent. In view of the rarity of the lesion, the review published by Howe (1965) is most valuable. His material consisted of six of his own cases and 54 from the literature published over the period 1929–63. The well-documented series of 66 cases of Hansen, Sapone and Sproat (1974), the 23 cases of Killey, Kay and Seward (1977), the 30 examples in 26 patients of Beasley (1976), the review of 161 cases including 67 new cases reported by Kaugars and Cale (1987), as well as the reviews of Mayer, Libotte and Ruppol (1967), Huebner and Turlington (1971) and Braun (1975), all provide valuable data on the condition.

In determining which cases to include Howe used the following criteria. The cyst should be single, have no epithelial lining and show no evidence of acute or prolonged infection. It should contain principally fluid and not soft tissue and the walls should be of bone which is hard though possibly thin in parts.

Age

The simple bone cyst occurs in young individuals. The age distribution of the 60 patients included in Howe's analysis is shown in **Figure 12.1**. The patients ranged in age from 2½ to 35 years and 46 of the 60 (78 per cent) were in their second decade. Killey, Kay and Seward also recorded a peak frequency in the second decade, but one patient was over 50 and another over 60. In the series of Hansen, Sapone and Sproat the age range was 7–75 years and more than half were in the second decade.

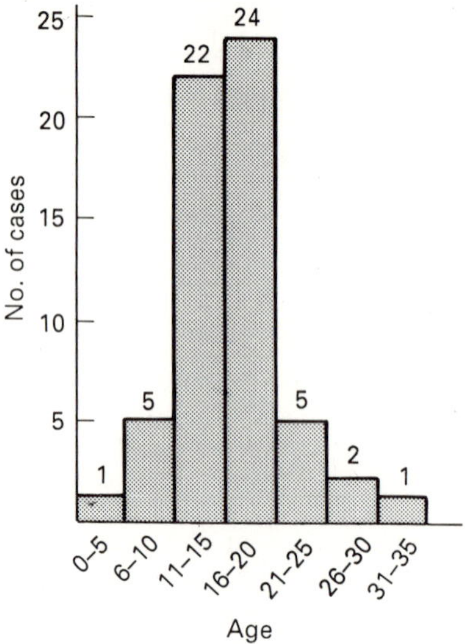

Figure 12.1. Age distribution of 60 patients with simple bone cysts of the jaws. (After Howe, 1965.)

In Beasley's study, 17 of 26 patients were in their second decade and 24 of them were younger than 40 years. The ages of the patients in the personal series of Kaugars and Cale ranged from 9–68 years with a mean age of 24.3 years.

Sex

Thirty-six cases in Howe's analysis were recorded in males and 23 in females, a male:female ratio of 1.6:1. Killey, Kay and Seward (1977), however, reported a frequency of 13 females and 10 males and there was an equal sex distribution in the series of Mayer, Libotte and Ruppol and Hansen, Sapone and Sproat. There were 16 males and 10 females in Beasley's sample from the Walter Reed Army Medical Center in Washington DC. In the most recent review done by Kaugars and Cale (1987), there was an equal sex distribution in both their literature survey and their own sample. They suggested however, that patients over 30 years were more likely to be black women.

Site

The overwhelming majority of solitary bone cysts of the jaws occur in the mandible and Howe stated that only one atypical case had been reported in the maxilla. This was confirmed by Mayer, Libotte and Ruppol. In the review of Kaugars and Cale 95 per cent of cases reported in the literature occurred in the mandible, as did all but one of their own 66 cases. In the report of Hansen, Sapone and Sproat (1974), however, about one-third occurred in the maxilla.

Almost all the maxillary cases have involved the anterior regions and the majority of the mandibular cases have been reported in the body and symphyseal area. Beasley (1976) described a number which occurred in the ramus as well as the body of the mandible. One of his cases involved the ascending ramus only, as did two examples described by Hosseini (1978–79), and one by Hall (1976). Cases reported by Persson (1985), Rubin and Murphy (1989) and Telfer *et al.* (1990) were found in the mandibular condyle. In the review of Kaugars and Cale, about one-fifth of their own and of reported cases occurred bilaterally and 10 patients in their literature review had multiple lesions. Five of these were either black or oriental women.

Clinical presentation

In Howe's survey, the majority of cases (60 per cent) were diagnosed fortuitously and almost all of these were chance radiographic findings. Swelling was the presenting symptom in 27 per cent, pain in 10 per cent, while 2 per cent complained of labial paraesthesia and in 2 per cent there were both pain and swelling. Over half the patients gave a history of significant trauma to the area and the time-lag between injury and diagnosis varied from 1 month to 20 years. Howe felt that trauma may play a role in at least some cases.

On clinical examination, 35 per cent had a mandibular swelling, most frequently buccal and labial, and only occasionally lingual. The related teeth were all vital in 67 per cent of cases. Of the 61 patients in the series reported by Hansen *et al.*, 44 (72 per cent) were completely symptomless and only eight reported definite symptoms. In Beasley's series, 77 per cent were symptomless and in only seven of his patients (27 per cent) was there a positive history of trauma. In the literature review of Kaugars and Cale 60 per cent of patients had symptoms, whereas in their own sample only 26 per cent did. There was a positive history of trauma in only six of their cases and they regarded the role of trauma in the development of the lesion as of minor importance.

Multiple lesions have been present in 11 per cent of reported cases (Kaugars and Cale, 1987).

Radiological features (Figure 12.2)

Careful interpretation of good radiographs is most valuable in the diagnosis. The cyst appears as a radiolucent area with an irregular but definite edge and slight cortication. An occlusal view shows the radiolucency extending along cancellous bone.

There is usually little effect on the buccal and lingual plates (Poyton and Morgan, 1965). Of the reviewed cases, 63 per cent showed some degree of marginal condensation but not as sharp or opaque as with radicular cysts. The radiological appearances of lesions in different parts of the mandible are similar. In 72 per cent of cases, usually in the posterior mandible, the cyst enveloped the roots of erupted teeth. Scalloping is a prominent feature of simple bone cysts and occurs both between teeth and away from teeth. The lamina dura may or may not be lost and occasional root resorption may occur. Bony septa may be present (Braun, 1975) and the lesions are sometimes interpreted as multilocular (Beasley, 1976; Gait, 1976; Markus, 1978–79; Gowgiel, 1979; Mitchell and Ward-Booth, 1984), which can lead to an erroneous diagnosis.

Pathogenesis

The pathogenesis of the solitary bone cyst is not known but there are a number of theories which have been examined. In 1951, Olech, Sicher and Weinmann

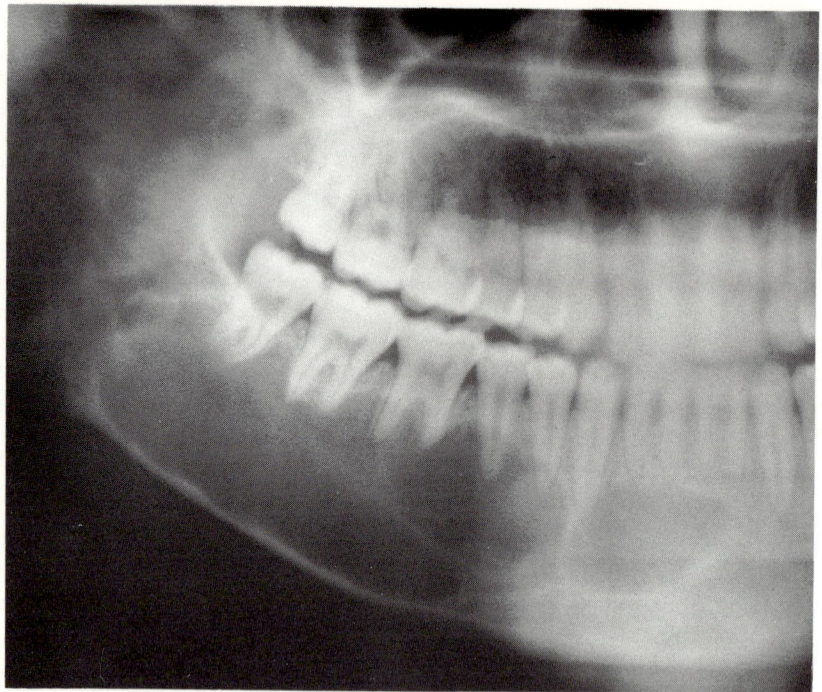

Figure 12.2. Radiograph of a simple bone cyst involving an extensive area in the right body of the mandible. This example has a well-defined margin with cortication. Interradicular scalloping is a prominent feature. (By courtesy of Professor C. J. Nortjé.)

suggested the following possible pathogenesis, based upon a traumatic aetiology, and Howe proposed an essentially similar natural history. Olech, Sicher and Weinmann introduced their hypothesis with the premise that following trauma to a bone, which causes intramedullary haemorrhage, only a failure of early organization of the haematoma in some of the marrow spaces and subsequent liquefaction of the clot can lead to the formation of a traumatic cyst. The crucial point, therefore, is the explanation of this failure. The assumptions which these authors postulated appeared to explain, they believed, all the peculiar features of the pathogenesis, location and age incidence of the simple bone cysts. These cysts seem to develop only after injury to those areas of bone where spongy bone containing haemopoietic marrow is enclosed in a heavy compact cortical layer. This would explain the most frequent sites in the metaphyses of long bones and in the mandible. It would also explain the fact that most simple bone cysts develop in young individuals.

There are arguments against this proposal, particularly the fact that it is difficult to establish a history of trauma in so many instances. Nevertheless, it seems that at least in some cases trauma may be the initiating factor. Trauma, or some other stimulus, leads to rupture of thin-walled sinusoids and intramedullary haemorrhage occurs.

According to Olech, Sicher and Weinmann, the primary haematoma will not be organized if it is not in contact with reactive and fibrous connective tissue and this will not be present if the intramedullary haemorrhage has led to necrosis of the bone marrow itself and related endosteum. The trabeculae of medullary bone are then slowly resorbed by osteoclastic activity on their opposite surfaces and by the time the viable connective tissue gains contact with the haematoma, the latter has liquefied. The breakdown of haematomas and their failure to organize, particularly if they are large, is however a well-known problem in surgery and it is perfectly conceivable that this can occur following intramedullary haemorrhage even in the presence of reactive and fibrous connective tissue. In his detailed histological study of 30 solitary bone cysts, Beasley (1976) observed areas of haemorrhage associated with necrosis and myxoid degenerative changes in a substantial number of cases.

Although the majority of solitary bone cysts are found at operation to contain only air or some other gas, the fact that some contain blood or serosanguineous fluid tends to support the concept of a haematoma breaking down. The breakdown products of haemolysis produce a local rise in osmotic pressure. Toller (1964) has confirmed experimentally that the osmotic tension of solitary bone cyst fluid was greater than that of the patient's blood. This in turn leads to a transudation into the cyst fluid. In the presence of intact cortical bone there is an increase in intraosseous pressure which leads to resorption of bone by osteoclastic activity and sometimes swelling by concurrent periosteal bone deposition. Occasional tooth displacement occurs. As transudation into the cysts occurs, the fluid is diluted so that intracystic pressure drops, but further bleeds may be responsible for progression of the lesion. Once no more bleeding occurs there will be gradual absorption of the serous fluid in the cavity, which becomes empty. The fact that the cysts are rarely found in patients over 30 years suggests that they are self-limiting and that many may undergo spontaneous regression. When the space is filled with blood as a result of surgical intervention, the defect heals and it has been suggested that a spontaneous haemorrhage into an empty cyst cavity may do the same.

This, however, is the main problem in accepting the pathogenesis described above. Essentially it proposes that on the one hand, intrabony haemorrhage is responsible for initiating and then maintaining the process, whereas on the other hand haemorrhage into the cyst cavity in the course of treatment leads to ready repair, and spontaneous haemorrhage is postulated as the reason for resolution without treatment. Olech, Sicher and Weinmann explained this by the fact that the new blood clot which fills the cyst cavity is in contact with healthy connective tissue of the flap from which the organization of the clot commences. When a pathological fracture occurs through a solitary bone cyst, they suggested that the reason for the cyst healing is not only the formation of a fresh blood clot, but also its contact with the vital connective tissue of the periosteum. Although no further evidence as to the pathogenesis of the solitary bone cyst has been published in the years since the paper by Olech and his colleagues, there are nevertheless aspects of their hypothesis which require further elucidation and I should like to see some experimental evidence that similar cysts can be produced by trauma.

A more recent suggestion has been made by Hosseini (1978–79). He proposed that solitary bone cysts might result from a failure of differentiation of osteogenic cells. Basing his hypothesis on an experiment done by Trueta in 1926 and referred to by him again (Trueta, 1968), Hosseini suggested that instead of developing into bone or cartilage, mesenchymal cells might form synovial tissue. The solitary bone cyst might therefore originate as multiple bursa-like synovial cavities which later coalesce to form a larger connective tissue-lined defect. Such an origin would account for the irregular outline of the lesion.

Pathology

When the cyst cavities are opened at operation, they are frequently found to be empty. In other cases, blood, serosanguineous or serous fluid may be present. In 58 per cent of Howe's sample, no visible lining was seen and in the other cases either a thin membrane, granulation tissue or blood clot were described. Ultrastructural study has confirmed the absence of any epithelium in the lining (Schwenzer, Ehrenfeld and Roos, 1985).

Histological features

The simple bone cyst consists of a loose vascular fibrous tissue membrane of variable thickness with no epithelial lining, although fragments of fibrin with enmeshed red cells may be seen. Haemorrhage and haemosiderin pigment are usually present and scattered small multinucleate cells are often found (**Figure 12.3**). Some cyst walls, possibly cases of longer standing, are more densely fibrous.

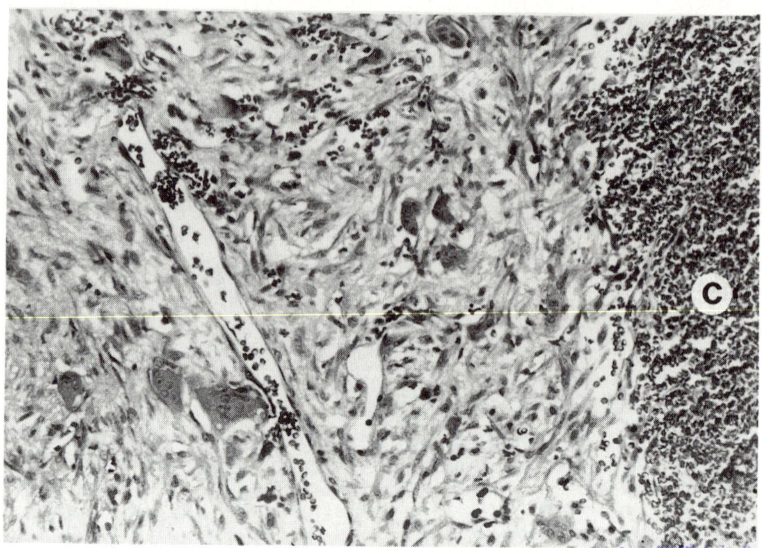

Figure 12.3. Lining of a simple bone cyst of the jaw. [C], cyst cavity. (H & E; × 180.)

The adjacent bone, when included in the specimen, shows osteoclastic resorption on its inner surface. Beasley (1976) described areas of haemorrhage associated with necrotic tissue or tissue showing myxoid degeneration. These occurred in cavities adjacent to areas of bone resorption. Thrombi were not observed in any of the specimens which he examined. Cases associated with florid osseous dysplasia or cemento-osseous dysplasia have been reported (Kaugars and Cale, 1987; Higuchi, Nakamura and Tashiro (1988).

Treatment

The treatment of solitary bone cysts is discussed in Chapter 18.

Lingual mandibular bone defect
(Stafne cavity, static bone cavity, latent bone cyst)

The lingual mandibular bone defect (**Figure 12.4**) is not a cyst. It does, however, produce a cystic appearance on radiographs, and as it is occasionally confused with the solitary bone cyst a brief note on the entity is included here. Of importance in the differential diagnosis is that the solitary bone cyst almost invariably lies above the inferior alveolar canal while the lingual mandibular bone defect lies below the canal.

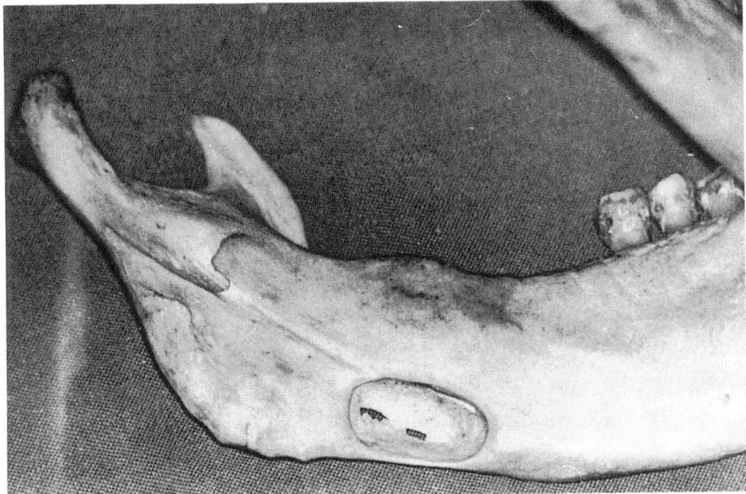

Figure 12.4. Developmental lingual salivary gland depression of the mandible. (By courtesy of Professor P. V. Tobias.)

A description of 35 cases was reported by Stafne in 1942 and since then the features have become well documented. The cavities are usually discovered fortuitously during radiographic examination. They appear as round or ovoid radiolucencies varying from 1 to 3 cm diameter below the inferior alveolar canal approximately in line with the position of the third molar tooth (**Figure 12.5**).

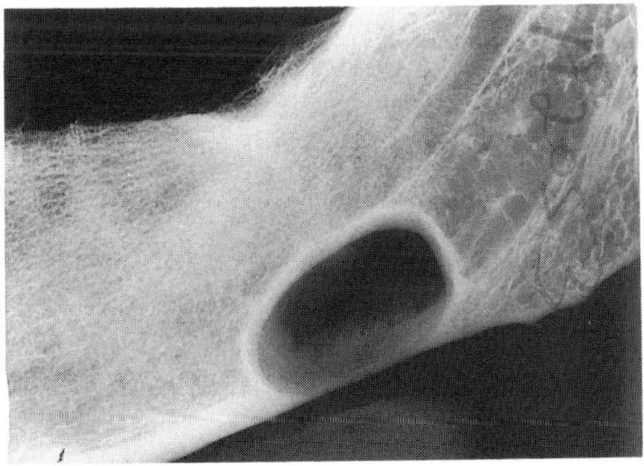

Figure 12.5. Radiograph of dry mandible illustrated in Figure 12.4. (By courtesy of Dr H. Mirels.)

Fordyce (1956) pointed out that apart from the outer distinct cortication, a second inner ring could frequently also be identified which encircles an area of more marked radiolucency.

Oikarinen and Julku (1974) found 10 examples in a survey of 10 000 orthopantomograms, a frequency of 0.1 per cent. All patients were males and with the exception of one 19-year-old, all were over the age of 40. In a similar survey Correll, Jensen and Rhyne (1980) discovered 13 cases in 2693 panoramic radiographs (0.48 per cent) taken in a Veterans' Medical Center where 96 per cent of patients are men. As the defect apparently occurs predominantly in males, this could account for a higher frequency than that shown by Oikarinen and Julku.

Most cases are located just anterior to the angle of the mandible. A few have been reported in the premolar-canine region but Correll, Jensen and Rhyne (1980) thought that those which had been described in the symphyseal area were not true examples of the entity. However, Buchner *et al.* (1991) evaluated 20 cases from the literature and added another four of their own. Histological examination of the contents of the defect in their four cases showed sublingual salivary gland tissue in three and adipose tissue in one. Eighteen of the other 20 reported cases showed salivary gland tissue consistent with sublingual gland origin. They supported the view that resorption of the bone was a reaction to pressure from a lobe of the sublingual gland and that the lesions are evident radiographically only when they are advanced.

Surgical exploration of these cavities has indicated that they represent developmental defects on the lingual aspects of the mandible which are occupied by a lobe of normal submandibular salivary gland. Stereosialography has confirmed that there is a close relationship between the mandibular defect and a lobe of the submandibular salivary gland (Oikarinen, Wolf and Julku, 1975). It seems likely that the salivary gland has an aetiological role in the development of the defect.

The defects are not necessarily congenital. Tolman and Stafne (1967) have shown that radiological evidence of their development may first appear after the patients have reached middle age. This is supported by well-documented evidence that the bone defect has been observed only very rarely in individuals below the age of 40 years. There has been the suggestion that the defect may increase very slowly with age, yet some examples in which follow-up radiographs have been done after a number of years have not demonstrated any change (Stafne, 1942; Oikarinen and Julku, 1974; Correll, Jensen and Rhyne, 1980). With regard to pathogenesis, the evidence tends to suggest that in some individuals, particularly middle-aged or elderly males, a lobe of the submandibular salivary gland may produce a localized pressure atrophy of the lingual surface of the mandible. Lello and Makek (1985) who reported an extensive review of the literature, suggested that the bone defect is the result of an ischaemic process in an area adjacent to the passage of the facial artery. Tensile muscle forces together with haemodynamic forces, they proposed, pulled the artery from the lingual cortex thus compromising its nutrition. This theory does not, however, take account of the relative rarity of lingual bone defects.

Chapter 13

Aneurysmal bone cyst

The aneurysmal bone cyst is an uncommon lesion which has been found in most bones of the skeleton, although the majority occur in the long bones and in the spine (Clough and Price, 1968). The term 'aneurysmal bone cyst' was suggested by Jaffe and Lichtenstein (1942) to describe the characteristic 'blow out' of the bone seen in radiographs of the lesion.

Clinical features

Frequency

The first report of aneurysmal bone cysts involving the craniofacial skeleton appears to be that of Bernier and Bhaskar (1958). In the following year, Bhaskar, Bernier and Godby (1959) described five cases. Gruskin and Dahlin reviewed the literature in 1968, and reported 13 cases including 2 of their own. Daugherty and Eversole (1971) reviewed 17 cases including their own and detailed analyses of the literature have been done subsequently by Steidler, Cook and Reade (1978-79), El Deeb, Sedano and Waite (1980), Struthers (1980); Struthers and Shear (1984 a and b); Gingell *et al.* (1984); and Toljanic *et al.* (1987). Aneurysmal bone cysts of the jaws are rare. When we did our 1984 studies we found that while approximately 650 cases involving the entire skeleton had been reported, we were aware of only 42 well-documented examples involving the jaws which had been recorded in the literature. Since then only a few more cases have been published. Twelve cases have been filed in our departmental archives over a 32-year period representing 0.5 per cent of 2616 jaw cysts (**Table 2.1**, p. 6). The data for age, sex and site recorded below, are those used in the publication by Struthers and Shear (1984a), derived from the 42 reported cases and four of our own specimens which had not been reported previously.

Age

The age distribution of 45 cases is shown in **Figure 13.1**. All but three patients were in the first three decades of life (93 per cent) with a peak in the second decade. Twenty-nine patients were younger than 20 years (64 per cent).

Sex

Twenty-eight patients were females (62 per cent) and 17 males.

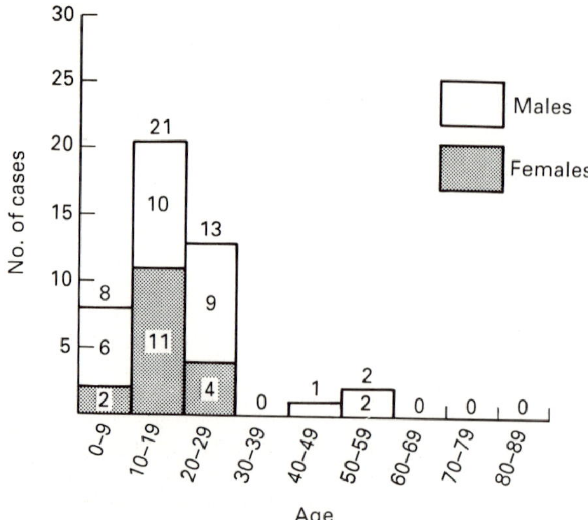

Figure 13.1. Age distribution of 45 patients with aneurysmal bone cysts of the jaws. (After Struthers, 1980.)

Site

Of the 46 cases, 28 were in the mandible (61 per cent) and 18 in the maxilla. One cyst was found close to the orbital floor and another in the zygomatic arch. The anterior region of the mandible was rarely involved. Most of the cases were located in the molar regions of the mandible and maxilla and a number of the mandibular cases extended posteriorly to involve the angle and ascending ramus.

Clinical presentation

Aneurysmal cysts of the jaws produce firm swellings which have been described as painful in fewer than half of the reported cases. The swelling and malocclusion frequently become progressively worse and the rate of enlargement is often described as relatively rapid. Occasionally there is a history of recent displacement of teeth, which remain vital. When the lesion perforates the cortex and is covered by periosteum or only a thin shell of bone, it may exhibit springiness or egg-shell crackling, but is not pulsatile. Bruits are not heard. According to the patients' histories, trauma does not seem to play a significant aetiological role. There may be some difficulty in opening the mouth if there is impingement of the lesion on the capsule of the temporomandibular joint.

Radiological features

The aneurysmal bone cyst produces a radiolucent area which produces an ovoid or fusiform expansion of the bone and may balloon the cortex. It is usually unilocular (**Figure 13.2**) but others have been described as having faintly discernible septation, or trabeculations, and some as being multilocular or honeycomb-like. Teeth may be displaced and root resorption has been described. Radiological differentiation from other expansile jaw lesions may be difficult.

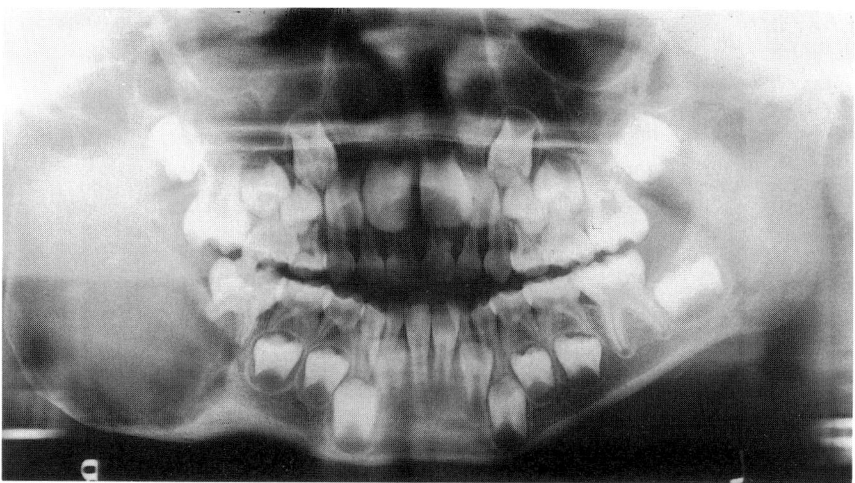

Figure 13.2. Radiograph of an aneurysmal bone cyst involving the angle and ascending ramus of the mandible. There is a ballooning expansion of the cortex. (By courtesy of Professor E. Raubenheimer.)

Pathogenesis

The pathogenesis of the aneurysmal bone cyst is controversial and a number of theories have been proposed. Although trauma has been postulated, there is little evidence to support this. A number of workers have subscribed to the view that the cyst results from a vascular disturbance in the form of sudden venous occlusion or the development of an arteriovenous shunt. This would usually occur in more vascular, newly formed parts of the immature skeleton and possibly arise, in some cases at least, in a pre-existing lesion (Clough and Price, 1968).

The concept that the aneurysmal bone cyst is a secondary phenomenon arising in a pre-existing bone lesion has gained considerable support, and there is undoubtedly good evidence to sustain it. As early as 1940, Ewing described what appears to be an aneurysmal bone cyst and suggested that it was a benign giant cell tumour modified by communication with large blood vessels. Jaffe (1950) proposed that the cyst may result from modification of some other lesion of bone, most of which may be destroyed by haemorrhage. Clough and Price (1968) described two cases, one of which contained areas with the appearance of fibrous dysplasia and the other with features of chondromyxoid fibroma. They suggested that the cyst may be either a primary occurrence or a secondary phenomenon in both benign and malignant lesions of bone.

Biesecker *et al.* (1970) showed evidence of an associated lesion of bone in 21 of 66 cases (32 per cent) of aneurysmal bone cyst. These were non-ossifying fibroma, chondroblastoma, giant cell tumour of bone, osteoblastoma, giant cell granuloma, fibrous dysplasia, myxofibroma and solitary bone cyst. They postulated that the primary lesion initiates an arteriovenous malformation in the bone and that its haemodynamic forces establish the aneurysmal bone cyst. In a similar study, Levy *et al.* (1975) reported 57 aneurysmal bone cysts associated with other lesions of bone. The most frequently associated lesions were solitary bone cysts, giant cell tumours and osteosarcomas, but the change was also observed secondary to non-ossifying fibroma, osteoblastoma, haemangioendothelioma and haemangioma. Some of their cases were secondary to fractures or other bone trauma. They acknowledged, however, that the aneurysmal bone cyst could develop as a primary lesion.

In their review of 53 cases of aneurysmal bone cyst of the jaws, El Deeb, Sedano and Waite (1980) reported that 11 (21 per cent) were associated with pre-existing lesions. These were ossifying fibroma (two cases), cementifying fibroma (one case), fibrous dysplasia (four cases) and giant cell granuloma (four cases). Robinson (1985) did a similar review, probably sampling much of the same material, and confirmed that of 58 cases of aneurysmal bone cyst of the jaws 13 were associated with other bone disease. His own case showed an associated cementifying fibroma.

In the review done in our department, Struthers (1980) and Struthers and Shear (1984b) concluded that an associated lesion could be identified in 33 reported cases. Two were ossifying fibromas, two cementifying fibromas, four fibrous dysplasias, 24 central giant cell granulomas and one was an osteosarcoma. Of our own five cases available at the time of the study, three were associated with tissue identical to that seen in the central giant cell granuloma of the jaws and two with ossifying fibroma. Two cases circulated by the WHO International Reference Centre for the Histological Definition and Classification of Odontogenic Tumours, Jaw Cysts and Allied Lesions were associated with ossifying fibroma and two with central giant cell granuloma.

Working on the hypothesis that the aneurysmal bone cyst is a secondary phenomenon which develops by breakdown of part of a pre-existing lesion of bone, histological material from 303 pathological lesions of bone of various kinds was studied to look for evidence of early changes which might indicate a potential for development into aneurysmal bone cyst (Struthers, 1980; Struthers and Shear, 1984b). As reference material the authors studied 19 established aneurysmal bone cysts from various parts of the skeleton, including the jaws, because in such lesions smaller blood-filled spaces and numerous microcysts are usually found at the periphery of the large blood-filled spaces. Changes of this kind were seen particularly in central giant cell granulomas. In a sample of 54 cases of central giant cell granuloma they observed such microcyst formation in 15 (28 per cent). In three of these the changes were strikingly similar to those seen in the aneurysmal bone cyst. The same changes were also recognized, although with a much lower frequency, in the fibrous dysplasias (8 per cent), ossifying fibromas (4 per cent) and cementifying fibromas (3 per cent) studied. One case of Paget's disease of bone showed the presence of large blood-filled spaces, as did several of the malignant lesions.

Struthers and Shear suggested that the initiating change in the primary lesion appeared to be the microcyst. They pointed out that the formation of microcysts in fibrous dysplasia had been described by Geschickter and Copeland (1949), by Jaffe (1953) and by Fisher (1976). The central giant cell granuloma has a propensity to form microcysts because of its loose, oedematous, fibrillar connective tissue stroma in which lie many thin-walled blood vessels and extravasated erythrocytes. Microcyst formation is facilitated by localized areas of necrosis in the stroma brought about by stagnation and ischaemia. The resulting microcysts are lined by stromal connective tissue and in giant cell lesions multinucleate giant cells may form part of their margins. They enlarge by further stromal breakdown and coalesce with each other. Enlargement will be aggravated if haemodynamic or osmotic forces become involved. Loss of stromal support leads to dilatation and

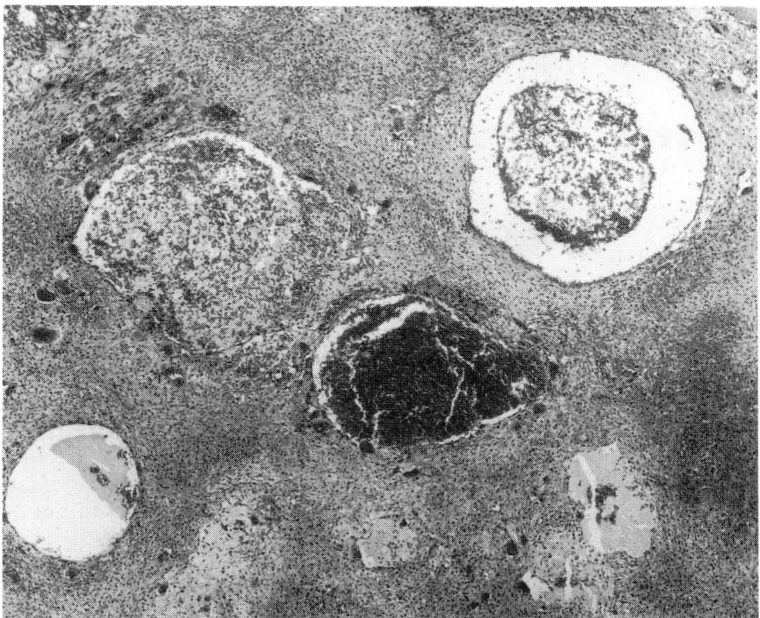

Figure 13.3. Dilated blood vessels and microcysts in part of an aneurysmal bone cyst. The intervening solid tissue suggests that the lesion has developed in a giant cell granuloma. (H & E: × 32.)

rupture of the thin-walled vessels and haemorrhage into the stroma and the microcysts. An association of dilated blood vessels and microcysts is frequently observed (**Figure 13.3**). Once a vascular connection is established between a larger vessel and a microcyst, haemodynamic pressure participates in its enlargement and little supportive resistance is offered if the surrounding stroma is loose and oedematous. The spaces now assume the dimensions of macrocysts which are surrounded by a layer of compressed stroma and these multiple expanding blood-filled cysts produce a pressure resorption of bone. Endosteal resorption of the cortical plates occurs ultimately and once these are breached a 'blow out' of the lesion, covered with periosteum, occurs. A layer of periosteal new bone may be deposited to form a thin shell covering the aneurysmal bone cyst (see **Figure 13.2**).

Struthers and Shear were of the opinion that a malignant lesion was less likely to produce the classic clinicopathological features of an aneurysmal bone cyst because of its tendency to break out of bone. Nevertheless of 42 fibrosarcomas which they studied histologically, six showed large blood-filled spaces; as did eight of 75 cases of osteosarcoma. They believed that the latter represented the telangiectatic form of osteosarcoma which several authors have described as resembling the aneurysmal bone cyst. The rare development of aneurysmal bone cyst in malignant lesions probably explains the so-called malignant form of the cyst occasionally reported in the literature (Levy *et al.*, 1975).

To conclude this discussion of the possible pathogenesis of the aneurysmal bone cyst, it should be stated that there are a number of authorities who dispute the theory that the cyst is a secondary phenomenon. Tillman *et al.* (1968) studied all tissue removed from 95 aneurysmal bone cysts and concluded that there was no evidence of precursor lesions in these cases. Similarly, Ruiter, van Rijssel and van der Velde (1977) did not identify other bone lesions in their series of 105 cases. Both groups of authors did, however, admit that areas may have been present which resembled other lesions. Schajowicz (1981) has stated that areas similar to those of the aneurysmal bone cyst may be found in many bone lesions but that they usually occupy only a minor portion of the process and that they are probably the result of haemorrhage.

Pathology

At operation an intact periosteum and a very thin shell of bone usually covers the cyst. When this is removed, dark venous blood wells up. Bleeding may be profuse and difficult to control until the cyst has been removed. The cyst contains variable amounts of soft tissue consisting of friable vascular tissue which subdivides the cavity into a number of blood-filled locules (**Figure 13.4**). Part of the lesion may contain areas of more solid tissue. These may represent either areas of repair or remnants of a pre-existing lesion. No direct communication with any vessels can be demonstrated at operation.

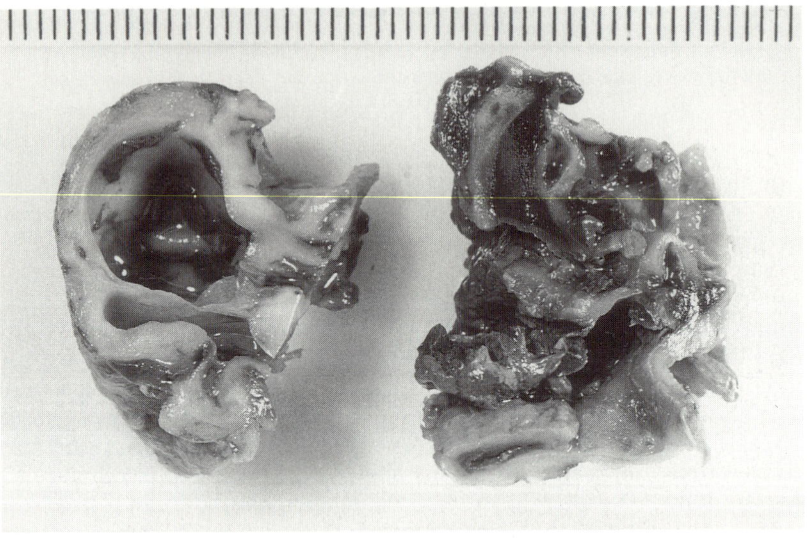

Figure 13.4. Section through parts of a gross specimen of an aneurysmal bone cyst of the mandible. Solid areas are interspersed with multiple cysts or locules.

Histological features

The lesions consist of many capillaries and blood-filled spaces of varying size lined by flat spindle cells and separated by delicate loose-textured fibrous tissue. Most cysts contain small multinucleate cells and scattered trabeculae of osteoid and woven bone. In some of the solid areas, sheets of vascular tissue, containing large numbers of multinucleate giant cells, fibroblasts, haemorrhage and haemosiderin, look very much like giant cell granuloma of the jaws (**Figure 13.5**). Other solid

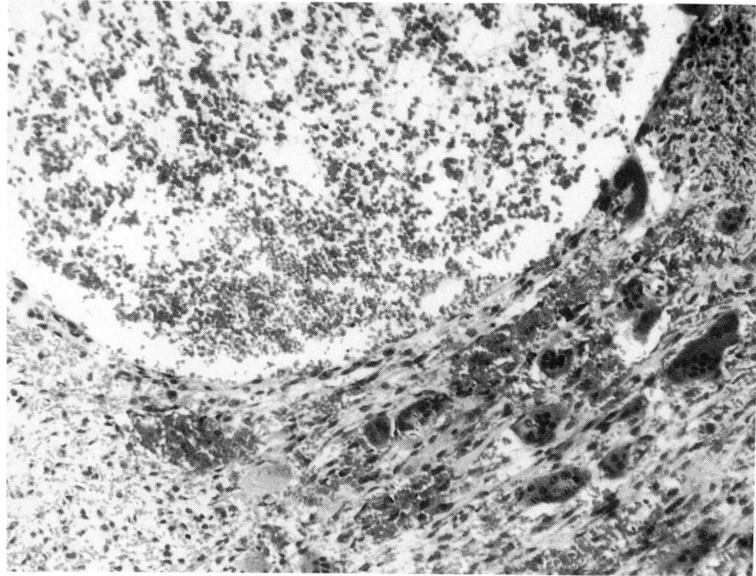

Figure 13.5. Aneurysmal bone cyst in which the solid areas have histological features identical to those of the central giant cell granuloma of the jaws. (H & E; x 100.)

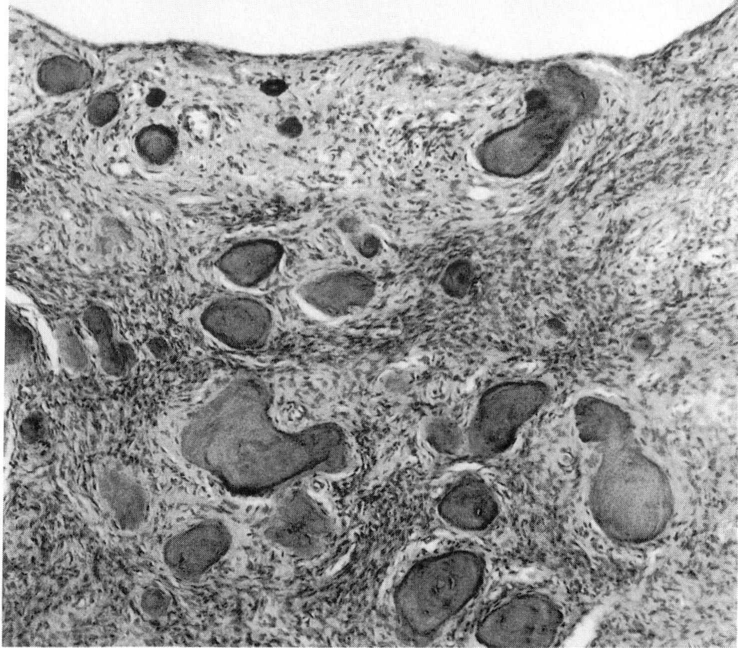

Figure 13.6. Aneurysmal bone cyst of the mandible. The solid areas show the features of cemento-ossifying fibroma and a portion of one of the many locules is present at the top of the photomicrograph. (H & E; × 100.)

areas may have the appearance of fibrous dysplasia, cemento-ossifying fibroma (**Figure 13.6**) and possibly other jaw tumours, and this gives credence to the view that the aneurysmal bone cyst may represent secondary change in a pre-existing lesion. The blood-filled spaces have no elastic tissue or smooth muscle around them. There are no cellular features suggestive of malignant neoplasia (Clough and Price, 1968) unless, of course, the cyst has developed in a malignant tumour.

Treatment

The treatment of the aneurysmal bone cyst must be determined by the nature of any associated lesion. According to El Deeb, Sedano and White (1980) the most frequent form of treatment in reported cases of aneurysmal bone cysts of the jaws has been curettage. Their review indicated a recurrence rate of 26 per cent for jaw cases. In the review done by Gingell *et al.* (1984) there was a 19 per cent recurrence rate with the jaw lesions including three cases with multiple recurrences. Recurrences also occur with the cysts involving other bones with rates ranging from 21 per cent to 44 per cent (Gingell *et al.*, 1984). Clough and Price (1968) reported continued growth even after careful curettage and bone grafting and recommended complete excision provided this would not interfere with function. One of the cases in our own series, which was associated with an ossifying fibroma, recurred twice following curettage. Thorough curettage of lesions associated with central giant cell granuloma are probably less likely to recur. As most aneurysmal bone cysts of the jaws appear to involve central giant cell granulomas, this would account for the successful conservative treatment recorded by a number of workers. There is no place for radiotherapy in the treatment of jaw lesions unless it is one of the very rare examples which may have developed secondary to a malignant tumour.

In view of the tendency for certain cases to recur, there should be a careful appraisal of each case after histological evaluation and patients should have periodic postoperative examinations.

Chapter 14

Cysts associated with the maxillary antrum

There are two cysts which are considered under this heading: the benign mucosal cyst of the maxillary antrum and the postoperative maxillary cyst or surgical ciliated cyst of the maxilla.

Benign mucosal cyst of the maxillary antrum

The mucosal cyst of the maxillary antrum has also been referred to as a mucocele, retention cyst, pseudocyst and intramural cyst, while uncertainty as to its pathogenesis has led in the past to its being termed 'mesothelial' cyst and 'lymphangiectatic' cyst. Allard (1982), Gardner (1984) and Gardner and Gullane (1986) have argued against the term mucocele for this lesion. Gardner and Gardner and Gullane preferred to call the entity 'pseudocyst', reserving the designation 'mucocele' for the postoperative maxillary cyst; and 'retention cyst' for lesions which are caused by blockage and dilatation of ducts of the seromucinous glands of the sinus and are therefore lined by epithelium. The preferred term of many authors appears to be 'mucosal cyst of the antrum', with secretory (retention cyst) and non-secretory types (Gothberg *et al.*, 1976; Shafer, Hine and Levy, 1983).

Clinical features

Frequency

This cyst probably occurs more commonly than was previously thought. Kwapis and Whitten (1971) have pointed out that more of them are being revealed with the increased use of panoramic radiographs of the maxilla. Their survey of a series of such radiographs disclosed the presence of round radio-opaque areas in the maxillary sinuses of 22 patients. Surgical exploration and subsequent histological examination were carried out on 14 of these and the features were consistent with the diagnosis of mucosal cyst of the maxillary sinus. Myall, Eastep and Silver (1974) surveyed 1469 orthopantographs and made a radiological diagnosis of mucosal antral cyst in 75 cases (5.1 per cent). A similar study by Casamassimo and Lilly (1980) on 4546 panoramic radiographs showed a lower frequency, 73 mucosal cysts (1.6 per cent) having been observed in their sample. Allard, van der Kwast and van der Waal (1981b) and Allard (1982), however, demonstrated 94 cxamples in a series of 1080 radiographs (8.7 per cent). The latter authors quoted the frequency in 11 other publications, which ranged from 1.4 to 9.6 per cent. Rhodus (1990) detected 54 (4.3 per cent) in panoramic radiographs of a sample of 1249 patients selected at random in a dental school patient population.

Age

The age distribution of 148 patients in the surveys of Myall, Eastep and Silver and Casamassimo and Lilly is shown in **Figure 14.1**. The great majority of cases were found in patients in the age group 21–30 years.

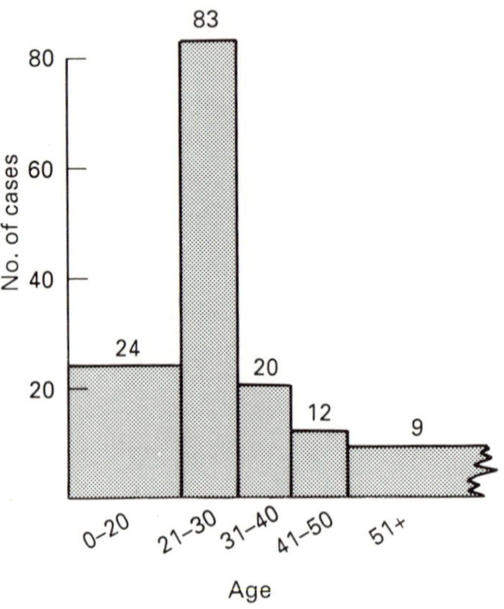

Figure 14.1. Age distribution of 148 patients with mucosal cysts of the maxillary antrum. (Data pooled from Myall, Eastep and Silver, 1974 and Casamassimo and Lilly, 1980.)

Sex

Of the 242 cases reported by Myall, Eastep and Silver, Casamassimo and Lilly and Allard, van der Kwast and van der Waal, 161 (68.1 per cent) occurred in males. The proportion of males in these three studies was roughly the same.

Site

In the series of Myall, Eastep and Silver, 43 of the 75 cases involved the antral floor (57 per cent). The cysts developed on the lateral wall in 24 cases (32 per cent) and the other antral surfaces were occasionally involved. In the great majority of cases only single cysts occurred, but in a few instances they were multiple and sometimes bilateral. In the study of Casamassimo and Lilly, 54 of their cases (74 per cent) involved the antral floor. In 14 of their patients (19 per cent) there was also a cyst in the contralateral sinus. Berg, Carenfelt and Sobin (1989) found that 24 of 27 mucosal cysts originated from a rather limited area at the sharp angle between the floor and frontal or lateral aspect of the sinus cavity, close to the alveolar process.

Clinical presentation

In many instances, the mucosal cyst of the maxillary antrum may be characterized by the absence of symptoms, the lesions being discovered only in the course of routine radiological examination. Patients may however complain of a wide range of symptoms such as a localized dull pain in the antral region, or fullness or numbness of the cheek, nasal obstruction, postnasal drip and a copious discharge of yellow fluid from the nostrils (Gothberg *et al.*, 1976). Sometimes an antral cyst may produce a swelling. One such case from our files occurred in a 32-year-old woman. She had a painless, fluctuant swelling of the left maxilla extending from the canine to the second molar which was noticed by her dentist during routine dental examination. She had not previously had any surgical procedure in the region. At operation a cyst was found arising from the lateral wall of the maxillary antrum and a diagnosis of retention cyst of the antrum was made histologically (**Figure 14.3**). Gothberg *et al.* found that the secretory type of mucosal cyst (retention cyst) was related to an increased frequency of symptoms and more frequently expanded into surrounding tissues.

A number of patients have reported allergies of various kinds but it is not clear whether the frequency is higher than in the general population. Rhodus (1990) found that a substantial number of his patients with mucosal cysts complained of allergy or sinusitis or both.

The presence of a cyst does not affect transillumination (Gothberg *et al.*, 1976).

Radiological features

The lesions may be discovered in the course of routine periapical radiography which includes the involved region. It is clear, however, that some examples are missed in dental views but are demonstrable in panoramic radiographs (Casamassimo and Lilly, 1980; Rhodus, 1990). When an antral cyst is suspected on intraoral radiography, supplementary panoramic radiographs are extremely useful in providing a view of the maxillary sinuses with little superimposition of adjacent structures. The cysts appear as spherical, ovoid or dome-shaped radio-opacities which have a smooth and uniform outline (**Figure 14.2**). They may have a narrow

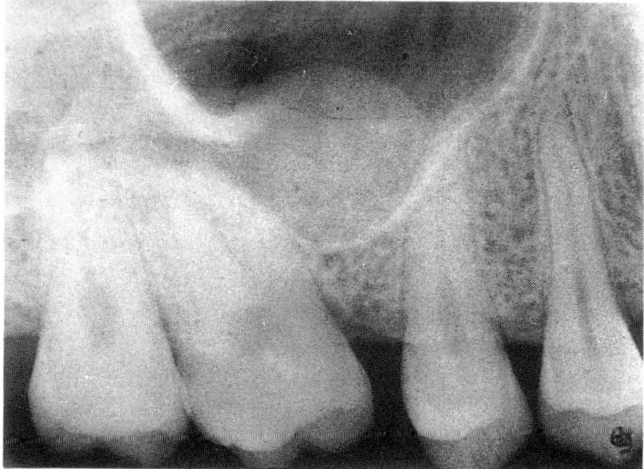

Figure 14.2. Radiograph of a mucosal cyst of the maxillary antrum. (By courtesy of Professor C. J. Nortjé.)

or broad base. They vary in size from minute to very large and may occasionally occupy the entire maxillary sinus (Killey and Kay, 1973). The smooth curved borders are well defined but not corticated. There is no resorption of adjacent bone and of particular importance is the persistence of the thin radio-opaque line of the antral cortex itself (Myall, Eastep and Silver, 1974).

Inflammatory lesions of the sinus must be considered in the differential diagnosis as well as the apical radicular cyst and the postoperative maxillary cyst. Superimposed anatomy such as an inferior concha may be another source of diagnostic error (Allard, van der Kwast and van der Waal, 1981b).

Follow-up radiological examination has shown that the cyst may persist without a change in size for a long time, and may eventually disappear spontaneously. Others slowly increase in size (Gothberg *et al.*, 1976; Casamassimo and Lilly, 1980).

Pathogenesis

The pathogenesis of the mucosal cyst of the antrum has not been definitely determined but a previous infection is frequently implicated. Kwapis and Whitten (1971) have suggested that severe inflammation around the ducts of the mucous glands of the antral lining may alter their integrity. When the patient sneezes, mucus can be expelled into the soft tissues through the wall of such an injured duct. Once this pathway for the extraglandular accumulation of mucus has been established, the process may continue until a cyst has developed. Gardner (1984) and Gardner and Gullane (1986) regarded these lesions as focal accumulations of inflammatory exudate that lift the antral mucosa away from the underlying bone. A possible relationship between the development of a mucosal cyst of the antrum with related endodontically treated teeth or periodontitis has been considered and Casamassimo and Lilly (1980) noted a trend toward larger cysts with increasingly severe periodontal disease. Gardner (1984) considered an association with periapical infection of adjacent maxillary teeth as a distinct possibility.

Berg, Carenfelt and Sobin (1989) suggested that because of the frequent location of the lesions at the sharp angle between the floor and the frontal or lateral aspect of the sinus cavity, close to the alveolar process, mechanical factors might be involved in the development of the cyst. Mucosal swelling, perhaps the result of previous common colds, may lead to mechanical stress to or rupture of the sharp angle tissue or its bony attachment. These authors found increased concentrations of IgG, IgA and C3d in the cyst fluid compared with the patients' serum ($P < 0.001$). The stimulus for this they thought was the presence of anaerobic organisms which could be of dental origin. They also found low concentrations of α_1-antitrypsin in the cyst fluid which suggested the possibility that a proteolytic process could lead to the expansion of the cysts.

Gardner (1984) suggested that the secretory type, or retention cyst, arose from a partial blockage of the duct of a seromucinous gland of the sinus.

Pathological features

When explored surgically, it is possible to demonstrate the intact and undisturbed cyst. It has a smooth blue surface, is thin-walled and contains mucinous material. Allard, van der Kwast and van der Waal (1981b) stated that it is almost always found in an otherwise healthy looking sinus whereas antral polyps will usually be seen in groups on inflamed oedematous mucosa.

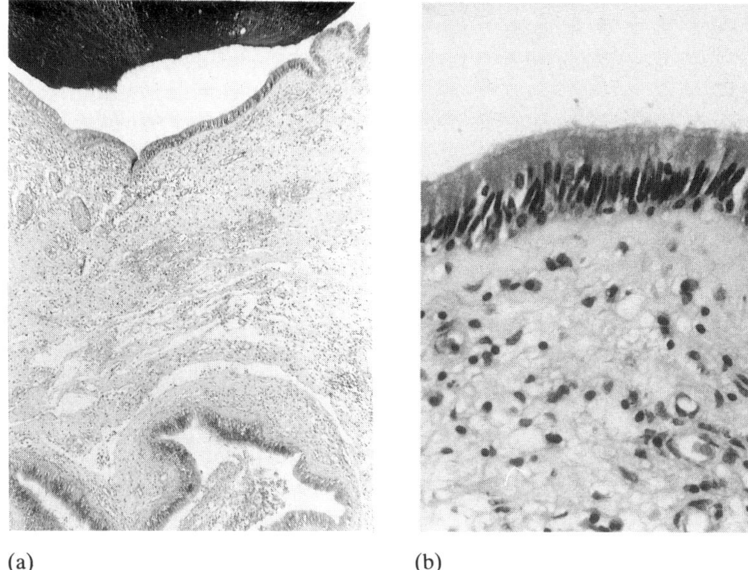

(a) (b)

Figure 14.3. (a) Mucosal cyst of the maxillary antrum. The cyst (top) illustrated here is of the secretory variety. It is lined by pseudostratified ciliated columnar epithelium and is filled with mucin. The lining of the maxillary antrum is seen below. (PAS; × 10.) (b) Mucosal cyst of the maxillary antrum. Higher magnification of part of the cyst lining illustrated in (a). (H & E; × 250.)

The microscopic features are very much like those of an oral mucocele. Usually no epithelial lining is present but in the case referred to above and illustrated in **Figure 14.3**, there was a mucin-containing cyst lined by pseudostratified ciliated columnar epithelium. The connective tissue wall of the cyst is infiltrated with varying numbers of chronic inflammatory cells and the lumen may contain inflammatory cells. The lesions which are not lined by epithelium are sometimes referred to as the non-secretory type and those lined by respiratory epithelium as the secretory type of antral cyst (Shafer, Hine and Levy, 1983). Gardner (1984) preferred the term 'retention cyst' for the latter type. The non-secretory type consists of loose, oedematous connective tissue and the lumen is lined by a layer of compressed fibrous tissue. In view of the definition of a cyst, there can be no justification for calling these lesions pseudocysts.

Treatment

As most of these cysts remain static and some regress spontaneously, and as they usually cause little discomfort, Kwapis and Whitten (1971) have recommended that surgical intervention is unnecessary. Killey and Kay (1973) tended to agree with this but suggested that if symptoms are present cannulation and drainage may be done. Large cysts, they felt, should be removed through a Caldwell–Luc approach. Allard, van der Kwast and van der Waal (1981b) indicated that only if specific or pertinent clinical features were present would they advise treatment, which, in their view, should be removal through a Caldwell–Luc approach. Rhodus (1990) agreed that most cysts resolve spontaneously over time but that their surgical removal may occasionally be necessary.

Postoperative maxillary cyst (surgical ciliated cyst of the maxilla)

The postoperative maxillary cyst is fairly commonly encountered in Japan but appears to be a rare lesion in most other parts of the world. Its name is derived from the fact that it is a delayed complication arising years after surgery involving the maxillary sinus.

Clinical features

Frequency

In our own department only four cases have been diagnosed over a 32-year period (**Table 2.1**) representing 0.2 per cent of 2616 jaw cysts, whereas Kaneshiro *et al.* (1981) reported a series of 68 patients with 71 lesions treated at the Niigata University Dental Hospital from 1967 to 1977. Similarly, Yamamoto and Takagi (1986) reported that in their hospital the postoperative maxillary cyst accounted for 19.5 per cent of all oral cystic lesions. They quoted similarly high frequencies in other reports in the Japanese literature. Maeda *et al.* (1987) studied 100 examples removed at their clinic over a 5-year period. Outside Japan, the only reports suggesting that the lesion may not be rare are those of Basu *et al.* (1985) and Smith *et al.* (1988) from the University of Birmingham Dental School, where 18 cases were diagnosed over a period of 3 years.

Age

The age distribution of 60 patients in the study of Yamamoto and Takagi (1986) is shown in **Figure 14.4**. The great majority of their patients were in the fourth and fifth decades and their ages ranged from 21 to 72 years. A very similar age distribution was shown by Kaneshiro *et al.* (1981) whose patients ranged in age from 27 to 63 years.

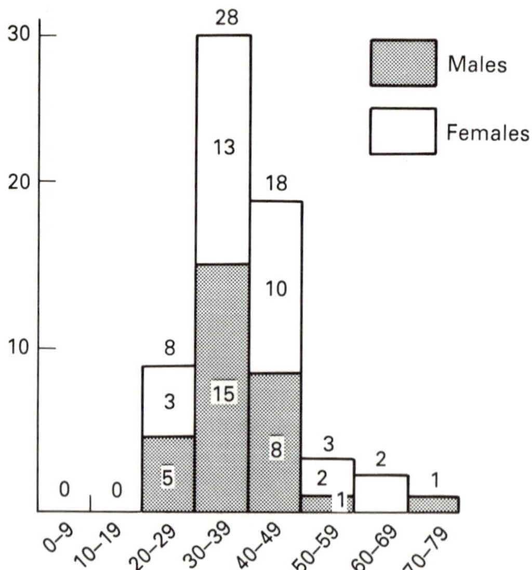

Figure 14.4. Age distribution of 60 patients with postoperative maxillary cyst. (After Yamamoto and Takagi, 1986.)

Sex

There was a preponderance of males to females (2:1) amongst the patients of Kaneshiro *et al.* (1981). In the sample of Basu *et al.* (1985) there were 11 females and seven males, while there was an equal sex distribution in the series of Yamamoto and Tagaki (1986).

Site

In the study of Yamamoto and Takagi, 24 cysts occupied half of the maxillary sinus, 19 were localized in the lower portion and 17 cases occupied the whole sinus. Most cases were located in the molar and premolar regions.

Clinical presentation

Gregory and Shafer (1958) drew attention to the development of these cysts in the maxillae of patients whose maxillary sinuses had been opened surgically during a Caldwell–Luc operation. They proposed the term 'surgical ciliated cyst of the maxilla'. Publication of large series from Japan as well as other reports have confirmed the association with previous maxillary surgery. In almost all cases it is an operation for maxillary sinusitis, particularly the Caldwell–Luc procedure including a nasal antrostomy, which is responsible, but the cyst can also result from gun shot injuries, fractures of the malar/maxillary complex and mid-face osteotomies (Sugar, Walker and Bounds, 1990).

The period between the original operation and the diagnosis of the cyst can be considerable. In the studies of both Kaneshiro *et al.* and Yamamoto and Takagi, the duration ranged from 10 to 29 years for 87 per cent of their patients. The shortest period was 4 years and the longest 49 years, with a mean of 18.3 years, in the experience of Yamamoto *et al.*

The patients may complain of pain, discomfort or swelling in the cheek or face, or intraorally in the palate or alveolus. Pus may be discharged.

Radiological features

Radiographs reveal a well-defined radiolucent area closely related to the maxillary sinus. In the series reported by Yamamoto and Takagi most cases were unilocular lesions with only four of them reported as multilocular. In 42 of their 60 cases buccal cortical bone was present. Surrounding bone sclerosis was evident in at least part of the bony margin in just over half of the cases. In the study of Kaneshiro *et al.*, the bony margin was missing in the lateral, posterior or upper walls in half of their cases. They showed that the diameter of 47 radiographically well-defined cysts in the Water's position was between 21 mm and 30 mm in 29 cases, less than 20 mm in 11 and more than 31 mm in seven cases. Occasionally the cystic area appears to encroach on the sinus itself but lack of communication between the two has been demonstrated by injecting the sinus with a radio-opaque material (Shafer, Hine and Levy, 1983). In the early lesions no destruction of bone is evident but as they enlarge the sinus wall becomes thinned and eventually perforated (Gardner and Gullane, 1986), and may resemble a malignant neoplasm (Basu *et al.*, 1985). Gradually the cyst expands beyond the original boundaries of the sinus.

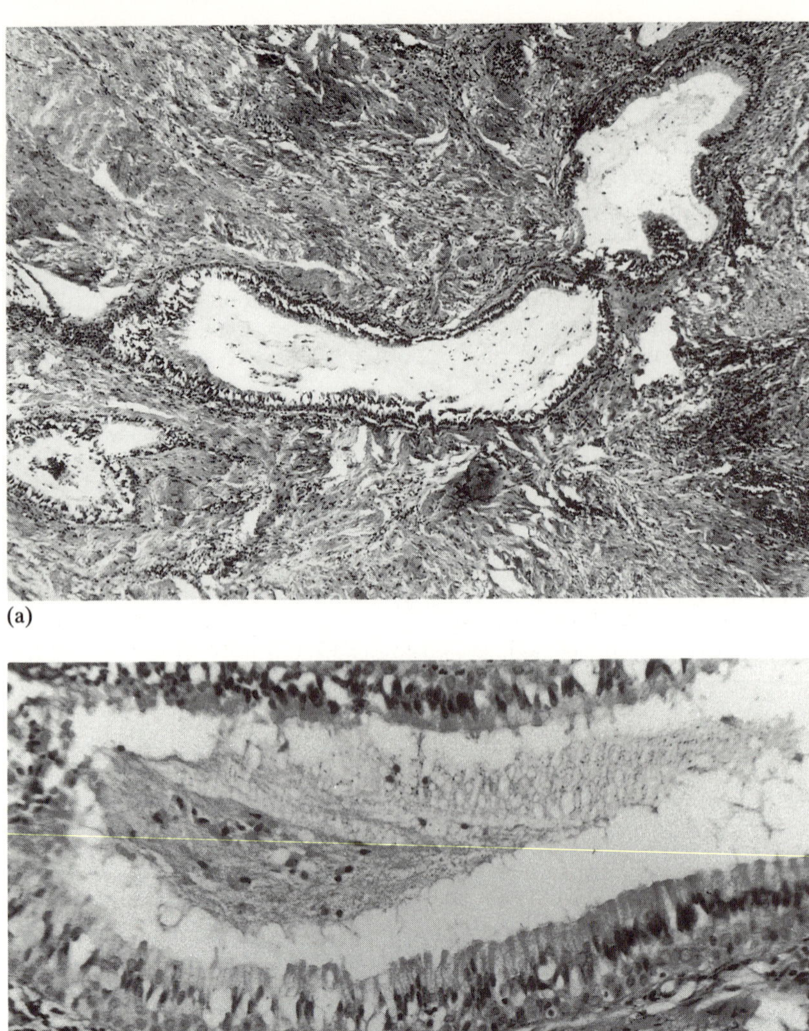

(a)

(b)

Figure 14.5. (a) Postoperative maxillary cyst. The cyst lining which is composed of pseudostratified ciliated columnar epithelium has ramified irregularly. (H & E; × 50.) (b) Postoperative maxillary cyst. Higher magnification of part of lining illustrated in (a). (H & E; × 230.)

Pathogenesis

The high frequency of postoperative maxillary cyst in Japan has been attributed to the large number of cases of maxillary sinusitis that occurred in Japan during and just after the Second World War that were treated by the Caldwell–Luc procedure because antibiotics were not available. It will be interesting to see whether the frequency in Japan declines in future years. Gregory and Shafer suggested that the cysts are derived from the epithelial lining of the maxillary sinus which is trapped in the wound during closure of the Caldwell-Luc incision, and subsequently begins to proliferate. By forming a closed sac which is unable to drain through the ostium into the nose, it constitutes a cyst or mucocele which enlarges and may resorb the bony walls of the antrum (Gardner and Gullane, 1986).

Pathological features

Histologically, the cysts are lined by pseudostratified ciliated columnar epithelium, with squamous metaplasia in chronically inflamed areas (**Figure 14.5**). Combinations of ciliated, cuboidal and squamous epithelium with varying numbers of mucous cells may be seen. Ciliated epithelium is the type most commonly encountered (Maeda *et al.*, 1987). The epithelium may be ulcerated in parts. The underlying connective tissue may be cellular or fibrotic (Gardner and Gullane, 1986). Foam cells, cholesterin clefts, haemosiderin and foci of calcification may be present.

Basu *et al.* (1985) described a well-defined acellular layer in the capsule, below and parallel to the surface, which was either hyaline or mucoid in appearance. Occasionally a cellular layer of fibrous tissue was interposed between this layer and the epithelium.

Basu *et al.* (1985) found wide variations in the protein levels of the cyst fluids, thus precluding any valuable preoperative information from this source for diagnostic purposes. However, in another study by the same group on the analysis of glycosaminoglycans in the fluid aspirate (Smith *et al.*, 1988), they demonstrated a characteristic electrophoretic pattern of hyaluronic acid and heparin sulphate, with lesser amounts of chondroitin-4-sulphate. This was different from the pattern they had previously shown in odontogenic cyst fluids (Smith, Smith and Browne, 1984), and might therefore be of diagnostic value. The presence of hyaluronic acid and chondroitin-4-sulphate in the fluids of this cyst was also demonstrated by Suzuki (1988). He concluded that hyaluronidase in the cyst fluid acts on the hyaluronic acid in the cyst wall which then passes into the cyst fluid.

Treatment

Sugar, Walker and Bounds (1990) have suggested that in most cases enucleation through an approach appropriate to the site is the treatment of choice, but marsupialization for unilocular cysts with a thin wall and extensive bony perforation was proposed by Yoshikawa *et al.* (1982). In the experience of Kaneshiro *et al.* (1981) recurrences may occur if the cyst is infected or if the wall is very thin and there is perforation of the bone, making enucleation difficult because of tight adhesion of the the cyst to adjacent tissues.

Chapter 15

Developmental cysts of the soft tissues of the mouth, face and neck

Dermoid and epidermoid cysts

Dermoid and epidermoid cysts may occur on the floor of the mouth. Dermoid cysts are lined by epidermis and skin appendages are present in the fibrous wall. Epidermoid cysts are lined by epidermis, but contain no appendages.

Clinical features

Frequency

Valuable reviews of these cysts have been written by Meyer (1955), Allard (1982) and Seward (1965). They quoted statistics from the Mayo Clinic which indicated that of 1495 'dermoid' cysts seen in an adult population over a 26-year period from 1910 to 1935, 103 (6.9 per cent) occurred in the head and neck region and only 24 (1.6 per cent) were found in the floor of the mouth. In a sample of 514 cases from the same source during the period 1936 to 1961 there was a higher frequency of 6.5 per cent in the floor of the mouth. Allard (1982) found 11 cases in the files of the Oral Pathology Department of his hospital out of a series of 8000 surgical specimens collected over 10 years. Howell (1985) traced five sublingual cases from three oral surgical units in England treated over a 9-year period.

Age

Although they may be present at birth (Yoshimura *et al.*, 1970; Yeschua *et al.*, 1977) and in old patients, the majority occur between the ages of 15 and 35 years. In a series of 76 oral cases collected from the literature, Allard (1982) found that 71 per cent occurred by the age of 30 years and 91 per cent by the age of 45 years. The duration of symptoms varied from 0 to 31 years.

Sex

Fifty-nine per cent of Allard's sample were found in males and 41 per cent in females.

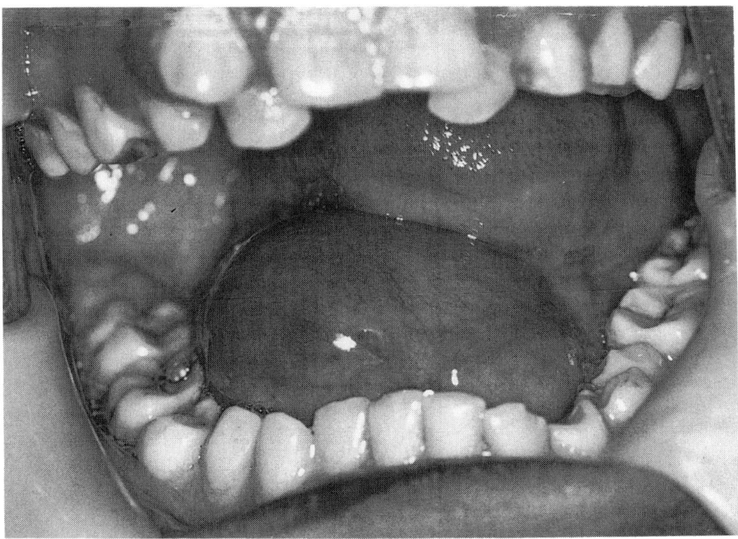

Figure 15.1. Dermoid cyst of the floor of mouth.

Site

The midline of the floor of the mouth is the commonest location of these cysts (**Figure 15.1**), which may also cause a swelling in the midline of the neck. In Allard's sample, 71 per cent occurred there of which about half had appendages in their walls (dermoid cysts) and half did not (epidermoid cysts). The remaining 29 per cent were evenly distributed in different parts of the mouth including four in the tongue which were all epidermoid cysts. Only two cases in this series were reported in the lateral part of the floor of the mouth.

Seward believed that dermoid and epidermoid cysts of the midline of the floor of the mouth always originate above the mylohyoid muscle, but may penetrate it. Some authors have differentiated between a sublingual or genioglossal type which is located between the geniohyoid muscle and the oral mucosa, and a geniohyoidal type which is positioned between the geniohyoid and mylohyoid muscle (Allard, 1982). The rare lateral type which is smaller, is located in the premolar-molar region and lies in the gutter formed by the mandible laterally and the genioglossal and geniohyoid muscles medially. It lies in the plane between the oral mucosa superiorly and the mylohyoid muscle inferiorly (Allard, 1982).

Issa and Davies (1971) have recorded an exceptionally rare example of a dermoid cyst which occurred in the coronoid region of the mandible in a 26-year-old woman. Another example of an intraosseous dermoid cyst was described by Craig, Holland and Hindle (1980). It occurred in the midline of the mandible in a 28-year-old man. The authors carefully assessed the possible pathogenesis of the lesion and concluded that it was of non-odontogenic origin. They suggested that an intraosseous dermoid cyst should be considered in the differential diagnosis of midline cystic lesions of the mandible.

Dermoid cysts also occur on the face. In a series of 231 cases in children about three-quarters were located above the shoulders (Pollard, Harley and Calhoun,

1976). The orbital and periorbital region was the area of the body most frequently involved, with 87 cases (37 per cent). Interestingly, the left eyebrow (50 cases) was affected very much more often than the right (20 cases). The neck, scalp, ear and nose were the other sites involved.

Clinical presentation

The intraoral swelling lifts the tongue (**Figure 15.1**) and may lead to difficulty in speaking, eating, breathing or closing the mouth. The swelling in the neck gives the patient a 'double-chin' appearance. The swelling may feel doughy or fluctuant. The cysts tend to be small in infancy and enlarge during adolescence.

Pathogenesis

The origin of dermoids and epidermoids of the floor of the mouth, like other developmental cysts, is controversial. Having examined and discarded a number of concepts, Seward (1965) suggested that the most likely site for their origin is anteriorly between the contributions from the mandibular arches to the tongue. The problem with postulating an origin from contributions of mandibular arches to the tongue or from the first pharyngeal pouch is that it implies endodermal derivation. This seems unlikely for a structure which contains skin adnexae. On the other hand, Hamilton and Mossman (1972) stated that by the 30th–32nd day of intrauterine life, the endoderm of the floor of the mouth can no longer be distinguished from stomodeal ectoderm and there is probably a considerable amount of intermingling of the two epithelia. The boundary line is, however, behind that part of the epithelium of the mandibular process which gives origin to the teeth.

Implantation keratinizing epidermoid cysts may occur in other parts of the mouth as a result of trauma (Ettinger and Manderson, 1973). These cysts are of limited size and remain small over many years. A definite history of trauma to the area 11 years before was recorded in a case of a midline cyst of the lower lip (Papanayotou and Kayavis, 1977).

Abrams, Andrews and Laskin (1977) described an implantation epidermoid cyst which occurred in the mandibular condyle following surgical treatment in the region 2 years previously.

Pathological features

As already indicated, both dermoid and epidermoid cysts are lined by keratinized epidermis. Occasional cases may have areas of pseudostratified ciliated columnar epithelium but cysts of the floor of the mouth lined predominantly by secretory epithelium are probably of salivary duct origin (Sadeghi and Bell, 1980). The dermoid cysts are characterized by the presence in the wall of one or more dermal appendages such as hair follicles, sweat glands or sebaceous glands (**Figure 15.2**). Hair is very rarely found. The lumen is usually filled with keratin.

Sewerin and Praetorius (1974) described the occurrence of keratin-filled epidermoid cysts of the vermilion border of the lower lip which they believed represent dilated excretory ducts of the sebaceous glands. Serial sectioning of material from their cases revealed an orifice which formed a direct connection between the cystic cavity and the surface. Consecutive sections also showed a

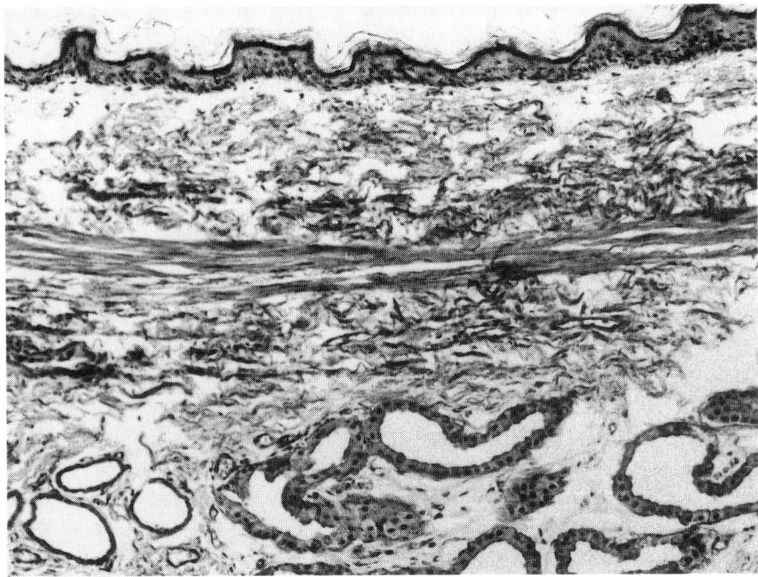

Figure 15.2. Dermoid cyst with dermal appendages in the wall. (H & E; × 100.)

sebaceous gland in the wall at one level and not at another and they emphasized that serial sectioning is obviously necessary before one attempts to label a cyst as either dermoid or epidermoid. In view of the ubiquity of sebaceous glands (Fordyce spots) in the oral mucosa, Allard (1982) speculated also that some so-called dermoid cysts are in fact epidermoid cysts with the fortuitous presence of Fordyce spots in the wall.

Olsen, Mostofi and Lagrotteria (1988) described a rare case of steatocystoma simplex in the maxillary buccal vestibule of a 65-year-old man. Histologically, the lesion consisted of a submucosal cyst lined by a thin stratified squamous epithelium containing sebaceous gland acini. No dermal appendages were found in the cyst wall.

Eppley, Bell and Sclaroff (1985) described the simultaneous occurrence of dermoid and heterotopic intestinal cysts in the floor of the mouth of a newborn boy. One cyst was lined by partly keratinizing, partly non-keratinizing stratified squamous epithelium with adnexal structures. The other was lined by non-ciliated columnar epithelium and contained within its wall, parietal and chief cells in some sections, and Paneth cells and goblet cells in others. A similar case was described by Arcand, Granger and Brochu (1988). A further account of oral alimentary tract cysts is given later in this chapter.

Ohishi *et al.* (1985) have described one of the rare varieties of teratoid cyst which occurred in the lateral part of the floor of the mouth of a 5-year-old boy. The cyst was lined by keratinizing stratified squamous epithelium, and sebaceous glands, sweat glands and cartilage were present in the wall, as well as other tissues compatible with the anatomical location of the lesion. Another rare variety of cyst was described by Miller and Houston (1989) in the cheek of a 26-year-old man. Histological examination showed that it was an ectopic apocrine cyst. The cyst was

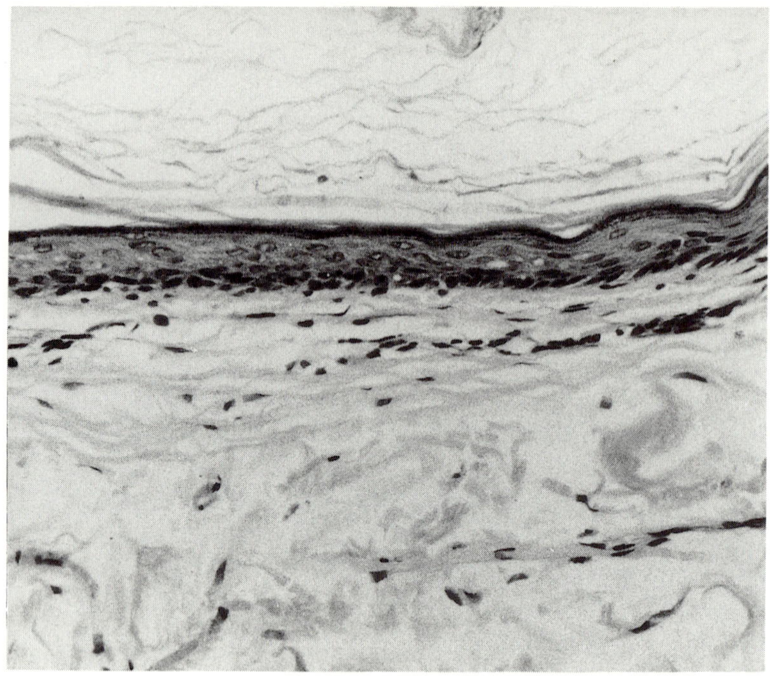

Figure 15.3. Epidermal cyst of the skin. There is a prominent stratum granulosum. (H & E; × 320.)

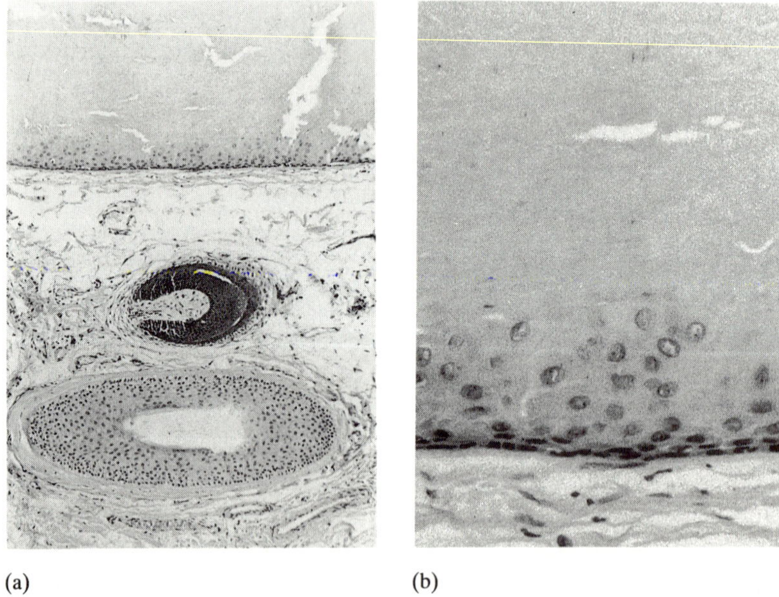

(a) (b)

Figure 15.4. (a) Trichilemmal (pilar) cyst of the skin. (H & E; × 50.) (b) Trichilemmal (pilar) cyst of the skin, showing the swelling of the superficial epithelial cells. There is no stratum granulosum. (H & E; × 270.)

lined by stratified squamous epithelium but in parts there were rows of secretory cells of variable height showing 'decapitation' secretion of the apocrine type.

A case has been reported of an epidermoid cyst in the mucosa of the cheek which contained in its wall an intradermal naevus and structures identical to Meissner's tactile corpuscles (Gutmann *et al.*, 1978).

Treatment

Treatment of epidermoid and dermoid cysts of the soft tissues is by surgical excision. A detailed account of the treatment of sublingual dermoid cysts is given in Chapter 18.

Keratinous cysts of the skin

Keratinous cysts may occur on the skin of the face, neck and scalp. Two varieties can be distinguished histologically. The commonest type is the epidermal cyst. These are often produced by traumatic implantation and hence are most frequently found on the hands and fingers. They are lined by keratinized stratified squamous epithelium with a prominent stratum granulosum (**Figure 15.3**). When part of the cyst lining ulcerates, a chronic inflammatory cell infiltration and foreign body type multinucleate giant cells are seen in the cyst wall.

The less common variety of keratinous cyst is the trichilemmal (pilar) type. These usually occur on the scalp, but rarely may be seen on the face, neck, trunk and extremities. They are lined by a stratified squamous epithelium but no stratum granulosum is formed (**Figure 15.4**). The superficial epithelial cells are swollen. The cornified layer of the epidermal cyst has a lower cystine content than stratum corneum of the skin and, moreover, citrulline is present. The trichilemmal cyst content is low in sulphur-containing amino acids and differs in this respect from hair cortex (Rosai, 1981). The term 'sebaceous cyst' which was used for this lesion is outmoded.

Lympho-epithelial (branchial cleft) cyst

The lympho-epithelial or branchial cleft cyst is a lesion whose pathogenesis has evoked considerable controversy, which is why it is referred to by two different names. Its location in the neck, in the parotid gland and intraorally, will be dealt with separately in this section and I shall use the two terms interchangeably.

Lympho-epithelial cysts of the neck

The commonest location of lympho-epithelial (branchial cleft) cysts is superficially in the neck, close to the angle of the mandible, anterior to the sterno-cleidomastoid muscle. They occur at all ages with a fairly equal distribution from the first to the sixth decades according to Rickles and Little (1967), but most commonly in the third decade according to Allard (1982). There is no sex predilection.

The neck lesions vary in size from small to very large (about 10 cm diameter). The most frequent symptoms are swelling, which may be progressive or intermittent, and pain. Sometimes attention is drawn to the lesions or they enlarge in response to a dental or upper respiratory tract infection. In view of their thick wall and fluid contents they impart, on palpation, a sensation similar to that of a partly-filled hot water bottle. They are demonstrable by ultrasound (Earl and Ward-Booth, 1985).

In a summary of the histological features of 689 branchial cysts of the neck reported in the literature, Allard (1982) found that in 96 per cent the cyst was lined by stratified squamous epithelium and the wall contained lymphoid tissue which was usually arranged in a follicular pattern. Cysts lined by ciliated or non-ciliated columnar epithelium or pseudostratified columnar epithelium were occasionally described.

The classic view of its pathogenesis in the neck has been that the branchial cyst develops from epithelial remnants of the branchial clefts and pouches. Bhaskar and Bernier (1959) postulated, however, that the neck cyst is not of branchial origin but that about 96 per cent of them in reality represent cysts in cervical lymph nodes. The cystic change occurs in salivary gland epithelium which is trapped in the nodes of the neck during embryogenesis. They proposed, therefore, that the lesion should be called 'lymphoepithelial cyst' rather than 'branchial cyst', supporting a suggestion that had been made by King (1949).

In their study, Rickles and Little (1967) concluded that several structures may give rise to the epithelium lining the cysts which occur in the neck. The few cysts found in the upper-neck region could develop from either salivary gland inclusions in parotid lymph nodes or from epithelial remnants of the upper portion of the branchial apparatus. The majority of cysts found in the midneck region could develop from epithelial remnants of the cervical sinus and/or the branchial pharyngeal pouches, both of which are part of the branchial apparatus. The cysts found in the lower-neck region may develop from remnants of the thymic duct or from the lower portion of the branchial apparatus.

Histochemical and ultrastructural studies by Howie and Crocker (1981) indicated that the epithelial linings of branchial cysts of the neck are similar to the crypt epithelium of palatine tonsils, suggesting that this epithelium might be the origin of the cyst linings. The immunohistochemical studies of Hirota *et al.* (1989) were unable to resolve the problem and they concluded that it is likely that cervical lympho-epithelial cysts are derived from both epithelial remnants of the branchial apparatus and from salivary inclusions in lymph nodes.

Lympho-epithelial cysts of the parotid gland

Lympho-epithelial cysts also occur in the parotid gland. A recent publication (Camilleri and Lloyd, 1990) indicated that about 70 cases have been reported in the literature. The age range was 16 to 69 years and there was a male:female ratio of 3:1. It is important that this lesion be differentiated from neoplasms, particularly cystic low-grade mucoepidermoid carcinoma and from cystic types of benign lymphoepithelial lesion (Weidner *et al.*, 1986). The latter authors reported five cases. All their patients consulted a doctor because of nodules in the parotid gland.

Histologically, all consisted of epithelial lined multilocular cystic spaces enclosed by dense lymphoid tissue composed of small lymphocytes, plasma cells and germinal centres. No subcapsular or medullary lymphatic sinusoids were seen. In three cases the epithelium appeared 'mucoepidermoid', being composed of variable mixtures of cuboidal cells and mucin-producing columnar cells. In these cases the epithelium was either stratified or composed of a single layer of cuboidal cells. In a few areas invagination of the epithelium into adjacent lymphoid or fibrous stroma formed small epithelial nests that were both solid and microcystic. In other areas the epithelium was papillary. In two lesions the epithelial component was entirely squamous and contained intercellular bridges. Mitotic figures were rare. All their patients were treated by superficial parotidectomy.

Hong *et al.* (1990) reported a case of a benign lympho-epithelial lesion with two large cysts in the parotid gland of a 60-year-old woman with Sjögren's syndrome. In view of the HLA-DR expression by the epithelium, the authors concluded that the cyst epithelium resulted from duct dilatation in response to an immune reaction.

AIDS-related bilateral lympho-epithelial cysts of the parotid associated with cervical lymphadenopathy

Holliday *et al.* (1988) reported an association between lympho-epithelial cysts of the parotid, cervical lymphadenopathy and infection by the human immunodeficiency virus. Their series consisted of 18 male patients ranging from 22 to 53 years, of whom 10 were homosexual and eight intravenous drug users. All patients had painless facial swellings and in four cases these were bilateral. Computed tomographic (CT) scans showed that 15 patients had multiple cysts in the parotid and in 14 of them the lesions were bilateral. All patients had multiple enlarged cervical lymph nodes. Eleven of 13 patients tested had antibodies to human immunodeficiency virus (HIV) and two of the others later developed AIDS. Fine needle aspirates showed benign lymphocytes and squamous or cuboidal epithelial cells. Histologically, the lesions consisted of cysts lined by cuboidal and squamous epithelium surrounded by lymphoid tissue with prominent germinal centres. The authors warned that the CT findings of multiple parotid cysts and cervical adenopathy may indicate, before the onset of opportunistic infections, that the patient is infected with the HIV virus. The patients should be referred for HIV testing and parotidectomy should be deferred.

Shugar *et al.* (1988) reported the same syndrome in nine homosexual males. CT and magnetic resonance scanning revealed that all but one of the patients had bilateral multiple intraparotid cysts and all had cervical lymphadenopathy. Fine needle aspirates were consistent with benign cysts and histological examination showed multiple cysts lined by epithelium suggestive of dilated salivary gland ducts. These were surrounded by a lymphoid hyperplasia containing enlarged germinal centres. In some specimens there was a uniform follicular hyperplasia. It would appear that the primary lesion is a lymphoid hyperplasia, as occurs in the cervical lymph nodes. Partial obstruction of salivary gland ducts within the hyperplastic parotid lymphoid tissue leads to the development of the cysts.

Elliott and Oertel (1990) reported 14 lympho-epithelial cysts of the salivary glands, 13 from the parotid, which were diagnosed in 11 patients. Thirteen of the cases had occurred within the past 6 years. Five patients were tested for evidence of HIV infection, and all were positive. Six patients had varying degrees of lymphadenopathy. The cysts were lined by stratified squamous epithelium and occasionally by cuboidal epithelial cells. Multinucleate giant cells with abundant eosinophilic cytoplasm were found in four cases in the lumen of the cyst or just below the epithelial lining or in the lymphohistiocytic infiltrate. Atrophy of surrounding salivary gland parenchyma with lymphocytic infiltration of the ductal epithelium suggested cell-mediated immune destruction of the epithelial cells of the ducts in response to infection by the virus.

Intraoral lympho-epithelial cysts

Intraoral lympho-epithelial cysts affect mainly the floor of the mouth and the tongue. Bhaskar (1966) reported a series of 24 intraoral lesions, 15 of which were in the floor of mouth and nine in the tongue. Most of the tongue cases involved the lateral margin. The age range was 15–65 years. No case occurred in the first decade and the majority were found in the third, fourth and fifth decades. Males (17 cases) were involved more frequently than females (seven cases). The cysts usually appeared as non-ulcerated, freely movable masses which had been present for periods ranging from 1 month to many years. Schiødt and Friis-Hasché (1972) reviewed the literature and their findings were essentially the same as Bhaskar's. Giunta and Cataldo (1973) reported a series of 21 of their own intraoral cases. The ages of their patients ranged from 7 to 65 years. There were 12 females and nine males. Seventeen of the cases (80 per cent) involved the floor of the mouth, two were in the soft palate and one each in the retromolar area and the mandibular labial vestibule. They ranged in size from 3 to 15 mm in greatest diameter, with an average of 6 mm. More than half of the cases were diagnosed clinically as mucoceles. All were treated by surgical removal without recurrence.

An analysis of 38 intraoral examples from their own files was done by Buchner and Hansen (1980). Their patients ranged in age from 14 to 81 years with most being in the third (nine cases), fourth (10 cases) and sixth (eight cases) decades. Twenty-three of their patients were males (61 per cent) and 15 were females (39 per cent). As in other series the most common location was the floor of mouth (50 per cent) followed by the ventral and the posterolateral surfaces of the tongue, each with 18.4 per cent. The remaining examples were found on the soft palate, anterior palatine pillar and buccal vestibule.

Allard (1982) did an extensive review of the literature and found 105 cases, to which he added three of his own. The youngest reported patient was 7 years and the oldest 81 years, with a peak frequency of 42 per cent in the third decade. Males were involved in 64 per cent of cases and females in 36 per cent. The floor of the mouth was involved in 69 per cent of cases, the tongue in 23 per cent, and other locations such as soft palate, buccal vestibule and anterior pillar of fauces in the other 8 per cent.

Most of the reported lesions were symptomless and were detected on routine examination, but a few patients complained of swelling or discharge. Their size ranged from 1–10 mm. The usual observation was of a round or oval swelling of the oral mucosa of normal colour except when large when they were yellow or white. The masses were submucosal and freely mobile. Some were described as firm, others as soft. The clinical diagnosis was frequently incorrect, many being described as mucoceles, lipomas or irritation fibromas.

With regard to pathogenesis, Bhaskar (1966) believed that as the oral cavity contains foci of lymphoid tissue it is possible that ectopic glandular epithelium within these foci can undergo cystic change and form the lympho-epithelial cyst of the oral cavity. Support for this view came from Vickers and von der Muhll (1966) who performed surgical autogenous transplants of hamsters' cheek pouch epithelium into their submandibular lymph nodes. In seven of nine experimental animals, inclusion cysts lined by keratinized stratified squamous epithelium formed within the lymph nodes.

Knapp (1970a and b) described what he called 'oral tonsils' and the possible role of these structures in the pathogenesis of the intraoral lympho-epithelial cyst.

These oral tonsils are normal structures in the oral mucosa which resemble the tonsils in Waldeyer's ring. They are 1–3 mm in diameter and are found in varying numbers on the soft palate, ventral surface of tongue and floor of mouth. Knapp postulated that lympho-epithelial cysts are in fact pseudocysts which develop in oral tonsils in which the crypt opening becomes plugged. Accumulation of retained material leads to formation of the pseudocyst. Buchner and Hansen (1980) were of the opinion that this pathogenesis was tenable in some, but not all lympho-epithelial cysts. Continuity between cyst and surface epithelium can be demonstrated in only some specimens, even in serial sections. It seems possible that both pathogenetic mechanisms may play a role in the development of intraoral lympho-epithelial cysts.

Further support for Knapp's hypothesis came from work by Howie and Crocker (1981). Their histochemical and ultrastructural studies showed that the epithelial linings of branchial cysts of the neck have many similarities to the crypt epithelium of palatine tonsils. They demonstrated that the epithelium of branchial cysts is a specialized tissue, not simply an inactive lining separating the cyst lumen from lymphoid tissue, in that, like tonsillar crypt epithelium, microvillous cells on its surface and an infiltrate of cells within intra-epithelial channels appear to be important in the function of antigen handling.

The studies of Toto, Wortel and Joseph (1982) supported the view that the intraoral lesion is a pseudocyst and that the epithelium could be of tonsillar crypt or of salivary duct origin.

The lympho-epithelial cyst in the mouth is usually lined by stratified squamous epithelium devoid of rete ridges and which may be keratinized (**Figure 15.6**). The keratotic layer is usually parakeratinized and only occasionally orthokeratinized (Buchner and Hansen, 1980). The majority of cysts in the neck are lined by stratified squamous epithelium. Many fewer, in both the neck and mouth, are lined by ciliated or non-ciliated pseudostratified columnar epithelium which may contain goblet cells and a few have a lining of simple cuboidal or flat epithelium (Rickles and Little, 1967; Buchner and Hansen, 1980). Areas of ulceration occur. The epithelium is closely enveloped by lymphoid tissue. In most cases the lymphoid tissue encircles the entire cyst (**Figure 15.5**) but in a few it is present in only part of the wall. In the majority of cysts the lymphoid tissue shows typical germinal centres (**Figures 15.5** and **15.6**) but in the others only a diffuse, dense infiltrate of lymphocytes may be present (Calonius, Hakala and Rapola, 1974; Buchner and Hansen, 1980). The lumen contains mainly desquamated parakeratotic cells (**Figure 15.6**).

Treatment

An account of the surgical treatment of branchial cysts of the neck is given in Chapter 18. The intraoral lympho-epithelial cyst is treated by local surgical excision.

Thyroglossal duct cyst

The anlage of the median lobe of the thyroid gland develops at about the fourth week of intrauterine life from a site at the base of the tongue which is recognized later as the foramen caecum. A hollow epithelial stalk known as the thyroglossal

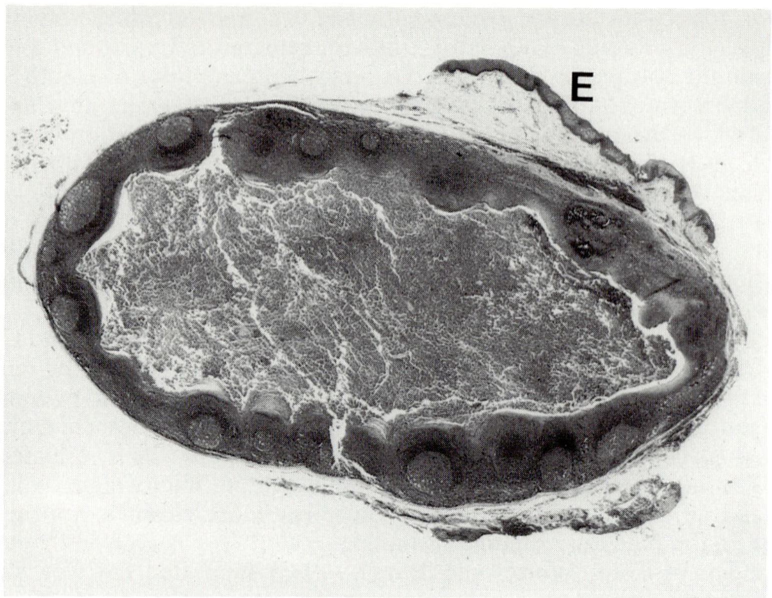

Figure 15.5. Lympho-epithelial cyst of floor of mouth. [E], oral epithelium. (H & E: × 10.)

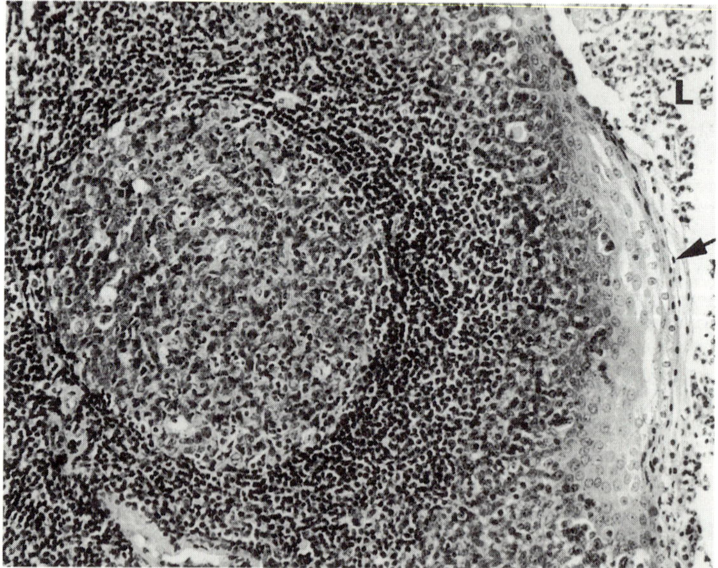

Figure 15.6. Higher magnification of lympho-epithelial cyst illustrated in Figure 15.5. The cyst is lined by stratified squamous epithelium (arrow). The lumen [L] contains desquamated parakeratotic cells. (H & E; × 150.)

duct, extends caudally and passes ventral to the hyoid bone to the ventral aspect of the thyroid cartilage where it joins the developing lateral lobes. The thyroglossal duct disintegrates by about the tenth week, but cysts may form from residues of the duct at any point along its line of descent. The aetiology is not known but inflammatory conditions which lead to reactive hyperplasia of the lymphoid tissue adjacent to the remnants of the thyroglossal tract and may stimulate the epithelial remnants themselves, have been mentioned, as has a blocked thyroglossal duct with an accumulation of secretion (Allard, 1982).

Allard (1982) undertook an extensive review of the literature which garnered 1747 cases, and found an equal sex distribution. In a slightly smaller sample of 1316 cases for which patient ages or decades were available, 32 per cent were younger than 10 years, 20 per cent were in their second decade, 14 per cent in their third and 35 per cent were older than 30 years.

The cysts are most commonly located in the area of the hyoid bone, and when they occur in the mouth, they do so either in the floor or at the foramen caecum. A proportion of thyroglossal duct cysts have an associated fistula. The cysts are usually in the midline and produce soft, movable, sometimes fluctuant, sometimes tender swellings. Sometimes they may be located laterally. Classically, they lift when the patient swallows or protrudes the tongue. If they are located high in the tract they may cause dysphonia or dyspnoea.

Histologically, they are lined by a pseudostratified columnar epithelium which may be ciliated, or by a stratified squamous epithelium. The latter type of epithelium is seen particularly in cysts close to the mouth. Thyroid tissue may be seen in the fibrous wall (**Figure 15.7**). Mucous cells may be present in the cyst wall and seromucous glands in the wall (Wampler, Krolls and Johnson, 1978), particularly if the cysts are located in the lingual area. In the same region prominent germinal centres may occur in the wall. Malignant change has occasionally been observed. A review of the literature on the subject revealed nine cases in which squamous carcinoma had developed (Lustmann, Benoliel and Zeltser, 1989).

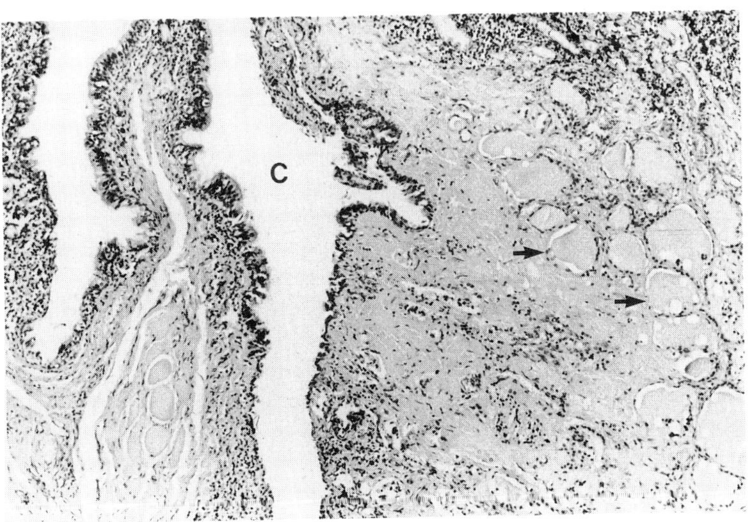

Figure 15.7. Thyroglossal duct cyst [C] lined by pseudostratified columnar epithelium. Thyroid tissue (arrows) is present in the wall. (H & E; × 45.)

Treatment

Surgical excision is usually advised for the treatment of thyroglossal duct cysts. The Sistrunk operation involves removal of a 1 cm block of tissue surrounding the duct and a 1–2 cm portion of the central part of the hyoid bone. The thyroglossal tract should also be traced down to the pyramidal lobe of thyroid gland and to the foramen caecum at the base of the tongue (Wampler, Krolls and Johnson, 1978). Reporting on a series of 16 thyroglossal duct cysts in patients over the age of 30 years, van der Wal *et al.* (1987) stated that there were no recurrences in eight patients who had been treated with the Sistrunk operation. The other group of eight were not treated for various reasons. Follow-up of these patients showed that the cyst had remained unchanged in one case, decreased in size in three and disappeared completely in the remaining four.

Anterior median lingual cyst (intralingual cyst of foregut origin)

The anterior median lingual cyst is a rare lesion. A case was reported by Fink (1963) which occurred in a 5-year-old boy. There was a fluctuant swelling of the anterior half of the dorsum of the tongue. It had been present since birth and had recurred after it had been incised and drained 2 years before. The cyst was enucleated.

On histological examination, it was lined in different parts by pseudostratified ciliated columnar epithelium and by cuboidal epithelium. The fibrous capsule showed a moderate infiltration of chronic inflammatory cells. The same histological features were present in a case of ours where the cyst occurred on the tongue of a 2-year-old girl and had been present since birth (**Figure 15.8**). A similar case was described by Quinn (1960) in a 9-year-old boy and this was lined by a parakeratinized stratified squamous epithelium.

Constantinides, Davies and Cywes (1982) described two cases of congenital intralingual cyst which displayed the same features as our own and that of Fink. The first occurred in a new-born infant boy who had a large, tense cystic swelling within the anterior half of the tongue. It did not interfere with breathing but made feeding difficult. At operation, after this cyst was removed, further dissection revealed a second cyst embedded in the base of the tongue extending into the neck. The authors considered that the lesion was in fact an hour-glass shaped cyst. Histological examination revealed that the cyst was lined mainly by stratified squamous epithelium but a there was a narrow extension lined by pseudostratified ciliated columnar epithelium and tall columnar epithelium. There was no recurrence after 7 years.

Their second patient was a 9-month-old girl with a large cystic mass on the ventrum of the tongue which had been present since birth. It prevented her from closing her mouth and eating was difficult. A large fluid-filled cyst was enucleated from the substance of the tongue. Histologically, the cyst was lined by stratified squamous epithelium and ciliated and non-ciliated cuboidal 'respiratory type' epithelium. The authors suggested that these were foregut cysts which resulted from some derangement during the development and differentiation of the primitive foregut. They pointed out that the proximal part of the foregut normally undergoes a type of dichotomy along its longitudinal axis, giving rise to a ventral and dorsal tubular structure. The ventral part evolves into the tracheobroncho-

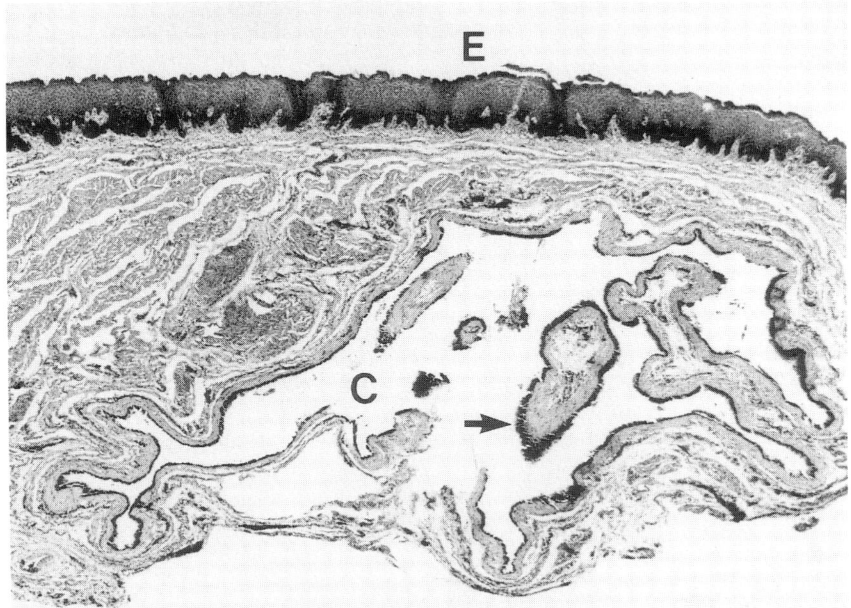

Figure 15.8. Anterior median lingual cyst (intralingual cyst of foregut origin) lined in part by cuboidal epithelium [C] and in part by ciliated pseudostratified columnar epithelium (arrow). [E], epithelium of tongue. (H & E; × 25.)

pulmonary tree, while the dorsal part develops into the oesophagus. The distal part of the primitive foregut gives rise to the stomach and duodenum. Cysts or duplications can be found anywhere along the path of the primitive foregut. The responsible mechanism is not known and although the cysts are commonly referred to as duplications they do not seem to imitate final structures developed from the foregut but rather to be the result of a cluster of cells being separated from the main body of cells which go on to form the final organ. They suggested that as their two cysts were lined by ciliated epithelium they should be regarded as cysts of foregut origin since ciliated epithelium is the hallmark of the primitive foregut.

Oral cysts with gastric or intestinal epithelium (oral alimentary tract cyst)

The rare occurrence of cysts in the mouth containing gastric or intestinal epithelium has been reported from time to time, and Gorlin and Jirasek (1970) have reviewed the literature. Fourteen cases, including one of their own, have been included in their analysis. More recent reviews have been published by Allard (1982) who collected 18 cases from the literature. Eppley, Bell and Sclaroff (1985) reported the simultaneous occurrence of dermoid and heterotopic intestinal cysts in the floor of the mouth of a newborn, and a similar case was decribed by Arcand, Granger and Brochu (1988).

Most cases have occurred in infants and young children. In Allard's survey, 12 patients were in the first year of life, three were between the ages of 2 and 11 years, and in two of the three adult patients the lesions had been present since childhood. The male to female ratio was 3:1. Eight cases were located in the anterior part of the tongue and two in the posterior part; three in the floor of the mouth, two in the anterior part of the neck and two in a submandibular salivary gland. The cysts may be enclosed entirely within the tongue or floor of mouth or may communicate with the surface.

The origin of the heterotopic gastric and intestinal mucosa is not known. Gorlin and Jirasek pointed out that in the 3–4 mm embryo the undifferentiated primitive stomach lies in the midneck region not far from the anlage of the tongue. Gastric mucosa has been shown to occur in the oesophagus of 7.8 per cent of infants and in 51 per cent of these the heterotopic tissue was located in the upper third. They suggested that in the sublingual region of the oral cavity and in the region of the apex and dorsum of the tongue, the ectodermal and endodermal epithelia fuse and mix. This may explain the presence of heterotopic gastric or intestinal mucosa. Cysts of the tongue and floor of the mouth could originate from the anterior portion of the primitive foregut (Constantinides, Davies and Cywes, 1982). Allard (1982) suggested that pluripotential embryonic cells may be responsible for the formation of the cysts in the zygomatic region.

Microscopically, the cysts may be lined partly by stratified squamous epithelium and partly by gastric or intestinal mucosa. Gastric mucosa is of the type seen in the body and fundus of the stomach. Both parietal and chief cells may be found. Gastric glands may be present. Some cysts have a muscularis mucosa. The cyst reported by Gorlin and Jirasek was lined with intestinal mucosa and Paneth cells, goblet cells and argentaffin cells were demonstrable. Another interesting feature of their case, which occurred on the floor of the mouth, was the presence of a tube which extended from the floor of the mouth into the cyst. The tube was lined by stratified squamous epithelium and adjacent sebaceous glands emptied into the tube.

Treatment

Treatment consists of surgical excision. Recurrences are rare but have been reported.

Cystic hygroma

The cystic hygroma is a developmental abnormality in which there is progressive dilatation of the lymphatic channels. It most frequently involves the face and neck although it can occur anywhere in the body.

It is often present at birth and most cases are diagnosed before the age of 2 years (Bayer and Hardman, 1976). Those which involve the facial tissues produce a swelling, often painless and usually compressible. The overlying skin may be blue and the swelling transilluminates. There may be a history of gradual or sudden enlargement.

Histologically, the cystic hygroma consists of dilated cystic spaces lined by endothelial cells.

Treatment should aim at complete surgical removal of the mass.

Nasopharyngeal cysts

Nasopharyngeal cysts are rare clinical entities which have been reviewed recently by Nicolai *et al.* (1989). They may be classifed as congenital or acquired, and midline and lateral. Retention cysts are the most frequent among midline cysts and are usually attributed to coalescence of the median recess of the pharyngeal tonsil. They are lined by ciliated or non-ciliated columnar epithelium with areas of squamous metaplasia in response to inflammatory stimuli. Lymphoid follicles are present in the wall. The cyst cavity is packed with epithelial debris.

Congenital midline cysts may arise either from the pharyngeal bursa (Tornwaldt's bursa) or from Rathke's pouch. Their clinical and histological features are similar to those of the retention cysts. Cysts arising from Rathke's pouch are exceedingly rare. They have a median base attached to the nasopharyngeal vault and lie anterior to the usual site of origin of the retention and pharyngeal bursa cysts. They are lined by stratified squamous epithelium, in keeping with their ectodermal origin.

Lateral nasopharyngeal cysts are usually of lympho-epithelial origin, and have been discussed previously.

Thymic cysts

Thymic cysts are rare clinical entities which arise in persistent thymic tissue which may occur in any location between the angle of the mandible and the midline of the upper neck to the sternal notch (Carpenter, 1982). Histologically, the cyst is lined by squamous and cuboidal epithelium and thymic tissue is present in the wall.

Chapter 16

Cysts of the salivary glands

Mucoceles

Mucous extravasation cysts and mucous retention cysts are often referred to collectively as mucoceles. Our practice has been to use the term 'mucous extravasation cyst' for those lesions in which mucus has extravasated into the connective tissues and in which there is no epithelial lining. The term 'mucous retention cyst' is employed to describe mucoceles which are lined by epithelium. Eversole (1987) preferred the term 'sialocyst' for the epithelial-lined lesion.

Clinical features

Frequency

Mucoceles of the mouth are very common. Their true incidence is difficult to determine as many patients endure them without seeking treatment, and of those diagnosed a large number are not surgically excised and do not reach a pathology department. Series of cases of mucoceles of the mouth have been reported by Bhaskar, Bolden and Weinmann (1956b), Standish and Shafer (1959), Gardner, Gallagher and Glaser (1963), Robinson and Hjørting-Hansen (1964), Cohen (1965), Cataldo and Mosadomi (1970), Southam (1974), Harrison (1975), Eversole, 1987, and Yamasoba *et al.* (1990). During the period 1958–78, our own department had collected 180 mococeles in 179 patients. Of these, 147 (82 per cent) were extravasation and 33 (18 per cent) were retention cysts. This represents a higher proportion of retention cysts than in the series reported by Cataldo and Mosadomi (4.0 per cent of 594), Standish and Shafer (6.2 per cent of 97), Cohen (9 per cent of 80), Southam (5.1 per cent of 236 mucoceles), Eversole (6.2 per cent of 1380 mucoceles), and Yamasoba *et al.* (2.9 per cent of 70 mucoceles of the lower lip); but similar to those of Chaudhry *et al.* (1960) (16.5 per cent of 66) and Robinson and Hjørting-Hansen (17.6 per cent of 125).

Age

The ages of the patients at diagnosis in a series of 151 of our cases is shown in **Figure 16.1**. The youngest patient was 8 months and the oldest 88 years, with a peak frequency in the third decade. Other studies have shown a peak frequency in the second decade and have included more cases in children up to the age of 9, but

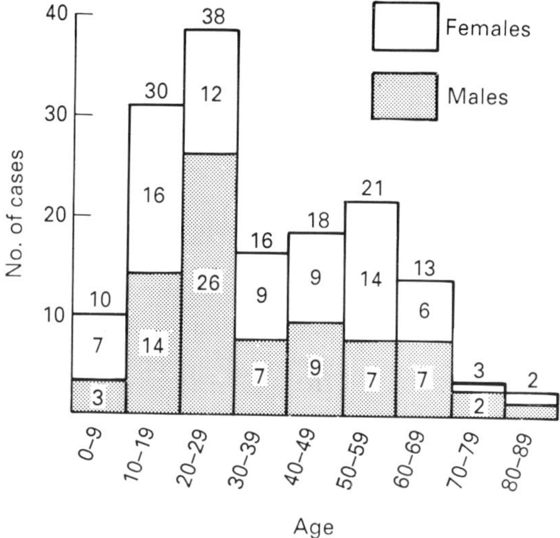

Figure 16.1. Age distribution of 151 patients with oral mucoceles.

all agree that most cases are seen before the age of 50. One example recorded by Standish and Shafer was present at birth and Poker and Hopper (1990) reported one which occurred in the tongue of a 10-week-old girl. In the large series of 594 cases reported by Cataldo and Mosadomi (1970) 16 (2.7 per cent) were in infants less than 1 year old. Southam found that all but one of the 12 retention cysts in his series were in patients over 50 years. Harrison (1975) analysed 400 mucoceles including 47 of his own cases and the remainder from the literature. He pointed out that extravasation cysts occurred most often in younger patients (84 per cent in the first four decades), whereas retention cysts occurred more frequently in older patients (85 per cent older than 40). In my own sample, 20 of 30 patients with retention cysts were older than 40 (67 per cent). This would probably account for the bimodal trend seen in **Figure 16.1**. In Eversole's sample of retention cysts (sialocysts) cases were rare before the third decade where there was a peak frequency, and there was a second peak in the seventh decade. His samples of reactive oncocytoid and mucopapillary sialocysts occurred in older patients.

Sex

In our material, the distribution was 95 males (52 per cent) and 88 females (48 per cent). In most studies there has been an equal sex frequency. Retention cysts are found somewhat more frequently in women than in men.

Race

A substantial proportion of our cases occurred in whites, an observation made also by Standish and Shafer, by Robinson and Hjørting-Hansen and by Eversole.

Site

The great majority of mucoceles are found in the lower lip. In our material, 83 cases (54 per cent) occurred in this site. By comparison, very few occurred in the upper lip (5 per cent). The distribution of the remaining cases is shown in **Table 16.1** and is similar to those in other reported series. In Harrison's study, 72 per cent of extravasation cysts were found in the lower lip whereas 39 of 40 retention cysts occurred elsewhere in the mouth. The same was found in Eversole's sample where the retention cysts were most often found in the floor of the mouth followed by buccal mucosa, lower lip, palate, tongue and upper lip.

Table 16.1 Site distribution of 155 mucoceles

Site	*Number*	*Percentage*
Lower lip	83	53.6
Upper lip	8	5.2
Floor of mouth and ventrum of tongue	30	19.4
Palate	17	11.0
Buccal mucosa	14	9.0
Retromolar	3	1.9
Total	155	100.1

Clinical presentation

Patients with mucoceles usually complain of a painless swelling which is frequently recurrent. They may have been present for only a few days but some patients tolerate them for months or even years before seeking treatment. The swelling may develop suddenly at mealtimes and many drain spontaneously at intervals. Some 10 per cent of patients are able to relate the development of the cyst to trauma. The mucocele may be only 1–2 mm in diameter but it is usually larger, the majority of them being between 5 and 10 mm in diameter. The ranula is invariably larger than this. The cyst reported by Poker and Hopper (1990) on the ventral aspect of the tongue of an infant, was 3 cm in diameter and interfered severely with normal feeding.

The swellings are round or oval and smooth (**Figure 16.2**). The superficial lesions are blue and fluctuant while the deeper lesions are the colour of normal mucosa and are firmer. The superficial cysts give few diagnostic problems but the deeper firmer lesions may be confused with the fibro-epithelial polyp or a small salivary gland tumour. A firm well-demarcated lesion of the upper lip is more likely to be a salivary gland tumour than a mucocele. Some have been diagnosed as lipomas.

Pathogenesis

The pathogenesis of the mucocele has excited a great deal of interest. For many years it was generally believed that obstruction of a salivary duct led to its dilatation proximal to the obstruction, with the formation of an epithelial-lined retention cyst. This concept was questioned by Bhaskar, Bolden and Weinmann (1956a) who carried out experimental obstruction of the excretory ducts of the submaxillary-sublingual glands in mice over periods ranging from 6 days to 9½ months. They

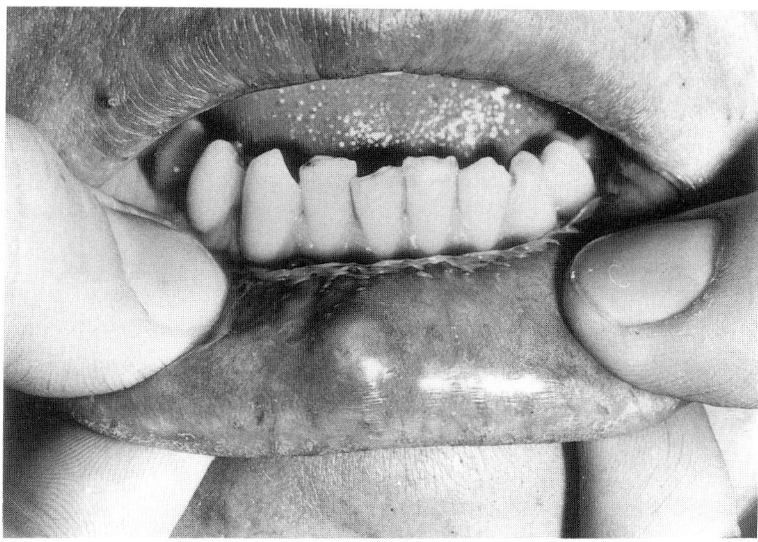

Figure 16.2. Mucocele of the lower lip. (By courtesy of Professor J. J. Pindborg.)

found that mucoceles did not develop although they did find microcyst-like spaces which they believed represented 'tangential cuts through the tortuous dilated ductal elements'. This study was followed by another series of experiments in which the right submaxillary excretory ducts of five young mice and six young rats were exposed and severed. The animals were sacrificed at intervals of from 1 to 9 days postoperatively and the glands were studied grossly and microscopically. They found that in six of the nine animals, severing of the duct produced typical mucoceles which were comparable to human lesions. In the early stages there was an accumulation of mucus in the connective tissue and with continuous pooling of saliva a clearly demarcated cavity developed which had no epithelial lining. They concluded that their experiments, when considered with the fact that mucoceles are found most frequently in areas exposed to trauma, such as the lower lip, indicated that a cut or a traumatic defect of a salivary duct was responsible for the production of mucoceles.

The failure to produce mucoceles following acute ligation of the main excretory ducts of the submaxillary and sublingual glands was confirmed experimentally by Standish and Shafer (1957). They did find, however, that when both the ducts and the arterial blood supply to the glands were ligated, thin-walled dilated ducts of cystic proportions occurred in some 8-, 12- and 16-week animals and appeared to be of submaxillary duct origin. In a later paper Standish and Shafer (1959) reinforced their view that the vast majority of so-called mucous retention cysts represent an extravasation phenomenon in which a ruptured duct allows the ready egress of mucus in the adjacent connective tissue. The smaller number of epithelial-lined mucoceles represent a partial retention phenomenon which is seen as a dilatation of the excretory duct and smaller lobular ducts with concomitant rupture and escape of mucus into the surrounding tissues.

Chaudhry *et al.* (1960) also concurred with these views but felt that complete severance of the minor salivary glands seemed an impracticable aetiological factor in the development of human mucoceles and that pinching of the duct seemed to be a more likely explanation for their formation. Their own experimental studies indicated that when the submandibular gland duct of the rat was cut or pinched with a haemostat, mucoceles may be formed by the escape of mucus into the surrounding tissues from the traumatized duct.

Experimental work done on cats (Harrison and Garrett, 1972) has, however, produced results which require that the effects of duct ligation be reappraised. These workers were at pains not to damage the chorda tympani and hence to avoid impairing the parasympathetic nerve supply to the glands. They therefore investigated the effects of duct ligation of the sublingual salivary gland of the cat. This gland secretes spontaneously, as do the minor salivary glands of man where mucoceles are most frequently found, and has a duct which may readily be tied anterior to the lingual nerve. They found that extravasation of mucus occurred in all glands up to 20 days after ligation. Ruptured acini were often observed in the first few days after ligation, but the ducts were not dilated and ductal ruptures were not seen. Ruptured acini were found only very occasionally after 2 days. These findings were reinforced in a later study by Harrison and Garrett (1975a). They suggested that following obstruction of the sublingual gland duct of the cat, continuing secretory activity in the gland results in rupture of acini and extravasation. If the macrophage and fibroblast reactions induced by the extravasated mucin are sufficiently intense in the first few days after ligation, then extension of the extravasated mucin and mucocele formation do not occur and the secretory acini become atrophic. If, however, the extravasation is too great to be contained in this way, a mucocele forms and the secretory acini remain active. Ultimately a balance appears to be achieved between the rate at which the secretions reach the mucocele and the rate of removal of fluid from the cavity of the mucocele. The fact that the minor salivary glands of man, like the cat sublingual gland, secrete spontaneously may be of significance in the pathogenesis of mucoceles of the oral mucosa.

A similar conclusion was reached by Praetorius and Hammarström (1974) based on a study of 200 mucoceles. They were of the opinion that trauma to the secretory acinar cells themselves led to their rupture and the formation of a pool of mucus, and that there need not necessarily be any rupture of the excretory ducts. They suggested that a mucocele formed in this way be termed the 'parenchymatous' type.

Mucoceles in humans may therefore follow trauma to a duct which is either pinched or severed; or trauma to the secretory acini, leading to the extravasation of mucus. Alternatively, complete ductal obstruction may lead to the development of a mucous extravasation cyst. The rarer mucous retention cyst which is lined by epithelium may possibly, from the very little evidence available, arise in some instances by partial or complete obstruction of the excretory duct by a salivary calculus, by congenital atresia of submandibular duct orifices (Hoggins and Hutton, 1974), by spontaneous dilatation (Southam, 1974) or by extraluminal causes such as periductal scar formation as a result of trauma. Factors which can lead to dilatation of the duct can also cause its rupture. The possibility of a different aetiology and pathogenesis for some retention cysts compared with the extravasation cysts is that more of the former appear to occur in an older age group, in females and in sites other than the lower lip.

The presence of eosinophilic oncocyte-like epithelial cells lining some retention cysts of the oral mucosa has led Southam (1974) to postulate that, in the absence of any evidence of duct blockage, these cysts may develop spontaneously in a duct lined by oncocytes. Alternatively, he suggested that they may represent a cystic type of papillary cystadenoma.

Pathology

Mucoceles are usually received in the laboratory excised with associated salivary gland and frequently a portion of oral mucosa is present on the superficial surface of the lesion. When the specimen is cut the cyst may be discrete, bound by a lining and filled with a gelatinous material. It may also be diffuse and have more liquid mucinous contents.

Histological features

Microscopically, three distinct morphological patterns of mucocele have been defined by Robinson and Hørting-Hansen (1964). The first two represent mucous extravasation cysts and the third, mucous retention cysts. Those designated 'poorly-defined cysts' consist of irregularly shaped, poorly-defined pools containing faintly eosinophilic mucinous material and numerous vacuolated macrophages which are sometimes called 'muciphages' (**Figure 16.3**). Some of these cysts are small and others extend widely into the connective tissue. There may be communication between the cyst and a duct (**Figure 16.4**). Those designated 'well-defined' cysts consist of two groups. Both are sharply circumscribed but they

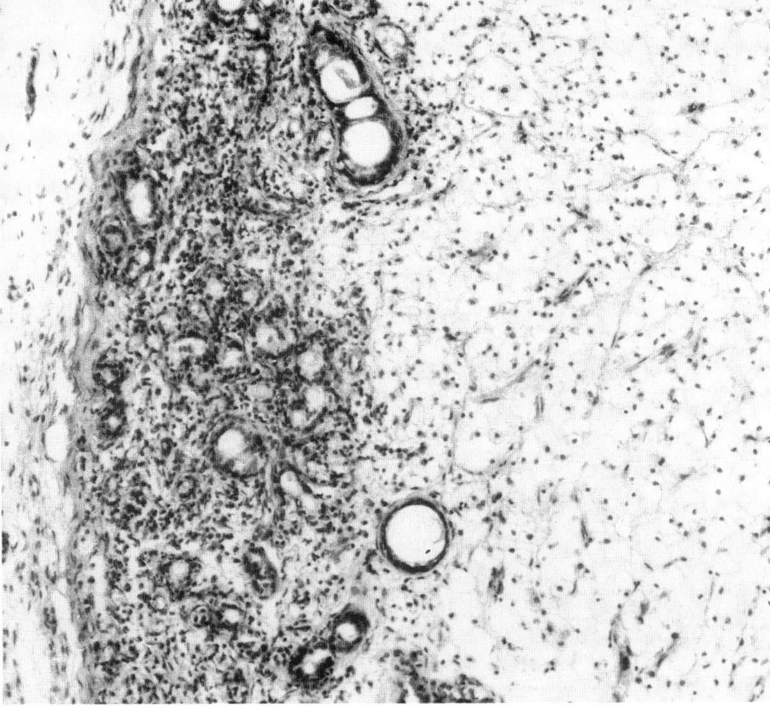

Figure 16.3. Poorly-defined mucous extravasation cyst filled with muciphages. (H & E; × 90.)

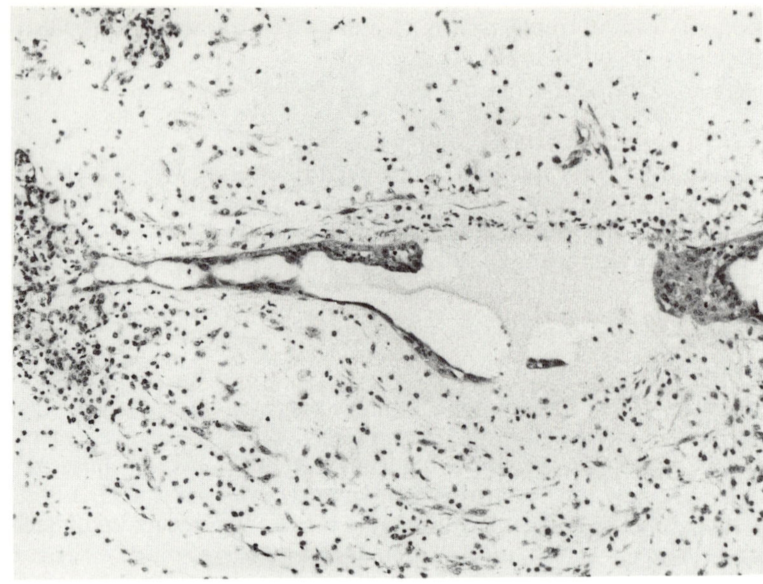

Figure 16.4. Ruptured duct with escaping mucus forming an extravasation cyst. (H & E; × 80.)

differ in that the periphery of the one consists of granulation tissue or condensed fibrous tissue or both, and is infiltrated by vacuolated macrophages, lymphocytes and polymorphonuclear leucocytes, including eosinophils (**Figure 16.7**). One or more dilated ducts may be present and sometimes a breach may be seen in a duct. The second group of well-defined cysts may be partially or completely lined by epithelium. The epithelium varies. It may consist of one or two layers of flattened cells or may be stratified squamous; or the lining may be of one or two layers of cuboidal cells or a thicker pseudostratified columnar epithelium (**Figure 16.5**).

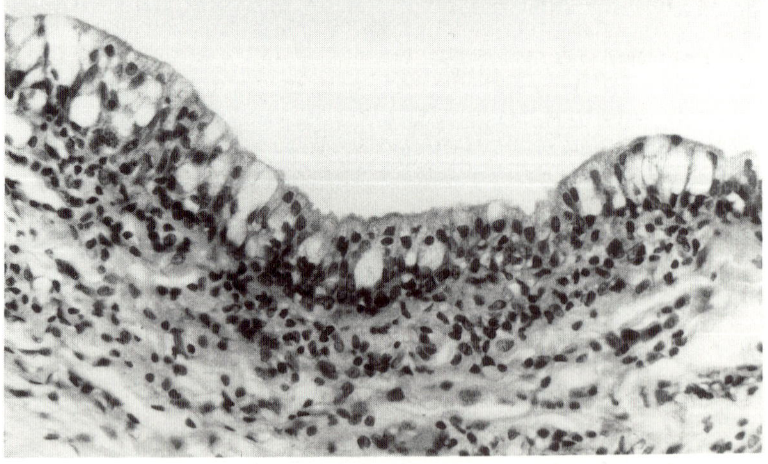

Figure 16.5. Mucocele lined by pseudostratified columnar epithelium with goblet cells. (H & E; × 235.)

Robinson and Hjørting-Hansen were able to demonstrate continuity between a cyst and a duct in 31 of their 150 cases (20 per cent). Granular eosinophilic oncocyte-like cells may be seen in the epithelial linings (Southam, 1974).

Eversole (1987) has done a detailed histological study of epithelial-lined mucoceles which he prefers to call sialocysts. He classified his sample of 121 cases into three subgroups: as mucous retention cysts (58 per cent), reactive oncocytoid cysts (34 per cent), and mucopapillary cysts (8 per cent). The microscopic criteria which he used for the diagnosis of the mucous retention cyst were the presence of a unicystic or multicystic cavity lined by non-oncocytic ductal epithelium with luminal mucous retention, no evidence of intraductal calcification and minimal inflammation in the wall. Of this subgroup, 82 per cent were unilocular while 18 per cent exhibited a tortuous or multicystic pattern. The lining epithelial cells were solely cuboidal in 52 per cent of examples, a combination of cuboidal and columnar cells in 22 per cent, cuboidal or columnar with mucous cells in 17 per cent, while in the remaining 9 per cent there were combinations of the above with foci of non-keratinizing stratified epithelium. None of these cysts recurred following excision.

Diagnosis of the reactive oncocytoid variety required the presence of oncocytoid metaplasia. They could be unicystic or multicystic and the lining cells were high columnar, often pseudostratified, with pronounced cytoplasmic eosinophilia. Seventy per cent were unicystic and the others showed multiple cystic foci. The adjacent minor salivary glands displayed mild sclerosing sialadenitis with ductal ectasia. Extralobular ducts were commonly lined by columnar oncocytes. In most cases the lining of the cysts was smooth but in about one-quarter of this group small papillary projections were present and the lesion then resembled the papillary cystadenoma. None of these cysts recurred following excisional biopsy.

Tal, Altini and Lemmer (1984) described a condition which they called 'multiple mucous retention cysts of the oral mucosa'. They reported two cases in which numerous minor salivary gland ducts, in one case more than 100, had dilated to form cysts. Histologically, there were numerous cysts and extensive ductal ectasia. Most of the small dilated ducts were lined by cuboidal and columnar oncocytes while the larger ones were lined by pseudostratified columnar epithelium containing mucus-secreting cells and many oncocytes. The duct orifices were dilated. In some areas there was a severe chronic inflammatory cell infiltration and the minor salivary gland tissue was replaced by fibrous tissue. The histological features in these cases closely resemble those of the reactive oncocytoid cyst but the extent of glandular involvement was remarkable.

There were 10 examples of the mucopapillary variety in Eversole's study. These were the rarest of the three varieties, and were large, tortuous and multicystic. They were lined by cuboidal and columnar epithelial cells with focal areas of squamous epithelium alternating with regions showing mucous metaplasia. Papillary projections lined with mucous cells protruded into the cyst cavities. Follow-up of this series ranged from 1–9 years and none recurred following complete local excision. These lesions have been described by a number of authors as papillary cystadenomas. Eversole disputed this diagnosis which implied that the lesions were neoplastic. Nevertheless, his interpretation of this lesion as a simple cyst must be regarded as controversial.

Ultrastructural findings on a naturally occurring mucocele in a cat suggested that the macrophages which are associated with the mucoceles ingest mucus and thereby form vacuoles (Harrison and Garrett, 1975b). Some lysosome-like structures

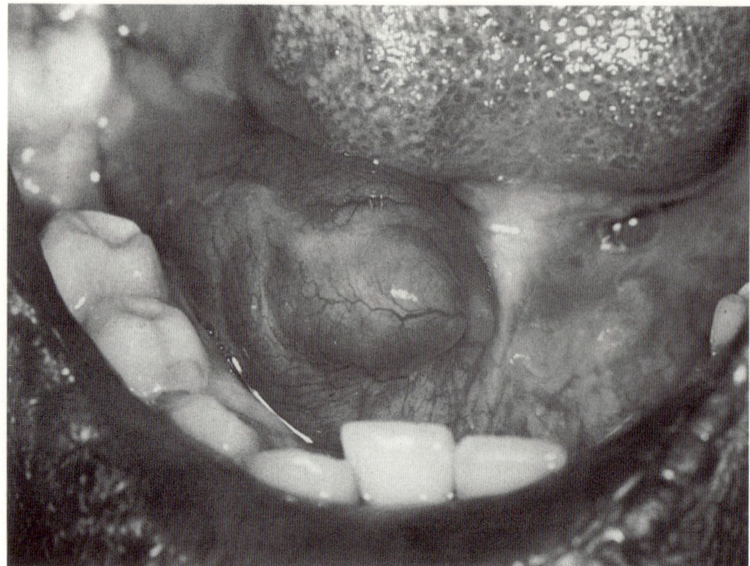

Figure 16.6. Ranula.

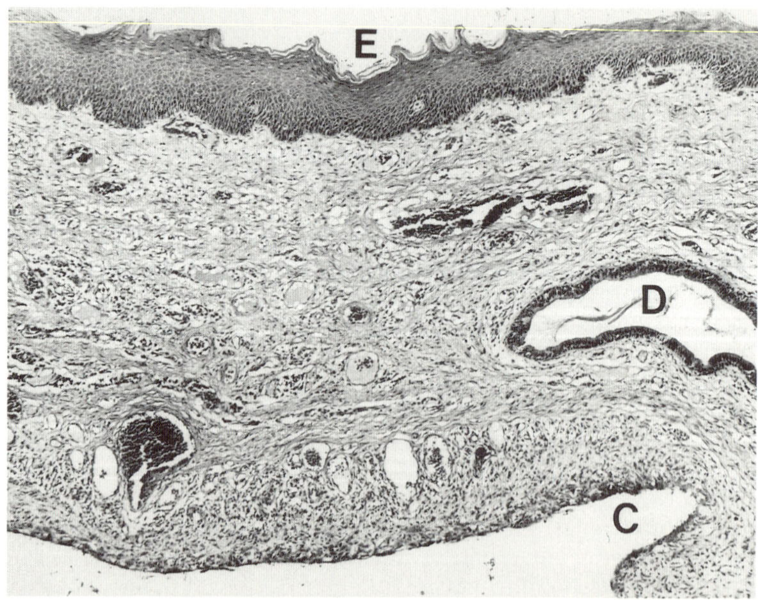

Figure 16.7. Ranula. The cyst [C] has a wall of granulation tissue containing inflammatory cells. [E], epithelium of floor of mouth; [D], dilated duct. (H & E; × 55.)

appear to release their contents into such vacuoles, presumably in an attempt to digest the mucus.

Treatment

Small mucoceles may require no surgical treatment provided that the patients find them no hindrance.

An account of the surgical treatment of mucoceles is given in Chapter 18.

Ranula

The term 'ranula' is used to describe those mucoceles occurring on the floor of the mouth (**Figure 16.6**). They are usually unilateral and because they produce a translucent blue swelling were likened to a frog's belly: from this the term 'ranula' was derived.

Ranulas have been classified as either superficial or plunging. The superficial variety may develop as a retention or extravasation phenomenon associated with trauma to one or more of the numerous excretory ducts of the sublingual salivary gland. Its pathogenesis and pathology are no different from those of the mucoceles elsewhere in the mouth. Significantly, the majority of these ranulas have no epithelial lining (**Figure 16.7**).

The pathogenesis and treatment of the plunging ranula have been controversial subjects. Roediger, Lloyd and Lawson (1973) have provided evidence to indicate that these ranulas are mucous extravasation cysts of sublingual gland origin which ramify diffusely into the neck. They recommended surgical removal of the sublingual gland through the mouth without any cervical approach, as the initial form of treatment. They argued that this removes the secreting source, thereby preventing recurrences, and also avoids the problem of a difficult neck dissection. Their observations and handling of the plunging ranula have been supported by McClatchey *et al.* (1984), de Visscher, van der Wal and Vogel (1989) and Galloway *et al.* (1989). Harrison, Sowray and Smith (1976) also referred to the persistent secretory activity of the sublingual glands. A deficiency or hiatus between the anterior and posterior parts of the mylohyoid muscle has been reported to be fairly common and herniated projections of the sublingual gland through these perforations may permit cervical mucous extravasation. Ectopic sublingual glands superficial to the mylohyoid may also provide a source for the extravasation (de Visscher, van der Wal and Vogel, 1989).

Congenital sublingual cysts may occur as a result of atresia of the submandibular duct orifices. In the two cases reported by Hoggins and Hutton (1974) it was possible to demonstrate that the cysts were, in fact, dilated submandibular ducts.

A further account of the surgical treatment of the ranula is given in Chapter 18.

Polycystic (dysgenetic) disease of the parotid glands

Seifert, Thomsen and Donath (1981) and Batsakis, Bruner and Luna (1988) have drawn attention to this condition which is probably of developmental origin. Its pathogenesis has been compared with the embryonic sequence of disturbances which lead to cystic malformations in other viscera such as the lung, pancreas, kidney and liver, although no such associated lesions have yet been reported in relation to the parotid gland lesion.

Although rare and only a few cases have yet been recorded, a consistent pattern has emerged. Clinically, it has occurred only in females; there was almost always bilateral parotid involvement; there was a history of fluctuating, non-tender parotid gland swelling for several years; overt clinical signs were delayed; and sialograms showed cystic alterations without involvement of the main parotid duct (Batsakis, Bruner and Luna, 1988).

Histological study of the series of cases reported by Batsakis, Bruner and Luna showed that the functional acinar parenchyma of the glands was almost completely replaced by a honeycombed, latticework-like multicystic lesion. Inspissated proteinaceous secretions were present in the cyst spaces. Small clusters of serous acini and occasional ducts lay in the intercystic fibrous septa. Often the cystic spaces appeared almost devoid of an epithelial lining because the cells were flattened and attenuated. Elsewhere the lining cells were cuboidal and often showed regressive hydropic changes and sloughing into the cysts. There was no squamous metaplasia and there was no evidence of inflammatory cells.

Familiarity with this disease should obviate the histological diagnosis of carcinoma. No surgery is necessary except for diagnosis and for cosmetic reasons if required.

Chapter 17

Parasitic cysts

Parasitic cysts occur in the mouth although they are rare. Valuable reviews have been published by Allard (1982) and Hansen and Allard (1984). Most of the reported cases of parasitic cysts in the mouth have been caused by the class Cestoda (flatworms and tapeworms). These include the genera *Echinococcus* and *Taenia*. There are two species of *Echinococcus, E. granulosus* and *E. multilocularis*; and two species of *Taenia*, *T. solium* and *T. saginata*. The class Nematoda (roundworms) produce oral lesions only exceptionally rarely. They include the genera *Trichinella, Gongylonema and Ascaris* with their respective species, *T. spiralis, G. pulchrum and A. lumbricoides*.

Hydatid cyst

Hydatid cysts occur in hydatid disease or echinococcosis. There are two species of the genus *Echinococcus, E. granulosus* and *E. multilocularis*. Hydatid disease is caused by the larvae of *E. granulosus*, the dog tapeworm. This tapeworm lives in the intestinal tract of the dog. Its ova are excreted in the faeces of the dog and may be ingested by the intermediate hosts, cattle, sheep and pigs. Man is also a susceptible intermediate host and, as dogs are common household pets, may accidentally ingest the ova.

The ingested ova hatch in the upper gastrointestinal tract from where the small embryos permeate the intestinal mucosa and are dispersed through the blood vessels and lymphatics to all parts of the body. The great majority of cysts are found in the liver, but others are found in the lungs, bones and brain. A few cases have been reported in the tongue. Perl, Perl and Goldberg (1972) have described a case in an 18-year-old black South African woman who complained of a painless swelling on the right side of the tongue which had been present for 3 months and was increasing in size. An intact unilocular cyst was removed which when cut in half revealed the presence of brood capsules. Five other reported cases were cited by Hansen and Allard (1984), which occurred in the tongue, cheeks and infratemporal fossa. Nandakumar and Shankaramba (1989) described a case in which a cyst had formed in the angle of the mandible of a 16-year-old male. The cyst was diagnosed at operation when the contents were accidentally spilled during enucleation and the presence of opaque, milky white particles were observed.

The hydatid cysts are initially of microscopic dimensions, but enlarge progressively. The mature cyst consists of three layers, one of host and two of

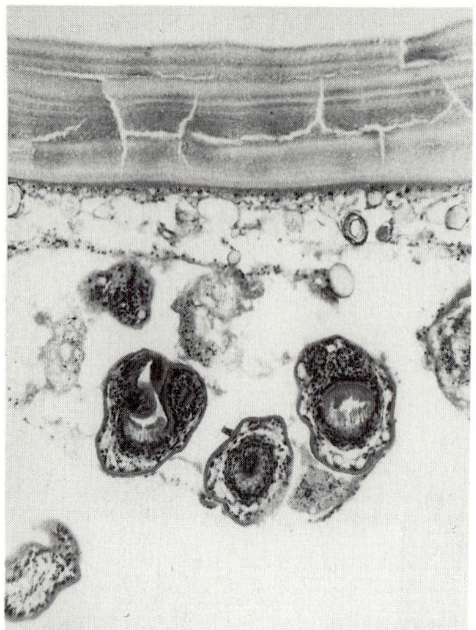

Figure 17.1. Hydatid cyst. Intermediate non-nucleated layer with germinative layer forming brood capsules on its inner aspect. The scolices are formed in these brood capsules. (H & E; × 100.)

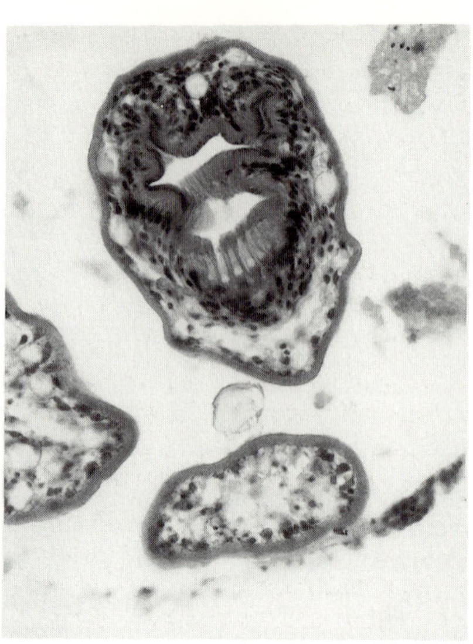

Figure 17.2. Scolex in the brood capsule of a hydatid cyst. (H & E; × 230.)

parasitic origin. The host layer consists of fibrous tissue in which there is an infiltrate of chronic inflammatory cells, eosinophils and giant cells. The intermediate layer is white, non-nucleated, and consists of numerous delicate laminations. It usually shrinks away from the outer fibrous layer when the tension within the cyst is relieved. Finally, there is the inner, nucleated germinal layer (**Figures 17.1**, **17.2**). The cyst fluid is relatively clear, albumin-free and contains the so-called 'hydatid sand' consisting of brood capsules and scolices. These brood capsules or daughter cysts develop originally as minute projections of the germinative layer which develop central vesicles and become minute cysts. Scolices of the head of the worm develop in the inner aspects of the brood capsules. It is when they separate from the germinative layer that they form the 'hydatid sand'.

Hydatid disease is common in sheep-raising countries such as Australia, New Zealand, Argentina and South Africa.

Cysticercus cellulosae

Man develops cysticercosis through the larval form, *Cysticercus cellulosae*, of the pork tapeworm *Taenia solium*. He can act as both the intermediate and the definitive host. The adult worm may be ingested in inadequately heated or frozen pork. Alternatively, man may ingest the cysticerci themselves from infested pork and these develop into the adult worm. This lives attached to the wall of the small intestine where, fully grown, it may reach a length of 7 m. Gravid proglottids or eggs begin to drop off and are passed in the faeces. In this way they may be ingested by man through contaminated food or from their own dirty hands, or they may be regurgitated into the stomach. In the stomach their covering is digested off and the larval forms are hatched. These penetrate the intestinal mucosa and are then distributed through the blood vessels and lymphatics to all parts of the body, where they develop into cysticerci.

There are very few reports of cysticercosis of the oral regions, but Rosencrans and Barak (1969) described a case which involved the lower lip and Timosca and Gavrilită (1974) have recorded five cases in Romanian patients. Two occurred subcutaneously in the neck, two deep to the cheek mucosa and one had multiple lesions involving the lip, cheek and skin. Three cases from our files have been reported by Ostrofsky and Baker (1975). One occurred as a swelling of the dorsum of the tongue in a 7-year-old child; another in the tongue of a 70-year-old man. The third was a firm mass 10 mm in diameter in the right cheek. Another two of our cases have been reported by Lustmann and Copelyn (1981). One occurred in the tongue of an 11-year-old boy and one in the tongue of a 25-year-old man. Hansen and Allard (1984) described four of their own cases, three in the lips and one in the cheeks. Their literature review identified 30 cases.

All the specimens examined in our laboratory have been intact cystic masses which, when cut, contained clear watery fluid and a coiled white structure apparently attached to the inner aspect of the cyst (**Figure 17.3**).

Histological examination of *Cysticercus cellulosae* shows a dense fibrous outer capsule which is derived from host tissue. This contains a fairly dense inflammatory cell infiltrate consisting predominantly of lymphocytes, plasma cells and histiocytes. On the inner aspect of this fibrous capsule, the nature of the infiltrate is different and consists of a dense aggregation of eosinophil and neutrophil polymorphonuclear leucocytes. A few foci of dystrophic calcification are present in this capsule, and some of these are concentrically laminated. Within the fibrous capsule is a delicate double-layered membrane consisting of an outer acellular hyaline eosinophilic layer and an inner, sparsely cellular layer. This membrane has

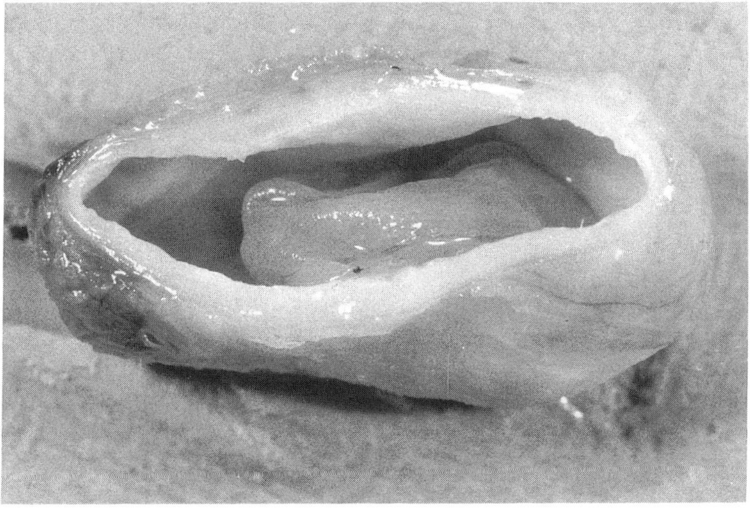

Figure 17.3. Gross specimen of *Cysticercus cellulosae* removed from tongue. (× 5.)

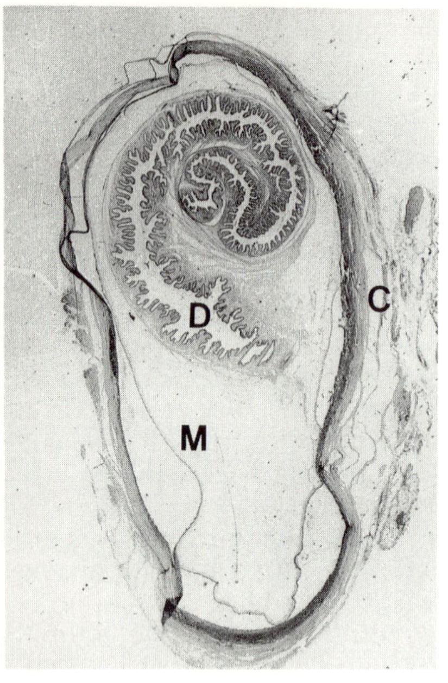

Figure 17.4. *Cysticercus cellulosae* containing the larval form of *Taenia solium*. [C], fibrous outer capsule; [M], double layered membrane; [D], duct-like invagination segment. (H & E; × 5.)

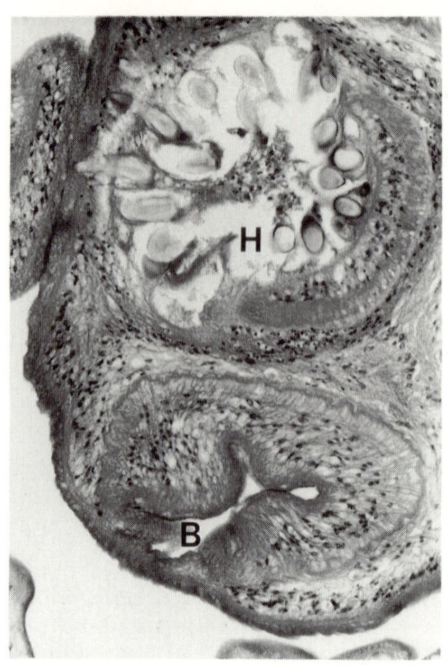

Figure 17.5. Scolex of larval form of *Taenia solium*. [B], bothria; [H], hooklets. (H & E; × 100.)

a loose attachment to the fibrous capsule and is readily torn away from it. The cyst lies within this membrane and contains the larval form of *T. solium* (**Figure 17.4**). At the cephalic extremity of the larva, the scolex with rostellum, bothria (suckers) and hooklets may be identified (**Figure 17.5**). Caudal to the scolex is the duct-like invagination segment lined by a homogeneous anhistic membrane.

Although *Cysticercus cellulosae* is harmless in the oral tissues, localization in the brain, heart valves and orbit occurs and produces important functional derangements. They may remain alive for many years. After their death a granulomatous reaction forms around the parasite, and calcifies.

Trichinosis

Trichinosis is caused by *T. spiralis* a roundworm parasite of rats and pigs. The reviews of Allard (1982) and Hansen and Allard (1984) revealed only two cases, one of which produced a tumour-like enlargement of the gingiva and the other a radiolucent area on the crest of the alveolar ridge. Microscopic examination showed an encysted form of *T. spiralis*. These reviews also identified two similar cases of oral lesions caused by the roundworm *G. pulchrum*.

Chapter 18

Treatment of cysts

Gordon R. Seward

Cysts of the jaws with an epithelial lining

The majority of epithelium-lined cysts of the jaws may be treated in a similar fashion. Enucleation of the entire cyst, including both the epithelial layer and the capsule with successful management of the resultant dead space is clearly curative. The free drainage of the liquid content of these cysts such that the cyst cavity remains empty of contents and in free communication with the mouth, is also curative. The cyst sac will shrink in size and new bone will be formed on its capsular aspect. The mechanism or mechanisms underlying such resolution are still to be fully resolved. At one time it was considered to be a simple question of decompression and removal of contents which had a greater osmolarity than the surrounding tissue and which consequently induced a positive internal hydrostatic pressure (see Chapters 2 and 11). It is now known that jaw cyst linings produce substances which stimulate the osteoclastic resorption of bone (see Chapters 5 and 11) and it is proposed that this is the primary cause of their enlargement. Nevertheless, the volume of the liquid contents of epithelium-lined cysts of the jaws is clearly related to the internal surface area of the sac. The surgically exposed lining is normally tensely filled by the contents and a papilliferous invagination into the cavity is not seen. Permanent drainage of the liquid contents results in shrinkage of the cyst lining. What is unclear is whether this is due simply to mechanical decompression or to the removal of a chemical stimulation of the bone resorptive abilities of the lining, or perhaps to both mechanisms.

Fortunately from the point of view of the operating surgeon successful, if empirical, treatment strategies have been developed. These will be discussed in relation to periapical radicular cysts; then the modifications in management of dentigerous cysts, keratocysts and other less common epithelium-lined cysts will be considered.

Regression of cysts without surgical treatment

There is good circumstantial evidence that some small radicular cysts will regress if the necrotic pulp remnants and/or bacteria are removed from the root canal of the causative tooth and the canal effectively filled. Circumscribed rounded zones of periapical bone destruction, perhaps up to 1.5 cm in diameter will be seen in some patients to reduce in size and resolve over a period of months. It is clear that this does not result from the drainage of the liquid contents through the canal as it occurs most successfully where the canal has been properly filled. Where root treatment of a tooth results in drainage of cyst contents through the canal and the lining is removed surgically subsequent to root filling there is often evidence of the early ingrowth of bone into the capsule, and this is the result of drainage. However, drainage through the canal is usually inadequate to produce complete healing. Indeed if the root canal is sealed between appointments drainage can only be intermittent. If the canal is left open and the apex widely perforated, the conditions required for the satisfactory filling of the canal are unlikely to be reached.

The evidence that there was a cyst present and that it regressed rests upon deductions made from the radiographic appearance, but since lesions of a modest size may respond in this way, the evidence is persuasive. This approach should be used with discretion and monitored by careful follow-up. Similar evidence comes from Oehlers' (1970) observations on the numbers, histological diagnosis and size of inflammatory periapical lesions seen about the teeth of matched series of Singaporeans before and after the removal of multiple diseased teeth. So, while continued drainage of the cyst contents results in the reduction in size of radicular cysts the reversal of chemical mechanisms of enlargement alone is the likely cause of healing in these particular circumstances.

As an occasional observation lateral dentigerous cysts located distally to the crowns of lower third molars may sometimes disappear following an episode of pericoronitis. Presumably the infection results in the drainage of the cyst into the pericoronal space beneath the operculum and perhaps also the destruction of the lining epithelium.

Marsupialization of dental cysts

The name of Partsch (1892) is normally associated with this operation although he also described enucleation of jaw cysts (1910) and it is unlikely that he was the sole originator or the only practitioner at the time using these methods.

Ready access to dental advice for a substantial proportion of the population is a relatively recent phenomenon even in Western societies, but as a result in the United Kingdom there has been a noticeable decline over 30 years in the size and number of jaw cysts seen even in busy departments of oral and maxillofacial surgery. Cysts with a volume of some 15–25 ml of contents or more are now rarities. Very large cysts which weakened the jaw were common in the past and were at one time treated by the insertion of a wide bore tube. This permitted the cyst to drain, and the cavity could be irrigated through the tube to try to control the accumulation of debris within and, of course, any infection. Making an opening into the cyst as large as is practical, and packing the cavity, is a more effective way of emptying the cyst. This is easy to accomplish where the patient is edentulous, or where the remaining teeth are extracted, and where a considerable opening can be made because the cyst is large.

The advantages of marsupialization are as follows:

(1) The procedure, at least for large cysts, is technically simple.
(2) Even quite large cysts can be dealt with under local anaesthesia as anaesthesia of the deeper recesses is not essential and this is particularly an advantage in the maxilla.
(3) Because the deeper parts of the lining are not disturbed closely adjacent important structures are not put at risk, namely, the blood vessels to the apices

of adjacent vital teeth, the inferior dental neurovascular bundle and the integrity of the linings of the antrum or nose.
(4) Marsupialization may be the best way to conserve the tooth of origin of a dentigerous cyst and to permit its eruption.
(5) It is probably the simplest way to treat a fracture complicating a large cyst of the mandible, because a ribbon gauze and Whitehead's varnish pack will splint the fragments. However, despite the presence of the cyst, a fracture will heal with subperiosteal callus if the jaw is immobilized. It is often proposed as the treatment of choice for very large cysts of the mandible as a means of reducing the risk of pathological fracture. In fact, it may be possible to enucleate such cysts through a smaller opening in the bony wall than is necessary for successful marsupialization so the problem revolves more around the management of a large intrabony haematoma.

The disadvantages of marsupialization are:

(1) The need for regular postoperative care, possibly over a substantial period of time. It is necessary to supervise healing so that the opening remains large in proportion to the underlying cavity.
(2) A rapid reduction in the size of the opening may be difficult to prevent. Indeed an opening into a large cyst in the ramus may present significant problems.
(3) Uneven reduction in size of the cavity may result in a slit-like cavity, difficult to keep clean.
(4) The change in voice which occurs when the cavity is not obturated and the accumulation of stagnant saliva and food debris in the cavity which leads to an unpleasant taste and smell.
(5) The need for greater attention to the details of surgical technique than is at first apparent to avoid complications.

The incision made when marsupializing a dental cyst is different from that made to permit primary closure after enucleation. A decision whether to pack the cavity or close the wound by suture must therefore be made preoperatively. The surgical cavity may be packed also after enucleation of the whole lining as a method of managing the dead space, so it is the intention to close the wound which is the important factor. Primary closure can only be undertaken following successful complete enucleation of the lining and with an appropriate flap design. It is valuable therefore to anticipate if there will be any difficulties in enucleating the lining.

Difficulty will be experienced:

(1) Where surgical access will be restricted for anatomical reasons.
(2) Because the cyst has been draining for some time and bone is actively growing into the capsule.
(3) If the cyst is chronically infected and the lining is friable or the lining is delicate because of the type of cyst.
(4) The cyst has penetrated the cortical plate at sites remote from the place of surgical access. It is easier to separate periosteum from lining than lining from periosteum, and easier to separate lining from the nasal mucosa than maxillary sinus mucosa. A small tear in nasal mucosa is usually repairable by suture. It is difficult to suture antral mucosa to produce a water-tight closure.
(5) The cyst involves the periodontal membranes of several teeth. The capsule is often adherent to periodontal membrane.

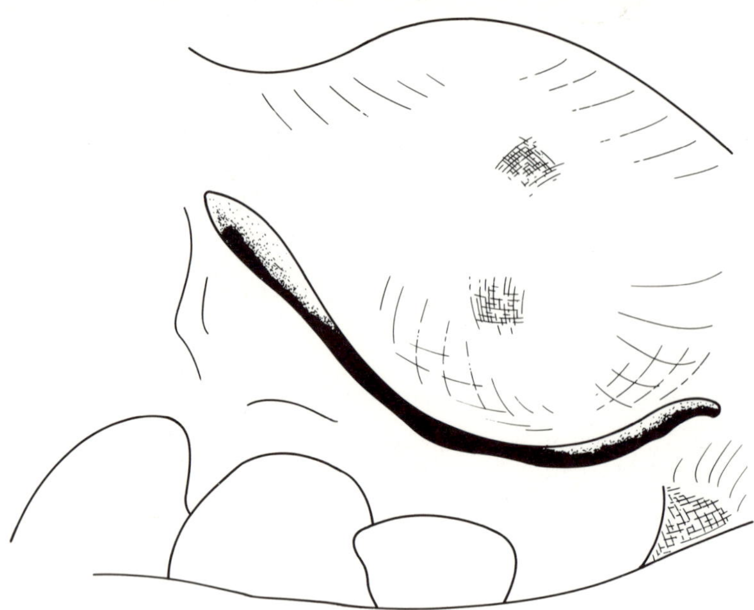

Figure 18.1. Illustration showing the U-shaped incision required to marsupialize a large radicular cyst on pulpless $\underline{|1}$. The root of $\underline{|2}$ is displaced distally.

Poor surgical access may mean that an adequate opening cannot be made for successful marsupialization. It may be better to change the surgical approach to improve access. Consideration of the other difficulties may favour marsupialization.

A U-shaped incision, based on the sulcus, outlines an area which is slightly smaller than the eventual bony opening into the cyst (**Figure 18.1**). This will leave a narrow rim of oral mucosa which can roll over the edge of the bone to become united to the cut edge of the cyst lining. The sulcus ends of the incision should be extended laterally to lie over unexpanded bone. Elevation of the periosteum starts at these points. This enables the operator to raise the flap in the correct tissue plane. It is unlikely that other than relatively large cysts will be marsupialized so it is probable that the cyst will have penetrated the bone. Provided elevation of the flap is started over intact bone it should be possible to continue elevation in the subperiosteal plane over the lining (**Figure 18.2**). Once the edge of the perforation is reached it is defined around the whole of its gingival aspect. This permits elevation of the flap from the surface of the protruding lining over a broad front. Pressure is applied to the undersurface of the periosteum just clear of its attachment to the underlying cyst, working backwards and forwards across the whole width of the flap.

If there is a sinus or sinus scar attaching the flap to the lining, separation of the flap should be continued on either side of it to define it closely. The sinus may then be separated with a scalpel held with the back of the blade flat against the lining.

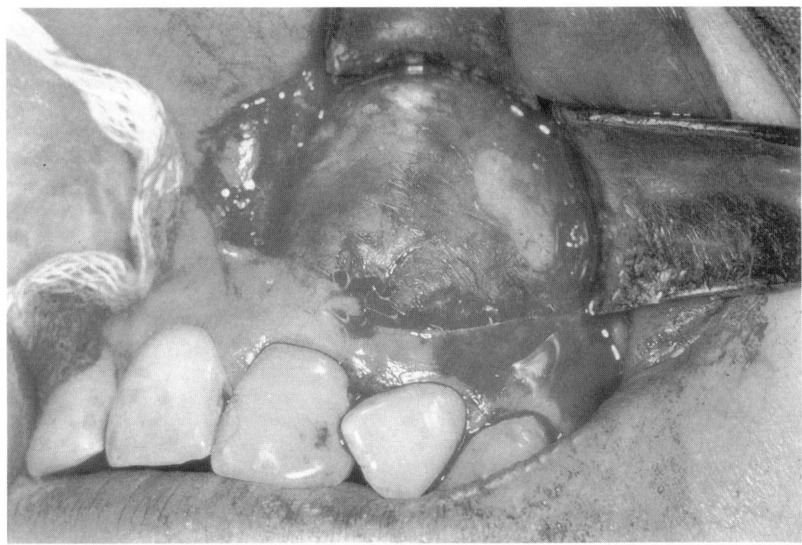

Figure 18.2. The same cyst after elevation of the flap. The large subperiosteal expansion is now seen. Little bone needs to be removed from the cortical perforation to make a suitable window.

Separation from the cyst lining should be continued at least until bone is again encountered and the whole periphery of the bony defect exposed. Elevation is advanced to the upper extent of the proposed surgical opening, under the hinge of the flap.

If there is no perforation in the outer cortex it will be necessary to remove bone with a large rose head bur until an extent of cyst lining has been uncovered. If, as is often the case, there is a natural perforation the cyst lining must be separated from the edge of the bone and the bone margin undermined. This way it is possible to remove further bone without risk of perforating the lining, particularly if bone nibblers are used. The bony opening should be made almost as wide as the maximum extent of the cyst, or as close to this as is possible without damage to adjacent structures.

A stab incision is made through the lining close to the edge of the bone with the point of a no. 11 scalpel blade. A no. 15 blade is inserted into the incision and the cut is continued, working from within outwards against the edge of the bone until a disc of lining has been removed flush with the bone edge (**Figure 18.3**). The specimen is sent for histological examination and the cavity irrigated gently with saline and inspected for any unusual features which would suggest a diagnosis other than a simple cyst.

A continuous 4/0 (2 metric) plain catgut suture may be run around the gingival aspect of the opening, joining oral mucosa to cyst lining. It is preferred that the related pulpless tooth should have been filled in an orthograde fashion preoperatively if the cyst is a radicular cyst. If this has not been done a retrograde filling may be placed at this point. If the tip of the root of such a tooth protrudes

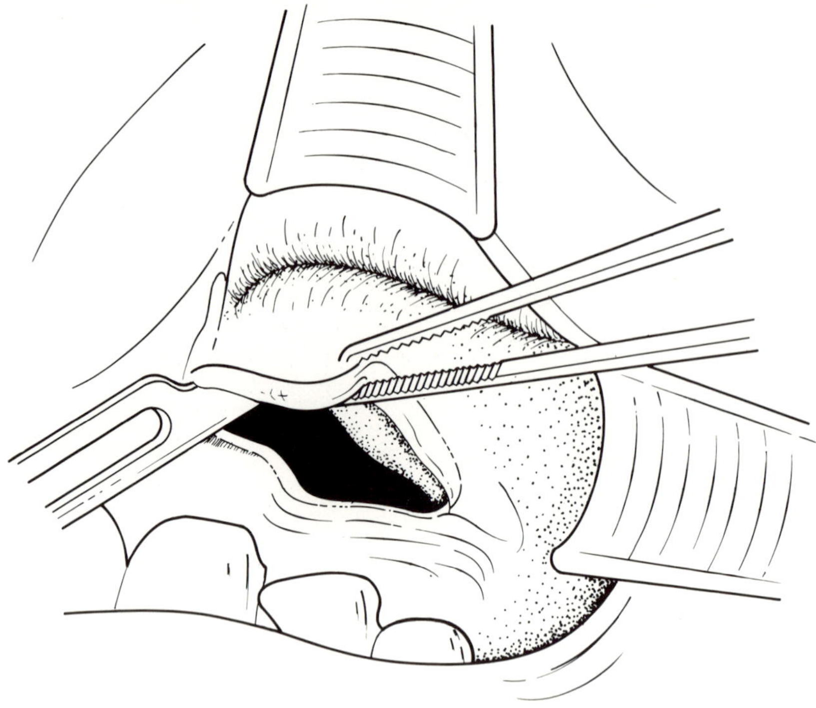

Figure 18.3. Diagram illustrating the method of removing the labial part of the lining.

through the lining it should be dressed down below the surface with a round bur as it is unlikely otherwise to be re-covered by soft tissue and then bone.

The flap is turned into the cavity and packed into place with ribbon gauze moistened with Whitehead's varnish (**Figure 18.4**). The cut end of the pack should be tucked in at the side of the pack so that it doesn't unravel. It does not matter if the flap overlies the cyst lining as the cyst epithelium will be destroyed and the flap will unite to the underlying capsule (Wassmund, 1935). Indeed in the maxilla the flap will reinforce the thin tissues where the cyst lining is in contact with antral or nasal lining. Wassmund would pass sutures from the flap edge through the palatal wall of the cyst to stretch it over the antral and nasal region.

The weaknesses of the marsupialization procedure are twofold: the difficulty in maintaining an adequate opening in many cases and the uncertainty about the speed and completeness with which the cavity will regress.

The size of the surgical opening is most stable where it is made through attached mucoperiosteum. Where the periphery is composed of mucosa supported by loose connective tissue wound contraction can reduce its size in as short a time as 48 h. (Wound contraction is due to contraction of existing connective tissue in a wound margin. A contracture is due to new collagen produced during healing.) The problem is greater still where the depth of soft tissue over the bone is substantial as over the anterior border of the ramus and where there is muscle in the edges of the opening.

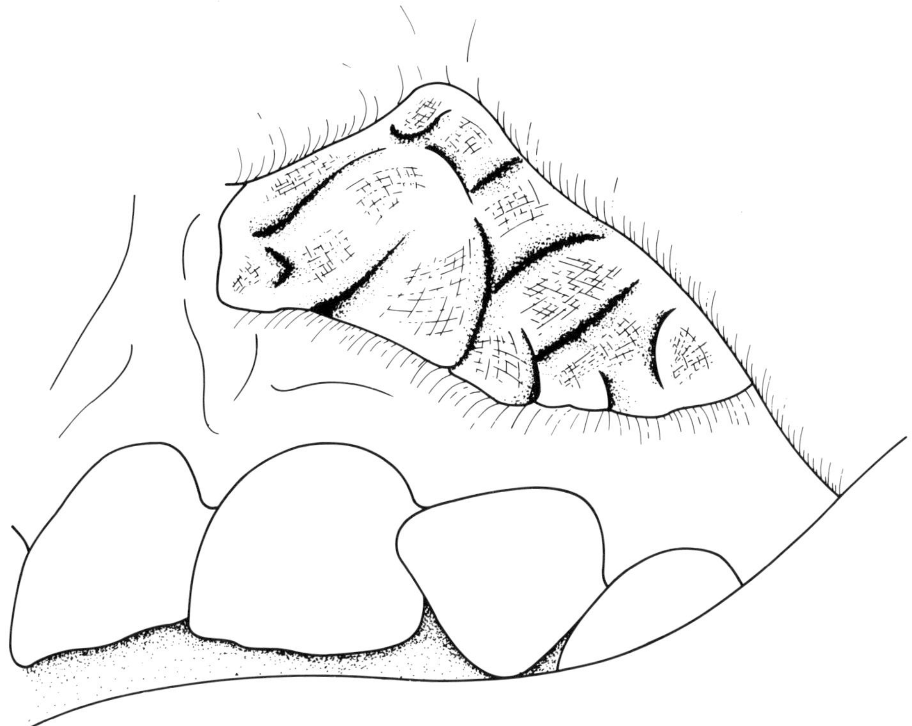

Figure 18.4. The ribbon gauze and Whitehead's varnish pack in place.

It requires some form of pack or plug to maintain the opening, but at the same time the obturator must not prevent reduction in size of the cavity. Constantly repacking the cavity is inconvenient. A silicone or acrylic plug can be fashioned and has the advantage that the deeper part can be trimmed while maintaining the diameter of the part in the opening.

Any plug must be retained sufficiently well not to be a hazard to the airway, particularly during sleep. However the patient must be able to remove it for a short while at regular intervals to irrigate and clean the cavity.

Mandibular cysts should not be marsupialized through the lingual plate as it is difficult to fit a satisfactory cyst plug and to irrigate the cavity from this side. Maxillary cysts should not be marsupialized through the palate as the normal contour of the plate may never be restored and satisfactory speech may be impossible without an acrylic plate.

Some cysts will fill in quickly if marsupialized. Very large cysts in both jaws predictably take many months and may never fill in completely. Because of the thick cortical plate in the mandible all benign cysts enlarge for a considerable distance along the medullary cavity before expanding subperiosteally. This behaviour is not just characteristic of keratocysts, but the belief that it is post-dates the time when large radicular and residual radicular cysts were common. These sausage-shaped cysts were often marsupialized to leave the crest of the ridge and the lingual wall. A denture was fitted on these and the buccal and labial flanges extended down to bear on the lower rim of the surgical opening. A permanently undercut ridge often remained.

In the anterior part of the maxilla the cyst lining may not become separated by bone from the palatal or nasal mucoperiosteum. A slit-like cavity results as healing progresses or a deep pit is left. It may be possible to excise the remaining lining, raising flaps about the periphery of the opening and performing secondary closure.

As healing progresses the lining shrinks in area but is probably never completely replaced by normal oral mucosa. Where the lining is noticeably different as seen with keratocysts or calcifying odontogenic cysts the residual patch of cyst lining may remain identifiable.

Enucleation and packing

Enucleation and packing carries most of the disadvantages of both marsupialization and enucleation and primary closure with few compensatory advantages. If the whole lining is enucleated adjacent anatomical structures are put at risk yet the advantages of primary closure are not achieved. Provided no damage is done by the enucleation it might be thought that healing by granulation of the whole cavity surface might provide a quicker reduction in size than after conventional marsupialization. In practice early epithelialization of the healing surface soon produces a cavity differing little from that which results when the lining is left.

It may be considered prudent to pack the cavity where access turns out to be more difficult than expected and the operator feels there may be fragments of retained lining. In practice this may not matter with radicular cysts and dentigerous cysts if the fragments are small but is clearly undesirable in the case of keratocysts. There is a practical problem in that the flap design for enucleation is different from that for marsupialization but the flap can be modified, and the part which rests on unoperated bone is sutured back in place while the rest is packed into the cavity.

The other indication is where a large cyst is chronically infected and unsuitable for enucleation and primary closure because of the certainty of wound breakdown. If normal marsupialization would leave an unsatisfactory opening liable to premature closure, enucleation and loose packing may be the answer, provided free drainage can be assured until all infection is under control.

Enucleation and primary closure

While it may be possible to modify an intraoral flap which has been designed with primary closure in mind to permit marsupialization it is rarely possible to produce a water-tight closure when the incision was designed for a marsupialization operation. Leakproof suture lines are normally produced by closing the wound in layers using continuous sutures. Eversion of the wound edge with a running horizontal mattress suture may increase the area of wound contact and ensure the integrity of the wound during the early healing phase. Bleeding within the wound must be controlled to prevent tension on the suture line. Where there is a dead space, ooze from the wall must be controlled before closure is started and a closed drainage system introduced to prevent any subsequent ooze overfilling the space.

Within the mouth an incision over the anterior border of the ramus can be closed in layers. There is rarely enough connective tissue of adequate strength beneath the mucosa in the buccal or labial sulcus to hold a suture line, even if periosteum is included. However, a continuous horizontal mattress suture of 4/0 chromic catgut can be inserted to close a horizontal incision in the sulcus because the tissues are elastic. The should evert the wound edge but should not be tight enough to act as a purse-string or threaten to strangulate the wound edge. To bring the wound edges together it is oversewn with a continuous plain suture of Vycril.

As it is not possible to close masticatory mucosa in layers a valve-like closure is effected. The incision is made well wide of the proposed bony opening to create a shelf of bone onto which the flap can be replaced (**Figure 18.5**). Haemorrhage into the cavity must be controlled before closure is started so that the blood clot is confined to the bony cavity and does not separate the flap from the bone. If this happens the valve-like arrangement is lost and early healing will only take place at the wound edge. Indeed tension may be created at the suture line and wound breakdown and infection of the haematoma supervene.

The size of the haematoma after successful enucleation and primary closure is dictated by the size of the bony cavity. The larger the haematoma, the longer the time before it is replaced by granulation tissue and the longer the period during which there is a risk that wound infection may occur. Normally once sound healing of the suture line has occurred the major risk of infection has passed. Initial healing is usually complete by 14 days after the operation. There should however remain no local means of ingress of infection. All suture materials should have been resorbed or should have been removed. Sutures should be disinfected with iodine before removal and cut close to the tissue surface to reduce the risk of drawing infected material into the wound. No roots or teeth with infected necrotic pulps, deep

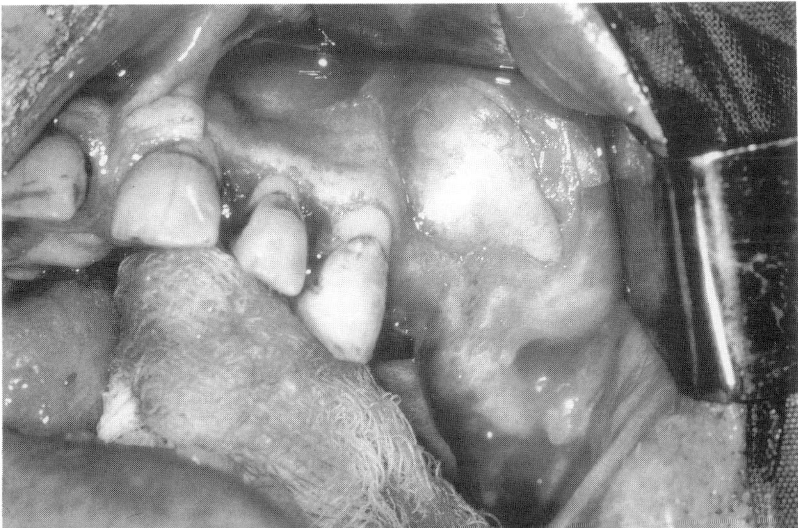

Figure 18.5. This photograph shows the design of flap appropriate for enucleation of the maxillary cyst, here seen presenting through a buccal cortical perforation.

periodontal pockets or gum flaps should be left near to the operation site and all known non-vital teeth should have been root-filled preoperatively.

At one time efforts were made to reduce the size of the blood clot by allowing the soft tissues to collapse through the opening in the outer cortical plate into the bone cavity (Brosch, 1957). This is particularly effective in reducing the size of a cavity in the ramus of the mandible. Unfortunately, the original bony contour may never be regained and a defect may be established which proves difficult to assess in the postoperative radiographs. The management of large maxillary cysts will be discussed in a further section.

As far as possible intraoral incisions are made 1–1.5 cm away from the anticipated outline of the opening to be made in the bone (**Figure 18.5**). The gingival margin of adjacent teeth will dictate the edge of the flap in this direction so this should be borne in mind during bone removal. Elevation of the flap and separation of the lining from the edge of any perforation in the cortex proceeds as before. Enlargement of the bony opening should be adequate to give good access to all parts of the cyst lining but with regard to the safety of related teeth and other anatomical structures (**Figure 18.6**). A Ward's periosteal elevator and a large bin-angled spoon excavator are two useful instruments with which to separate the lining from the wall of the bony cavity. The aim should be to remove the lining in one piece, without tearing it. To begin with it is best if the cyst remains tense. As the separation progresses deeper into the cavity some of the contents should be aspirated so that the lining can be adequately displaced to make it possible to see

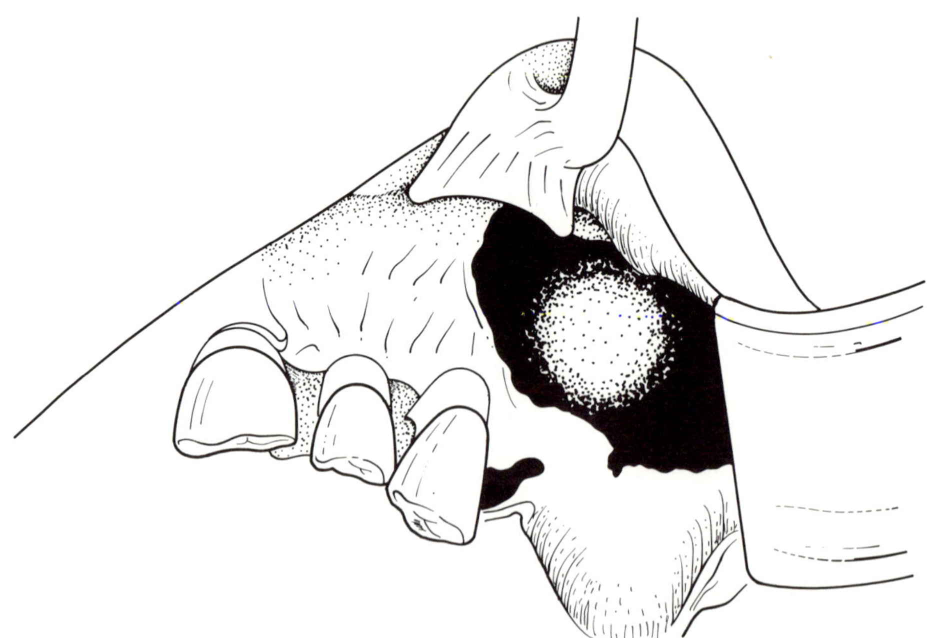

Figure 18.6. The opening in the bone has been enlarged and the cyst lining has been enucleated. A residual cyst from ⌊4 root.

the line of attachment. All places where separation is easy should be explored first. As soon as it becomes apparent that the cortex is perforated on the lingual or palatal side, then the mucoperiosteum should be raised from this aspect also until the entire periphery of the perforation is freed. In general it is easier to raise the periosteum from the cyst lining than to dissect the lining off the periosteum from within the bony cavity.

The lining will be difficult to separate from the periodontal membranes of markedly involved teeth. The most difficult situation is where the cavity extends lingually or palatally to the roots. The spoon excavator is a good instrument to use in this situation. Both the excavator and the Ward's periosteal elevator should be used with the convexity facing the lining. Away from difficult areas the edge of the instrument can be applied firmly to the bone. Consideration should be given to how the blood supply reaches the apices of adjacent vital teeth. Often, even when it appears radiographically that apices have been denuded of bone, a thin layer will still cover them. In other cases separating the lining in the direction of the apical vessels will peel it off without damage. Every effort must be made to visualize the line of attachment to the underside of the nasal mucosa so that the lining can be worked off systematically. Often there is still a tenuous layer of subperiosteal new bone over the dome of cysts which invaginate the antrum, which is fortunate as once the cyst lining is adherent to the sinus mucosa, successful dissection without tearing the antral lining is unlikely.

In the mandible it is the inferior dental neurovascular bundle which gives most cause for concern. Examination of rotational panoramic tomograms, lateral true occlusal films and a posteroanterior (PA) jaws view will enable the operator to work out its position in most cases. Usually it is displaced downwards and laterally. Units with a Scanora will be able to take hypocycloidal tomograms, both in cross-section and buccolingually, of restricted fields concentrated on the cyst, which will help sort out anatomical relationships. It is rarely necessary, or advantageous, to use computed tomographic (CT) scans.

The aim should be to free the cyst lining from all other parts except the area of the bundle. Dissection should proceed from front to back along the line of the nerve, never across it. Instruments will automatically come to lie between the lining and the nerve with this approach. Buccolingually, periosteal elevators will tend to follow the bony wall and pass under the bundle, so tearing it,

If the lining is tough it may be grasped with dissecting forceps and partly lifted out of the cavity to improve access to the deeper recesses. If it is friable such a move is hazardous. Great care with retraction, displacement, dissection and suction are required to avoid leaving portions of lining behind. The more delicate the lining the more generous the exposure must be. For a cyst in the ramus the relative advantages and disadvantages of an intraoral or submandibular approach should be considered.

Once enucleation is complete the cavity is freely irrigated with saline solution, sucked dry and inspected. The neat removal of an intact cyst sac will leave little cause for concern. If it has become torn, the cavity can be loosely packed while the lining is arranged on a swab and inspected. Areas where it is suspected that lining may have been retained should be irrigated, dried and inspected with a good light. Gentle teasing of the surface with a periosteal elevator will help, but damage to important structures should be avoided.

Next, the cavity is packed with ribbon gauze which is left in place for 5–10 min. Abseal (Ethicon Ltd), a paste of fibrin and collagen is applied to cancellous areas

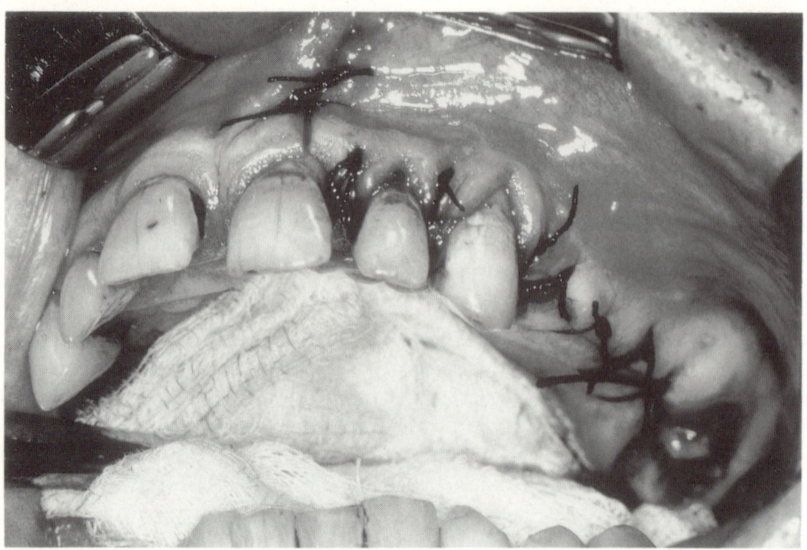

Figure 18.7. Wound closure for the same cyst. Note that the suture line is well away from the opening in the bone and there is no distension of the sulcus by blood clot.

or any patches which persistently ooze. Once haemostasis is adequately assured the wound may be closed (**Figure 18.7**). A Minivac drain may be passed from a large mandibular cyst out through the neck. Once closure is complete, firm pressure is applied to the flap for a further interval of time to try to ensure adherence to the underlying bone. If possible a postoperative gauze pack with tails is moistened with saline and applied over the flap for the early postoperative period.

Sutures are removed 7–14 days postoperatively dependent upon the degree to which local tissue activity puts tension on the flap.

Enucleation of cysts through the palate

Radicular cysts arising from upper lateral incisors and dentigerous cysts on supernumeraries in the upper incisor region and on canines tend to enlarge beneath and towards the nose and ultimately bulge the palate downwards. The major part of the cavity is on the palatal aspect of the roots of the teeth and their blood supply runs through the bony wall labial and buccal to the cavity. Only a limited opening can be made from the labial aspect without risk of damage to the teeth.

In such cases a palatal approach is the obvious direct route. A palatal flap, therefore, is raised from around the necks of the maxillary teeth and reflected backwards well clear of the posterior limit of any bony expansion. In creating an adequate exposure it is usually necessary to remove bone over the cyst to within a few millimetres of the alveolar margin. This does not matter because palatal flaps seal back onto the underlying bone very well as they are non-elastic and do not tend to contract away at the edges. The periodontal membranes and roots of adjacent teeth must not be uncovered and the margins of the alveolar bone must not be damaged (**Figure 18.8**).

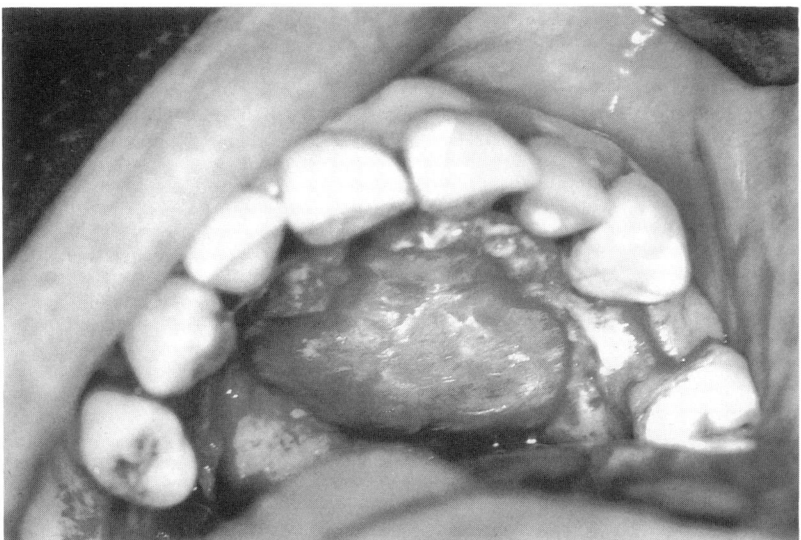

Figure 18.8. A palatal flap has been reflected and bone has been removed to expose the lining of a cyst, arising from pulpless |2 and lying mainly in the palate.

The cyst lining is enucleated in the usual way. The spoon excavator may need to be used to separate it from the periodontal membranes of adjacent teeth and care will be required in peeling it off the nasal and antral extensions. In the case of a radicular cyst, root filling must be completed preoperatively as there is clearly no possibility of placing a retrograde filling. If there is an extension on the labial aspect of the lateral incisor root this may give trouble and warrant an additional limited lateral approach.

If an impression is taken preoperatively a simple acrylic palatal plate can be prepared with cribs on suitable cheek teeth. After haemostasis has been achieved in the usual way and the flap sutured back into position the plate is inserted with a small amount of softened black gutta-percha attached to the underside (**Figure 18.9**). This will correct the contour of the palate where it was previously expanded. The plate is removed, the gutta-percha is chilled and it is reinserted to confine the blood clot within the bony cavity. It should be worn for 1 week. As has been indicated, healing of the palatal flap margins proceeds very quickly (**Figure 18.10**).

The advantages and disadvantages of enucleation and primary closure

The advantages are clear; once the surgical wound has healed the patient finds the mouth returned to normal and is unaware of the relatively slow resolution of the intrabony cavity. Healing within the cavity takes place from all aspects, instead of just the inner half as when a cyst is marsupialized, and the contour of the jaw is largely preserved.

The major disadvantage is the enhanced risk to adjacent structures. A realistic assessment of this risk must be made and discussed with the patient preoperatively. Adequate warnings of possible complications must be given and a record of these made in the notes. If, for example, the risks of anaesthesia of the lower lip or of the

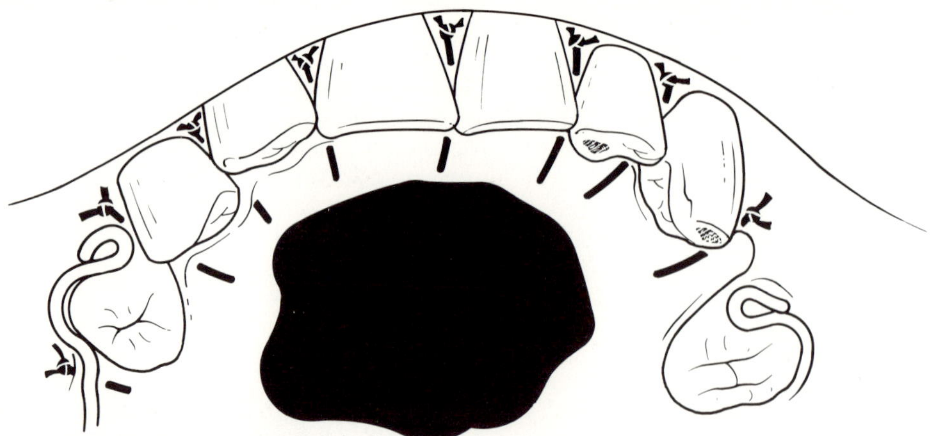

Figure 18.9. Diagram to show the palatal plate, relined with gutta-percha.

need to root-fill many teeth are considerable, it may be appropriate to marsupialize the cyst. The pros and cons of alternative treatment should be discussed and the reasons for your preference made clear.

Postoperative follow-up

Initially the cavity will be filled with firm blood clot. During the first few weeks, although granulation tissue will be growing into the clot, the centre will liquefy and the region of the bony deficit will feel softer. It will become firm again as more

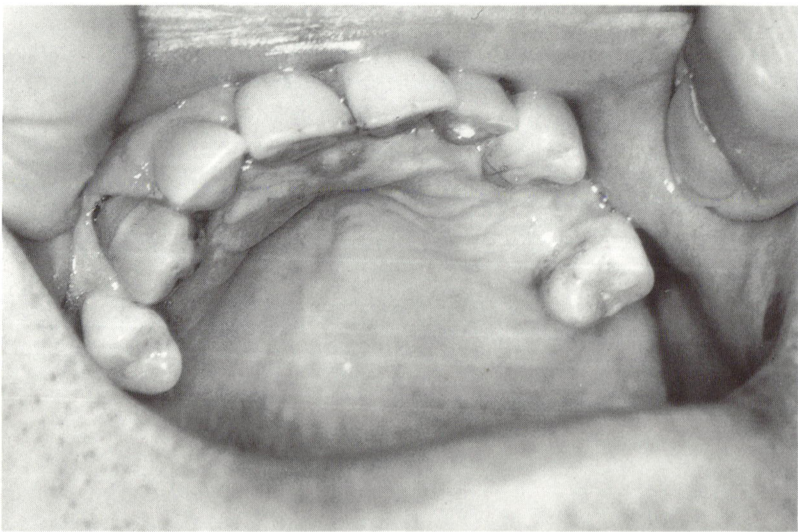

Figure 18.10. A photograph taken 2 weeks postoperatively to show the excellent contour of the healed palate at this stage. |2 was root-filled preoperatively.

granulations are formed and subperiosteal new bone is deposited. If substantial amounts of cortex have been removed to gain access to the cyst, subperiosteal new bone may be deposited over other aspects of that part of the jaw. Usually new bone trabeculae can be detected radiating inwards from the circumference of the cyst from about 3 months onwards. Depending upon the size of the cyst it will take 6–18 months or even longer for complete healing to occur, as seen in serial radiographs.

The patient is reviewed weekly for the first 3 weeks; then after a further month, at 6 months postoperatively and then annually, depending upon evidence of complete healing and the need for subsequent follow-up. With keratocysts the follow-up should be for a minimum of 5 years.

Treatment of large cysts of the maxilla

While the thinnest continuous layer of subperiosteal new bone remains over the dome of the cyst where it invaginates the maxillary sinus, it is likely that the operator can enucleate a cyst with care without penetrating into the antrum. Because closure of a tear in the antral lining so as to produce a leak-free suture line is difficult, infection of the blood clot is likely to follow. Successful enucleation and primary closure of a sizeable maxillary cyst wound is followed by a remarkable degree of remodelling which re-establishes the contours of the maxillary sinus. Paradoxically, marsupialization of a large cyst tends to result in a cavity which only partially fills in so that a permanent obturator is required to permit normal-sounding speech and to prevent food accumulating in the cavity.

Very large maxillary cysts almost fill the maxillary sinus and bulge the floor of the nose upwards to the inferior concha. The latter may be dislocated upwards and the cyst may extend under the opposite side of the nose. The cartilaginous nasal septum resists resorption by the cyst creating a groove between the two nasal bulges. The antral lining is pushed upwards and backwards so that a slit-like recess is created behind the cyst which may become infected from time to time. This is an additional hazard to a large blood clot in an operated maxillary cyst cavity.

A variety of procedures which open the cyst cavity into the maxillary sinus or nose have been described (Seward and Seward, 1968). The following account involves what are thought to be the best features from these.

The incision needs to be long enough to permit the flap to be raised well up on the maxilla without undue tension. It must also provide for sound closure in the region of the surgical opening in the bone. It therefore runs from behind the tuberosity forwards, either through the buccal gingival crevice but including the interdental papillae, or to the palatal aspect of the crest of any edentulous ridge. In the region of the canine it is usually reasonable to carry the incision up into the labial sulcus and then across to the opposite lateral incisor/canine region. The palatal gingival margin is incised in a similar fashion but only as far forward as the lateral incisor on the same side. It is likely that the palate is expanded and not unlikely that there is a perforation of the palatal cortex. The palatal mucosa is therefore raised from the bone being careful not to perforate any cyst lining which is encountered, or damage the greater palatine nerves and vessels. It is rarely necessary formally to reflect the palatal mucosa to do this.

The buccal flap is raised next. Large perforations of the outer cortex will be encountered and the usual care should be exercised in separating the periosteum from the capsular aspect of the cyst (**Figure 18.11**). Reflection is continued until the

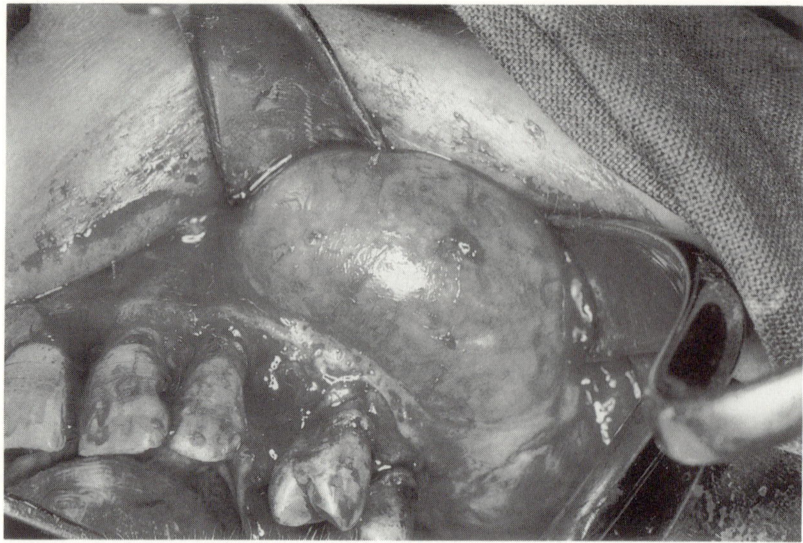

Figure 18.11. Photograph of a large cyst of the maxilla after reflection of labial and palatal flaps. A strap of bone separates two separate cortical perforations.

whole of the margin of such perforations has been uncovered. The periosteum is raised further over the anterolateral surface of the maxilla until the infraorbital foramen is identified. Elevation is continued laterally over the zygomatic-alveolar crest, but once clear of any perforations further exploration over the back of the maxilla behind the zygomatic prominence is unnecessary.

Removal of the cyst lining follows the usual routine. The lining is successively separated from the edges of the buccal perforations as they are enlarged to gain access to the cyst. Any teeth which are to be extracted should be removed before bone removal over the cyst weakens the alveolar process. The pattern of bone removal should respect the apices of teeth to be conserved, the infraorbital nerve, and if possible the anterior superior dental nerve as it runs in the rim of the anterior bony aperture of the nose. It is usually possible to create a substantial opening which makes enucleation of the lining straight forward. Extension palatally to the roots of standing teeth can prove tedious but the separation of the nasal mucosa should not be a problem because this can be done, if necessary, through the anterior bony aperture of the nose as well as through the opening in the cyst wall. As the antral aspect is separated a tear into the antrum is of no lasting consequence. Once the lining has been removed the partition between cyst and antrum is finally penetrated. This is done most safely out towards the zygomatic extension. Any bone in the partition must be removed but antral mucosa can be turned down against the inside of the cyst cavity. Care must be taken not to strip the antral mucosa off the residual normal walls of the sinus (**Figure 18.12**).

Cyst lining should not be left behind because it is not ciliated and will create a nidus of desquamated squamous cells in the floor of the cavity. The object is that the new combined antral and cyst cavities will be lined by proliferating respiratory epithelium.

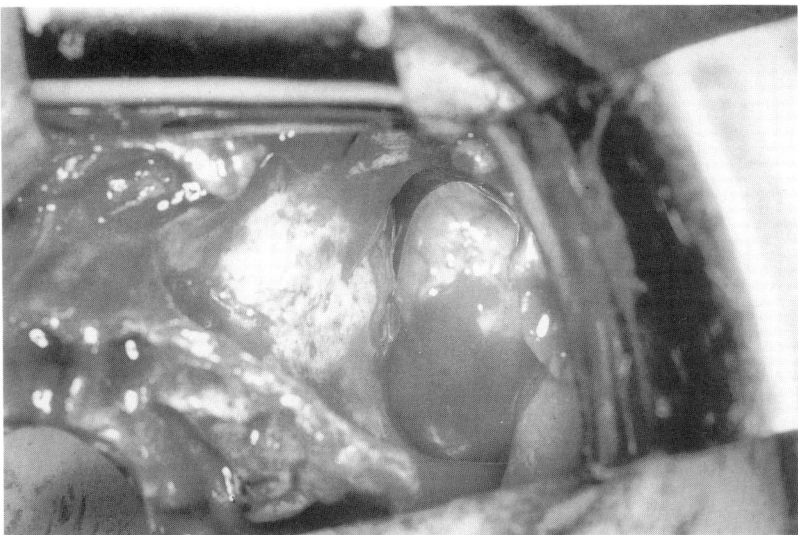

Figure 18.12. The bone separating the two cortical perforations has been removed, the lining enucleated and the dome-shaped partition between the cyst cavity and antrum removed. The antral recess is seen in front of the retractor.

If a large blood clot were to accumulate in the cavity it would become infected and threaten healing of the oral suture line or even the vitality of the alveolar bone. This can be prevented by creating a temporary inferior meatus antrostomy and draining the cavity. Vaseline ribbon gauze can be threaded into the cavity through the nose and carefully and methodically folded from the antrostomy towards the back of the cavity. It should not be packed tightly and should be drawn out through the nose on about the third postoperative day. The risk is that the pack will become caught up on a bony edge or will be incorporated in a suture so that it cannot be removed through the nose.

A safer alternative is to pass a wide bore polythene tube from the antrum out of the antrostomy (**Figure 18.13**) and the nostril and then fasten it to the ala with a suture. In addition a Minivac drain can be inserted via the sulcus beyond the incision and carried back above the sulcus (**Figure 18.14**). The oral wound is closed carefully after haemostasis. It is easy to smooth the margins of any sockets and advance the buccal flap to cover them. An intraoral postoperative pack is applied over the operation site until the patient is awake. An external pressure dressing can be applied to the cheek.

Sutures are left for 14 days and prophylactic antibiotics are given.

The treatment of specific cyst types

Dentigerous cysts

Cysts developing in the growing child will enlarge much more rapidly than in the adult. It is therefore important for clinicians to investigate properly teeth which fail to erupt at the expected time. A distinction must be made between the widening of

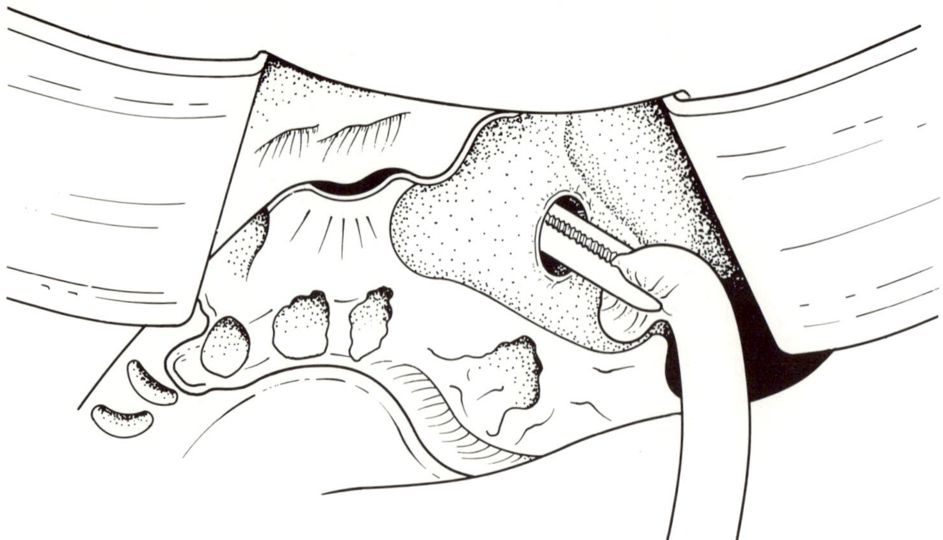

Figure 18.13. Diagram showing how the drainage tube is drawn out through the inferior meatus anstrostomy.

the follicular space which normally accompanies imminent eruption and the early stages of dentigerous cyst enlargement. If a dentigerous cyst is discovered in a young person there are two reasons for early surgical intervention: the first is the speed with which the cyst may enlarge and the other that the involved tooth should be given the best chance of eruption. In particular every effort should be made to preserve space for the missing tooth in the arch. In general if it is hoped that the tooth will erupt it is best to marsupialize the cyst. If for any reason it is decided to enucleate the lining, but conserve the tooth, it should be remembered that in young persons the tooth will be easily displaced from its socket. Great care will need to be exercised to dissect the lining away from the crown of the tooth. A scalpel will be needed to cut it away or the tooth will be avulsed. The cavity should still be loosely packed unless it is relatively shallow, otherwise the tooth may become buried. An orthodontist should be involved from the beginning to preserve space in the arch, upright any teeth tilted by the cyst, and to guide the tooth into place as it erupts.

Dentigerous cysts found in adults more often involve third molars rather than canines, premolars or first molars. Not only is the tooth of origin unlikely to erupt in an adult but there is rarely any point in attempting to conserve a third molar. Both in the ramus and the tuberosity region a dentigerous cyst appearance in a radiograph may be shared by an extrafollicular envelopmental keratocyst and an ameloblastoma. More will be said about this in discussing the management of keratocysts.

With a dentigerous cyst arising from a lower third molar there is often a portion of the cavity related to the roots of the second molar and a portion in the ramus anterior to the inferior dental canal and reaching up to the base of the coronoid process. Because of the difficulty in maintaining an opening through the thick soft

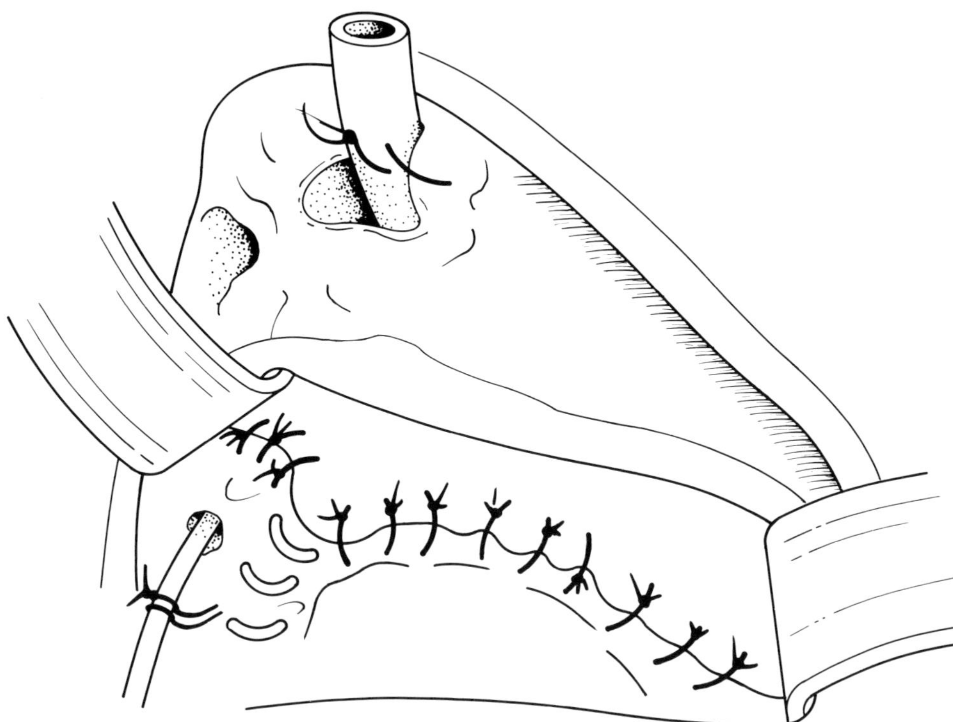

Figure 18.14. Same case as Figures 18.11–18.13. The drain has been secured to the ala of the nose by a suture which transfixes the drain and the oral wound sutured. A Minivac has been threaded along the sulcus. This drain will not hold a vacuum but will provide a closed system.

tissues over the anterior border of the ramus enucleation is the best treatment. It is important to determine from radiographs the relationship of the anterior component to the roots of the second molar. If the cavity is lingual to the second molar, and an intraoral approach is made, enucleation of the lining from this part will be very difficult unless the second molar is extracted. The relationship of the inferior dental bundle to the cyst and to the unerupted third molar must be established. If the canal is at the neck of the tooth the dislocation of the third molar without damage to the inferior dental nerve may be difficult. The shape of the roots and the position and angulation of the tooth are also important. A simple root shape may mean easy elevation; an unfavourable root shape or hypercementosis in a person of middle age or older may mean its removal will be difficult.

In some patients wide access is easy, but if there are unfavourable features and poor access, serious consideration should be given to making a submandibular incision with exposure of the lateral surface of the mandible.

Dentigerous cysts in the maxilla in adults or older teenagers are usually in relationship to upper third molars. The third molar disappears from its expected position in the tuberosity and is found high in the maxilla; sometimes just under the orbital floor. Further radiography demonstrates the cyst largely filling the maxillary sinus from behind forwards. It is important to study the floor of the maxillary sinus in periapical films. Even if it is not apparent in other views these may show a narrow slit of sinus cavity trapped over the apices of the cheek teeth. The antrum may be unintentionally opened if this is not appreciated.

A large flap should be raised. An adequate opening should be developed in the bone with caution. Avoid cramped access. Do not be surprised if the cyst expands backwards towards the pterygoid space. Enucleation and primary closure should be the aim. Marsupialization is not appropriate. Fortunately, delivery of the unerupted tooth is usually easy.

If real problems develop, open forwards into the anterolateral wall of the sinus and remove the partition between the cyst and the antrum as this will greatly improve access. The cavity is drained into the nose as previously described.

It is important to obtain an aspirate from the cyst either shortly before treatment or after raising the flap as some will turn out to be keratocysts. In the latter circumstance great care must be taken to enucleate all the lining. Unexpected daughter cysts may be uncovered perforating into the pterygoid region. It is following surgery on dentigerous cysts of the maxilla that postoperative maxillary cysts may develop.

Keratocysts

Keratocysts have a tendency to recur (Seward, 1962b; Pindborg and Hansen, 1963; Browne and Miller, 1969; Browne, 1970). In attempting to formulate a rational attitude to treatment, comparisons have been made with ameloblastomas on the grounds that both lesions can be multilocular, both can form small daughter cysts at the periphery of large cysts, and the rate of cell division of the epithelium of keratocysts is greater than of other benign odontogenic cysts. However, the differences are significant; ameloblastomas have a much higher recurrence rate after enucleation than keratocysts and the great majority are more aggressively invasive. If a keratocyst is marsupialized, not only does the cavity reduce in size but the epithelium shrinks in area. Ultimately it becomes a small stable patch on the surface. Recurrence is no more likely with marsupialization than after enucleation. With an ameloblastoma, after an initial period during which the bony cavity reduces in size, tumour tissue fills the visible cavity and fungates through the opening. In both cases unwise surgery which breaches the enveloping periosteum without removing all the abnormal tissue can lead to recurrence in the soft tissue (Emerson, Whitlock and Jones, 1972), but this is more invasive in the case of the ameloblastoma and can ultimately bring about the patient's death by infiltrating, for example, the base of the skull. In a small, but significant proportion of cases, ameloblastomas metastasize; keratocysts do not kill patients.

When further keratocysts arise in a patient's jaws a distinction must be made between recurrence and the development of a fresh cyst or cysts.

Keratocysts develop from dental lamina remnants. The factor which results in reactivation of the resting groups of epithelial cells may affect a local group of cell nests. A single cyst may develop or a local cluster of cysts, or again if the first cyst is enucleated a further cyst or cysts may arise in the same location from the activated group of cell nests. Harnische (1961) recognized the presence of groups of odontogenic epithelial cells from a backward extension of the dental lamina in the mucosa of the retromolar region. Stoelinga and Peters (1973) attributed some recurrences of keratocysts in the anterior part of the ramus to these cell nests and advocated their excision in continuity with the cyst lining. Recurrence can also occur from the epithelium in the residual gubernaculum between an extrafollicular envelopmental cyst and the overlying mucoperiosteum. The contents of any opening or canal in the crest of the adjacent alveolar bone must be curetted out (Cantatore, 1957).

The lining of keratocysts is thin and easily torn so that fragments are retained and give rise to a recurrence. Recurrence in the soft tissues or in the bone grafts after resection of part of the jaw may result from fragments which adhere to the periosteum (Scholfield, 1971; Emerson, Whitlock and Jones, 1972; Persson, 1973; Attenborough, 1974). It is possible that viable particles of lining are forced into cancellous spaces by vigorous curettage. It is conceivable that the cyst contents contain viable desquamated cells which could graft within tissue planes.

The developing dental lamina has the ability to burrow into the tissues. It is not surprising therefore to find epithelial strands arising from the lining epithelium and penetrating into the cyst capsule. There is no direct linkage with the frequency of these and liability to cyst recurrence, even if the cyst is marsupialized. What is not known is how often they give rise to daughter cysts and, further, whether or how often they penetrate as far as the adjacent medullary spaces to give rise to daughter cysts or recurrent cysts outside the limits of the original capsule.

In some patients a greater extent of the residual dental lamina gives rise to keratocysts. This can lead to multilocular cysts in a short segment of jaw, a multilocular cyst involving a considerable part of the jaw (usually the mandible) or multiple cysts either occurring within a short space of time or over years. Cysts arising afresh in adjacent parts of the residual dental lamina cannot be avoided by any reasonable operative procedure.

Attempts have been made to devitalize the cells of the cyst lining before enucleation by instilling Carnoy's fluid (Voorsmit, 1986), a powerful histological fixative. Attempts have been made similarly to devitalize any fragments of lining left in the cavity after enucleation or any out-growths of epithelium in the adjacent medullary bone, either by swabbing the cavity with Carnoy's fluid (Voorsmit, Stoelinga and van Haelst, 1981) or by freezing the bony wall (Webb and Brockbank, 1984). Such techniques are likely to do uncontrolled damage to the tissues and to leave necrotic tissue in the walls of the wound and do not find favour with the author. A greater attention to detail in operative technique will reduce markedly the proportion of cysts which recur and careful follow-up will pick up recurrences before their removal becomes a major procedure.

Since enucleation is a satisfactory procedure both for keratocysts and other benign odontogenic cysts an accurate preoperative differential diagnosis between the two is of less importance than a differentiation between keratocysts and ameloblastomas. Fortunately aspiration of cyst contents is a good way to distinguish keratocysts.

The key to success is gentle, complete enucleation with adequate access. Sometimes the cyst will expand on the lingual or palatal aspect of certain teeth. An approach from both sides of the alveolar process may be helpful. With the more anterior teeth it may be possible to root-fill a tooth and do an apicectomy to create better access. Extraction of selected teeth will provide more room, but may be avoided by accepting a less than ideal exposure, recognizing that a recurrence is a possibility. If a submandibular approach will provide better access and vision this should be the choice. Lining is easily left where the cyst perforates the cortex and becomes adherent to the periosteum. Sharp dissection with a scalpel, removing both lining and periosteum should be employed rather than risk tearing the lining.

With multilocular cysts be sure to open all the bony compartments. In the rare cases in which there is a multitude of cysts involving a substantial part of the jaw, Bramley (1974) recommended excision of the appropriate portion of mandible. The jaw should be exposed through a submandibular incision to ensure good access. If necessary periosteum is left over any bony perforations to avoid tearing the cyst lining. The overlying tissues are raised using a scalpel to dissect in a plane just outside the involved periosteum. However the major bony cavity should be opened and the cyst lining uncovered before the patient is finally committed to a resection. Sometimes a large cyst with a lobulated wall will look like a complex multilocular cyst. It can be helpful to pack off the soft tissues below the mandible with damp swabs to prevent contamination.

Extra-follicular envelopmental cysts require removal of the involved tooth in adults as in the case of dentigerous cysts. In growing children selected teeth may be permitted to erupt by marsupializing the cyst (**Figure 18.15**). Marsupialization is also appropriate to conserve other unerupted teeth or adjacent standing teeth which would be damaged by enucleation. Be sure to deal with the tissue in any gubernacular canals (Cantatore, 1957). Similarly it is worth excizing a narrow strip of retromolar mucosa as advocated by Stoelinga and Peters (1973).

Careful follow-up after the treatment of keratocysts for a minimum of 5 years is essential. Life-long follow-up of Gorlin's syndrome patients (see Chapter 2) is advisable because of the sequence of problems which occur throughout life.

Nasopalatine duct cysts

These are usually enucleated after raising a palatal flap. The long spheno-palatine nerve may be spread out over the upper surface of the capsule on one or both sides and may need to be cut to free the lining. These nerves may need separate anaesthetization if the procedure is carried out under local anaesthesia. The technique follows that described under enucleation of cysts through the palate. Nasopalatine duct cysts rarely reach a large size although exceptions have been reported (Nortjé and Farman, 1978). Small, symptomless ones can be watched as they may not enlarge even over many years.

Contour defects of bone

It is rarely essential to chip bone graft cyst cavities (Holtgrave and Spiessel, 1975). Subperiosteal new bone will soon strengthen the jaw and bone will start to fill in quite large cysts. Chip bone grafting should only be done where there is a real risk of mandibular fracture postoperatively or where the contour of the alveolar bone will be unsatisfactory as a foundation for dentures. Flap design and wound closure need to be meticulous. A small wound breakdown and loss of clot may prove a prolonged inconvenience. If bone chips have been inserted even their partial loss may negate any advantage of the procedure. Cancellous bone from the iliac crest is the best material to use as a graft.

Attempts have been made to use resorbable materials both as a scaffold for

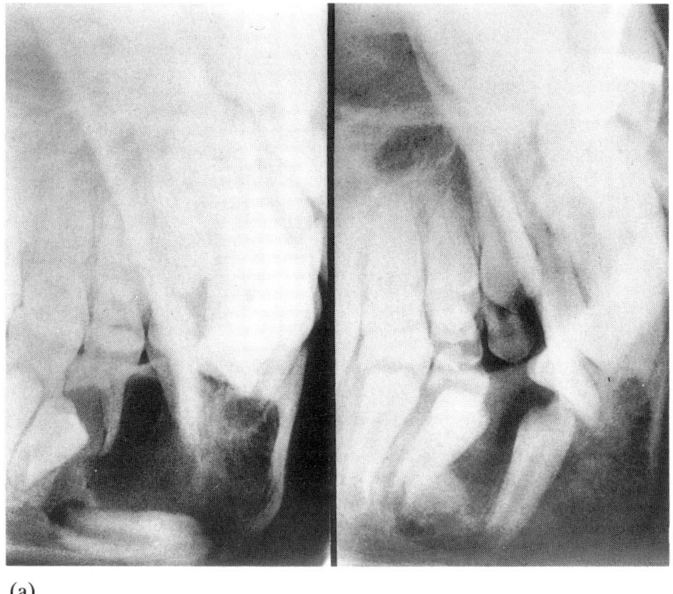

(a)

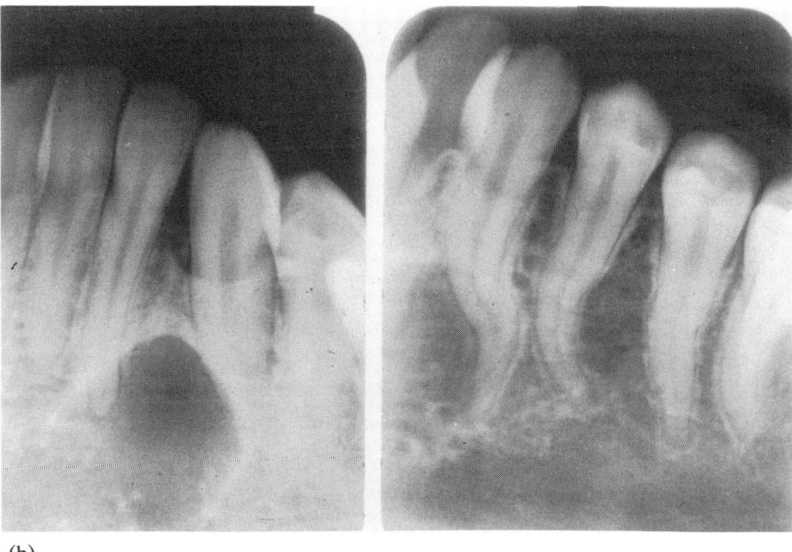

(b)

Figure 18.15. (a) A large extrafollicular envelopmental keratocyst on $\overline{|3}$ was marsupialized. $\overline{|34}$ were brought into the arch as they erupted and $\overline{21|12}$ up-righted with a fixed orthodontic appliance. (b) There is a limited recurrence. Notice its relationship to the gubernacular canal in the inter-radicular septum.

ingrowing granulation tissue and as a support to the soft tissues, so maintaining bony contours. Fibrin clot is difficult to beat as a scaffold for granulation tissue. Not only is it biodegradable, but breakdown of the fibrin and trapped red cells provides a local supply of amino acids for the growing granulation tissue. Most materials suggested for this role actually impede the growth of granulation tissue as they are more difficult to remove than clot. Some may however act as haemostatics and ensure that the clot is confined to the cavity in the bone.

Only preparations of decalcified bone matrix are likely to form an alternative to cancellous bone grafts to speed the formation of bone.

Nasolabial cysts

An incision is made in the labial sulcus over the cyst. Although the cyst lies supraperiosteally it often adheres to the periosteum and the latter may be incised around the cyst to facilitate its elevation from the surface of the bone.

Gentle dissection with a scalpel will free the soft tissues of the nasolabial region from the cyst sac. At this point it will be left attached to the mucosa of the inferior meatus of the nose. Patience is required to separate it as it is often firmly adherent to the nasal mucosa. Any tears should be repaired with fine horizontal mattress sutures inserted from the wound aspect. They will tend to invert the edges towards the nose. Because the wound cavity will collapse there will not be a sizeable haematoma and a leaky suture line is of no consequence. The oral wound is closed after careful haemostasis with diathermy and a pressure dressing applied for some hours.

Solitary bone cysts

Careful aspiration of the larger ones using two needles to avoid producing a negative pressure will produce a yellow liquid which will clot on standing. If a bloody aspirate is obtained it should be put into an anticoagulant tube and spun to get rid of the red cells. The supernatant plasma and fluid should be tested for bilirubin. This is often high and accounts for the yellow colour. Clearly, small haemorrhages occur into the cyst and the breakdown products of haemoglobin are unable to escape from the cavity.

The cyst should be approached by raising a suitable flap. A piece of the outer bony wall is outlined and removed and sent for histological examination to confirm the diagnosis. The rest of the inside of the cavity should not be scraped to avoid damage to the inferior dental nerve or the tiny neurovascular bundles to adjacent teeth. If it is lightly packed haemostasis is soon achieved and the wound can be closed. This is all that is usually necessary in adults to provoke healing. In children or teenagers the cavity may fill in completely or there may be a residual radiographic defect or the cyst may recur. Once the diagnosis has been established beyond doubt by the operation the lesion can be kept under observation. After some years it may regress as the child becomes an adult. If it does not regress it can be re-opened and packed. A layer of surgicel should be placed to line the wall and protect it from the pack. The rare, large, multilocular bone cyst should be removed piecemeal to saucerize the affected area.

Soft tissue cysts

Intrabony cysts can be enucleated because of the abrupt change in density of the tissues at the boundary between the capsule and the bone. This change in physical properties is less where the cyst lining protrudes into the soft tissue, hence the difficulties in dissection where the cortex is perforated.

Most cysts in the soft tissues enlarge because of an accumulation of desquamated epithelial cells or glandular secretions within the cyst cavity. Surgical tissue expanders have shown how skin and thin muscle layers can be progressively stretched and will increase in surface area over a slowly enlarging mass. Consider also the anterior abdominal wall over the pregnant uterus. Most cysts start at some depth inside the body and exploit planes of loose connective tissue to enlarge. Where they arise in relation to thick, active muscles these eventually squeeze the cyst out from under one or other of their borders. Soft tissue cysts are usually lined by epithelium but are covered by a capsule which exhibits dissectable layers of loose connective tissue. Dissection of the cyst sac is through the loose connective tissue around it. A layer should be chosen which is close enough to the connective tissue supporting the epithelium to ensure the cyst's safe removal but not so close that the cyst is ruptured and the dissection made difficult.

Midline sublingual dermoid cysts

The majority of midline sublingual dermoid cysts lie between the genial muscles and extend backwards into the tongue. Even when there is a substantial submental swelling when the mouth is closed the cyst will be found above the mylohyoid. A separate subcutaneous rounded swelling may be felt in some cases. This is usually a lymph node following infection of the cyst. A separate submental cyst has been recorded but is most unusual. A point of differential diagnosis for a superficial cyst is a high thyroglossal cyst in the region of the hyoid bone.

An incision in the midline from just below the tip of the tongue (Seward, 1965) through the line of the lingual frenum to the back of the mandible will mostly provide adequate access as the mucous membrane is elastic and will stretch with retraction (**Figure 18.16**). Not a lot is gained by dividing the floor of the mouth laterally from the anterior end of the incision, anterior to the sublingual glands. In the case of a very large cyst it may be necessary, should the anaesthetist have difficulty in intubating the patient, partially to aspirate it. Otherwise the dissection proceeds more comfortably if it has not been decompressed. An appropriate plane of dissection is more easily established. The cyst wall is freed by scissor and finger dissection, retracting the genial muscles in segments to provide access to each part of the surface in turn. The aim is to get beyond the greater diameter of the cyst and to dislocate it forward (**Figure 18.17**). If this proves impossible it may be necessary to open the neck. An incision is made horizontally above the hyoid bone, curving up a little towards the ends parallel to the lower border of the body of the mandible. Skin and platysma are raised to the lower border of the mandible. The submandibular fat is divided in the midline and the underside of the mylohyoid exposed. This in turn is divided from chin to hyoid in the midline. The exploring finger will encounter the cyst. Access is usually disappointing but sufficient to complete separation of the cyst and its displacement out of the oral wound.

Before the submental region is opened another manoeuvre can be tried. The cyst is opened at its upper surface and the contents sucked out. Several sutures are each

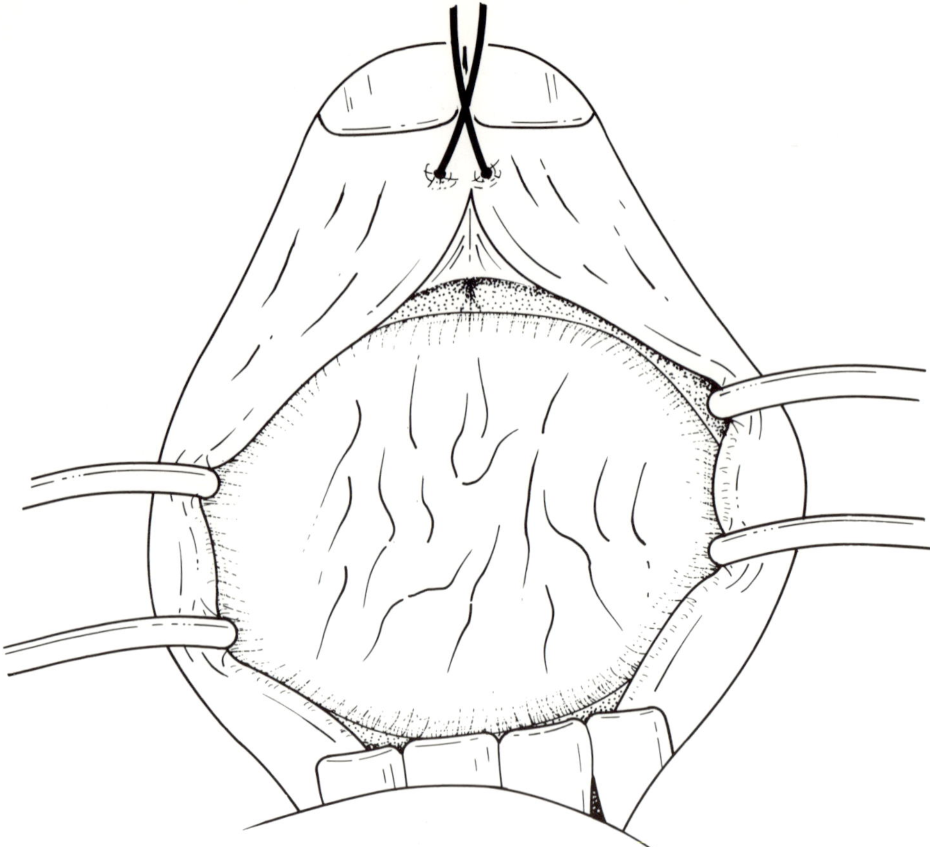

Figure 18.16. Diagram of a sublingual dermoid cyst as it appears through the median sublingual incision.

passed twice through the cyst sac close to the opening to provide traction and a finger inserted into the cavity. This may guide dissection of the remaining points of attachment. Any vessels encountered crossing to the cyst wall should be ligated if possible before they are divided. An aneurysm needle is a useful instrument with which to do this. Haemostasis is achieved after the enucleation is completed and a vacuum drain passed out through the submental region before closure. Any evidence of postoperative haemorrhage must be treated seriously in case a threat to the airway develops.

Lateral sublingual dermoids

Small ones can be excised through an incision in the floor of the mouth medial to the sublingual plica. The submandibular duct and the lingual nerve which may cross above it must be sought and conserved. As the cyst increases in size it emerges behind the mylohyoid muscle and presents in the submandibular region. In such cases it is best removed from this aspect so that the facial vessels can be controlled.

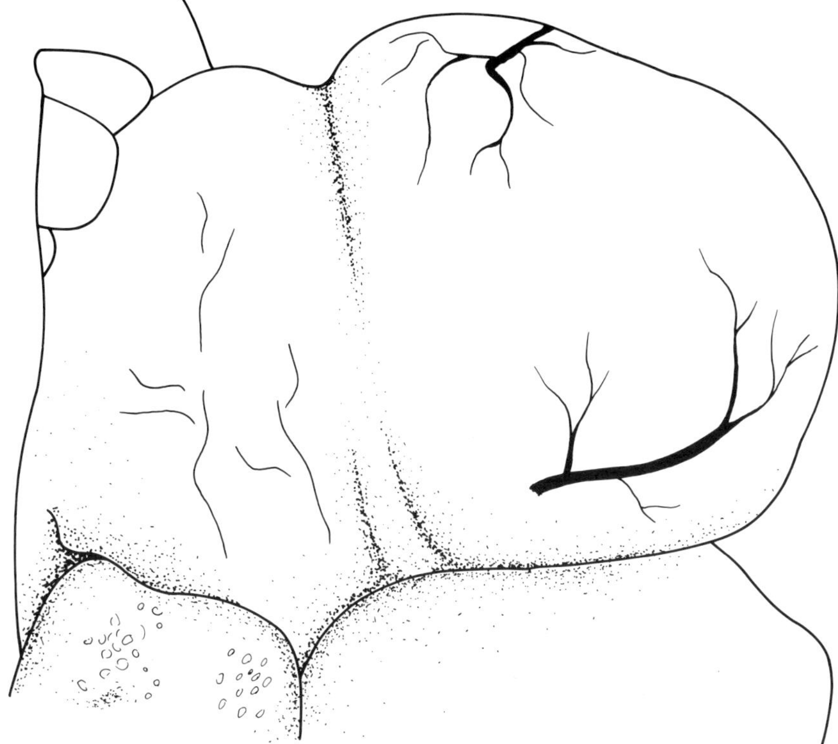

Figure 18.17. Illustration made once the bilobed cyst had been dislocated out of the wound. The operator's finger is below and behind the cyst.

The lower pole of the submandibular gland is mobilized backwards and the posterior part of the mylohyoid muscle defined. If, once the posterior border of the latter has been raised, adequate exposure cannot be gained by retraction, the muscle can be divided a little above the hyoid bone (**Figure 18.18**). After removal of the cyst and, if necessary, the submandibular gland haemostasis is assured and the wound closed in layers with vacuum drainage in the usual way.

Lympho-epithelial (branchial) cysts

The most frequent branchial cyst is the one which presents from deep to the anterior border of the upper third of the sternomastoid muscle. A horizontal incision is made in or parallel to skin creases across the middle of the bulge. It is deepened through the platysma and flaps raised upwards and downwards immediately deep to this muscle.

Next, the anterior border of the sternomastoid muscle is defined, mobilizing the great auricular nerve on its surface and as it crosses to the surface of the parotid gland. This will give sufficient mobility for retraction of the muscle. The upper end

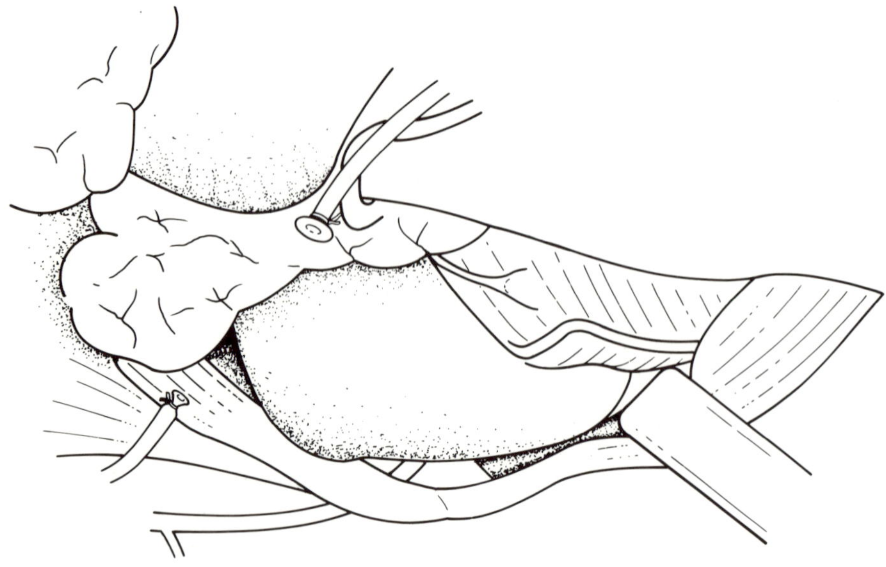

Figure 18.18. A lateral sublingual dermoid cyst has been exposed in the right submandibular region. The mylohyoid muscle has been divided low down after retracting the anterior belly of digastric. Note the nerve to the mylohyoid is inserted higher up on the muscle. The lower pole of the submandibular salivary gland has been raised and turned backwards.

of the external jugular vein will probably lie superficial to the cyst and should be taken well below the parotid and retracted upwards. The cervical branch of the facial nerve usually emerges from the gland just in front of the vein.

The anterior border of the sternomastoid is mobilized and raised on retractors and dissection started close to the surface of the cyst. As the upper part is freed the posterior belly of the digastric will be encountered and its lower border should be followed downwards towards the tendon. Some cysts pass deep to the digastric at the upper pole. The external jugular vein will be encountered on the deep surface of the cyst and must be separated carefully (**Figure 18.19**). With a large cyst, expect to encounter the vascular supply to the upper part of the sternomastoid muscle, entering the deep surface towards the back of the muscle and about a quarter of the way down its length. The accessory nerve will be crossing the internal jugular vein to join the sternomastoid artery and veins and penetrate the muscle. It must not be damaged. Once the lower pole of the cyst is freed it can be dislocated forwards and gently manipulated, holding it with a swab. Retraction of the adjacent tissues and displacement of the cyst will permit dissection of the upper end. Watch out for the external carotid and its branches beneath the upper pole. Haemostasis and closure in layers with vacuum drainage proceeds as usual.

Mucous extravasation cyst

Mucous extravasation cysts do not have an epithelial lining. After a time a defined delicate connective tissue capsule will be formed. Those in the lip, usually the lower

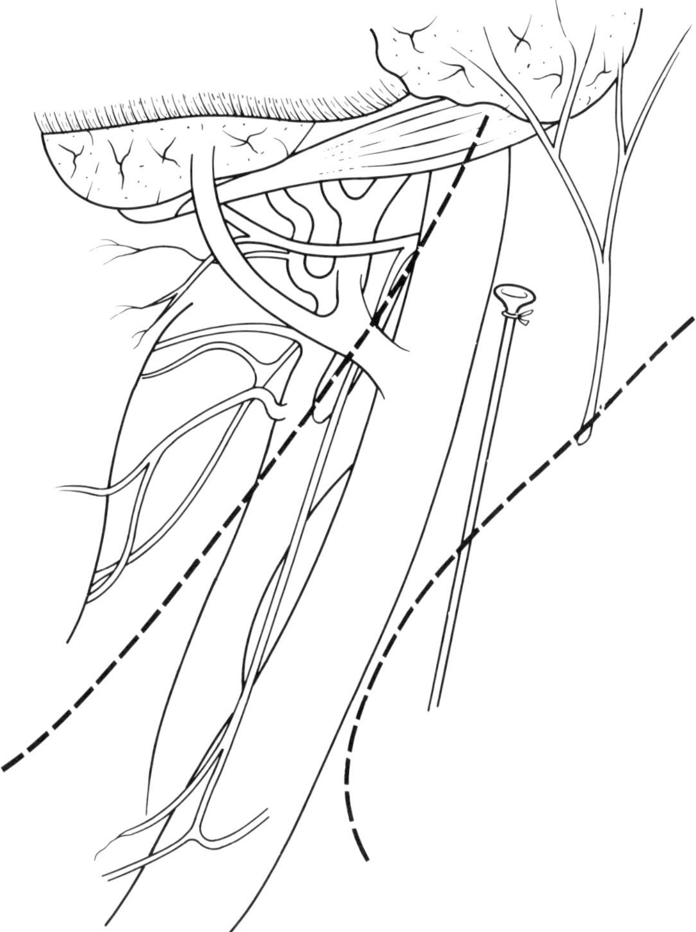

Figure 18.19. Illustration showing the anatomy deep to a branchial cyst. The sternomastoid muscle is indicated by the broken line. In the upper part of the neck the branches of the internal jugular and external carotid are shown. The internal and external laryngeal nerves are also shown but should not be at risk.

lip, can be approached through a vertical incision. This is made just into the mucosa over the convexity but a little deeper above and below. It is raised with a scalpel from the surface of the cyst, elevating the flaps with skin hooks. It is useful if the cyst can be reasonably well defined before it ruptures because this helps to identify the related minor salivary glands from which it is arising. Any mobilized cyst capsule and the underlying glands are removed. The connective tissue is closed with fine catgut to ensure haemostasis and the mucosa closed with mild eversion with interrupted 4/0 soft gut. Eversion is necessary if the red margin is involved to avoid a notch forming as the scar contracts.

Ranulas are large mucous extravasation cysts involving the floor of the mouth. They are exposed by an incision between the submandibular duct and the sublingual plica. Wharton's duct is often an opaque cord passing over the surface of the ranula and must be freed gently. Again the sac is of delicate connective tissue only and is difficult to free without rupture. Since the important part of the operation is the removal of the sublingual gland mass its rupture is of little account. The lingual nerve should be sought where it crosses deep to the submandibular duct towards the tongue opposite the first lower molar. The nerve can be followed laterally, firstly to conserve it, secondly to start mobilization of the sublingual gland mass. The sublingual branch of the lingual nerve lies deep in the groove between the sublingual glands and the mandible. The sublingual veins lie between the gland and the hyoglossus as it enters the tongue and will be encountered as the lingual nerve and Wharton's duct are dissected. In a plunging ranula the saliva spills over the posterior border of the mylohyoid muscle to form a cystic swelling in the neck. Once more the sublingual glands are removed. The neck swelling is emptied by aspiration with a syringe and with a sucker over the back of the mylohyoid through the mouth.

As a rare entity the submandibular gland can be a source of a ranula. As the floor of mouth swelling is explored its relationship to this gland, rather than the sublingual, becomes apparent. The gland is excavated by the cystic accumulation of saliva leaving a thinned-out shell and it will be necessary to make a further submandibular incision to remove it.

References

Abaza N. A., Gold L. and Lally E. (1989) Granular cell odontogenic cyst: a unicystic ameloblastoma with late recurrence as follicular ameloblastoma. *Journal of Oral and Maxillofacial Surgery* **47**, 168–175.

Abrams A. A. and Howell F. V. (1968) The calcifying odontogenic cyst. *Oral Surgery, Oral Medicine, Oral Pathology* **25**, 594–606.

Abrams M. B., Andrews J. E. and Laskin D. M. (1977) Epidermoid (implantation) cyst after temporomandibular joint surgery. *Journal of Oral Surgery* **35**, 587–589.

Abrams A. M., Howell F. V. and Bullock W. K. (1963) Nasopalatine cysts. *Oral Surgery, Oral Medicine, Oral Pathology* **16**, 300–332.

Ackermann G. L., Altini M. and Shear M. (1988) The unicystic ameloblastoma: a clinicopathological study of 57 cases. *Journal of Oral Pathology* **17**, 541–546.

Ackermann G., Cohen M. and Altini M. (1987) The paradental cyst: a clinicopathologic study of 50 cases. *Oral Surgery, Oral Medicine, Oral Pathology* **64**, 308–312.

Ackermann K. (1976) Pathogenese odontogener Zysten. *Zahnarztliche Praxis (Munchen)* **27**, 128–129.

Aguirre A., Takai Y., Meenaghan M., Neiders M. E. and Natiella J. R. (1989) Lectin histochemistry of ameloblastomas and odontogenic keratocysts. *Journal of Oral Pathology and Medicine* **18**, 68–73.

Ahlfors E., Larsson A. and Sjögren S. (1984) The odontogenic keratocyst: a benign cystic tumor? *Journal of Oral and Maxillofacial Surgery* **42**, 10–19.

Albers D. D. (1973) Median mandibular cyst partially lined with pseudostratified columnar epithelium. *Oral Surgery, Oral Medicine, Oral Pathology* **36**, 11–15.

Allard R. H. B. (1982) Non-odontogenic Cysts of the Oral Regions. *MD Thesis,* Free University of Amsterdam, Naarden: Drukkerrij Los BV.

Allard R. H. B., van der Kwast W. A. M. and van der Waal I. (1981a) Nasopalatine duct cyst. Review of the literature and report of 22 cases. *International Journal of Oral Surgery* **10**, 447–461.

Allard R. H. B., van der Kwast W. A. M. and van der Waal I. (1981b) Mucosal antral cysts. Review of the literature and report of a radiographic survey. *Oral Surgery, Oral Medicine, Oral Pathology* **51**, 2–9.

Allison R. T. (1974) Electron microscopic study of 'Rushton' hyaline bodies in cyst linings. *British Dental Journal* **137**, 102–104.

Allison R. T. (1977a) Microprobe and microradiographic studies of hyaline bodies in odontogenic cysts. *Journal of Oral Pathology* **6**, 44–50.

Allison R. T. (1977b) Hyalin material bounding dystrophic calcification in the epithelial lining of odontogenic cysts. *Journal of Oral Pathology* **6**, 113–121.

Al-Talabani N. G. and Smith C. J. (1980) Experimental dentigerous cysts and enamel hypoplasia: their possible significance in explaining the pathogenesis of human dentigerous cysts. *Journal of Oral Pathology* **9**, 82–91.

Altini M. and Cohen M. (1980) The follicular primordial cyst (odontogenic keratocyst). *Journal of Dental Research* **59D**, 1915 (Abstr.).

Altini M. and Cohen M. (1982) The follicular primordial cyst (odontogenic keratocyst). *International Journal of Oral Surgery* **11**, 175–182.

Altini M. and Cohen M. (1987) Experimental extra-follicular histogenesis of follicular cysts. *Journal of Oral Pathology* **16**, 49–52.

Altini M. and Farman A. G. (1975) The calcifying odontogenic cyst. Eight new cases and a review of the literature. *Oral Surgery, Oral Medicine, Oral Pathology* **40**, 751–759.

Altini M. and Shear M. (1992) The lateral periodontal cyst: an update. *Journal of Oral Pathology and Medicine*. In press.

Anniko M., Anneroth G., Bergstedt H. and Ramström G. (1981) Jaw cysts with special regard to keratocyst recurrence. A long-term follow-up. *Archives of Oto-Rhino-Laryngology* **233**, 261–269.

Arcand P., Granger J. and Brochu P. (1988) Congenital dermoid cyst of the oral cavity with gastric choristoma. *Journal of Otolaryngology* **17**, 219–222.

Arendorf T. (1981) Prostaglandin E2 and bone and root resorption in hamsters. *Journal of the Dental Association of South Africa* **36**, 317–322.

Arey L. B. (1965) *Developmental Anatomy*, 7th edn, Philadelphia and London, Saunders, p. 205.

Arwill T. and Heyden G. (1973) Histochemical studies on cholesterol formation in odontogenic cysts and granulomas. *Scandinavian Journal of Dental Research* **81**, 406–410.

Atkinson M. E. (1972) A histological study of tooth grafts in an inbred strain of mice. *Journal of Oral Pathology* **1**, 115–124.

Atkinson M. E. (1976) A histological study of odontogenic cysts formed following mouse molar tooth transplantation. *Journal of Oral Pathology* **5**, 347–357.

Atkinson M. E. (1977) An autoradiographic study of experimental odontogenic cyst formation in the mouse. *Journal of Oral Pathology* **6**, 382–386.

Attenborough N. R. (1974) Recurrence of an odontogenic keratocyst in a bone graft. Report of a case. *British Journal of Oral Surgery* **12**, 33–39.

Babál P., Soler P., Brozman M., Jakubovsky J., Beyly M. and Basset F. (1987) In situ characterization of cells in periapical granuloma by monoclonal antibodies. *Oral Surgery, Oral Medicine, Oral Pathology* **64**, 348–352.

Baker A. W. W. (1891) Notes on the pathology of a dentigerous cyst. *Journal of the British Dental Association* **12**, 61–65.

Bartlett P. F., Radden B. G. and Reade P. C. (1973) The experimental production of odontogenic keratocysts. *Journal of Oral Pathology* **2**, 58–67.

Basu M. K., Rout P. G. J., Rippen J. W. and Smith A. J. (1985) Post-operative maxillary cyst. *IRCS Medical Science* **13**, 562.

Batsakis J. G., Bruner J. M. and Luna M. A. (1988) Polycystic (dysgenetic) disease of the parotid glands. *Archives of Otolaryngology Head and Neck Surgery* **114**, 1146–1148.

Bayer R. A. and Hardman F. G. (1976) Intraoral surgical management of cystic hygroma. *British Journal of Oral Surgery* **14**, 36–40.

Beasley J. D. (1976) Traumatic cyst of the jaws: report of 30 cases. *Journal of the American Dental Association* **92**, 145–152.

Benn A. M. L. (1991) The role of deciduous teeth in the pathogenesis of odontogenic cysts. *MSc (Dent) research report*, University of the Witwatersrand, Johannesburg.

Benn A., Ackermann G. L. and Altini M. (1990) The role of deciduous teeth in the pathogenesis of odontogenic cysts. *Journal of Dental Research* **69**, 1092 (Abstr.)

Berg O., Carenfelt C. and Sobin A. (1989) On the diagnosis and pathogenesis of intramural maxillary cysts. *Acta Otolaryngology (Stockholm)* **108**, 464–468.

Bernier J. L. and Bhaskar S. N. (1958) Aneurysmal bone cysts of the mandible. *Oral Surgery, Oral Medicine, Oral Pathology* **11**, 1018–1028.

Bhaskar S. N. (1965) Gingival cysts and the keratinizing ameloblastoma. *Oral Surgery, Oral Medicine, Oral Pathology* **19**, 790–807.

Bhaskar S. N. (1966) Lymphoepithelial cysts of the oral cavitiy. *Oral Surgery, Oral Medicine, Oral Pathology* **21**, 120–128.

Bhaskar S. N. (1972) Nonsurgical resolution of radicular cysts. *Oral Surgery, Oral Medicine, Oral Pathology* **34**, 458–468.

Bhaskar S. N. and Bernier J. L. (1959) Histogenesis of branchial cysts: a report of 468 cases. *American Journal of Pathology* **35**, 407–423.

Bhaskar S. N., Bernier J. L. and Godby F. (1959) Aneurysmal bone cyst and other giant cell lesions of the jaw. *Journal of Oral Surgery* **17**, 30–41.

Bhaskar S. N., Bolden T. E. and Weinmann J. P. (1956a) Experimental obstructive adenitis in the mouse. *Journal of Dental Research* **35**, 852–862.

Bhaskar S. N., Bolden T. E. and Weinmann J. P. (1956b) Pathogenesis of mucoceles. *Journal of Dental Research* **35**, 863–874.

Biesecker J. L., Marcove R. C., Huvos A. G. and Miké V. (1970) Aneurysmal bone cysts. A clinicopathological study of 66 cases. *Cancer* **26**, 615–625.

Binkley G.W. and Johnson H.H. (1951) Epithelioma adenoides cysticum: basal cell nevi, agenesis of the corpus callosum and dental cysts. *American Medical Association Archives of Dermatology and Syphilology* **63**, 73–84.

Binnie W. H. and Rowe A. H. R. (1974) The incidence of epithelial rests, proliferations and apical periodontal cysts following root canal treatment in young dogs. *British Dental Journal* **137**, 56–60.

Blair A. E. and Wadsworth W. (1968) Median mandibular developmental cyst. *Journal of Oral Surgery* **26**, 735–738.

Bodin I., Isacsson G. and Julin P. (1986) Cysts of the nasopalatine duct. *International Journal of Oral and Maxillofacial Surgery* **15**, 696–706.

Borg G., Persson G. and Thilander H. (1974) A study of odontogenic cysts with special reference to comparisons between keratinizing and nonkeratinizing cysts. *Swedish Dental Journal* **67**, 311–325.

Bouyssou M. and Guilhem A. (1965) Recherches morphologiques et histochimiques sur les corps hyalins intrakystiques de Rushton. *Bulletin du Groupement International pour la Recherche Scientifique en Stomatologie et Odontologie (Bruxelles)* **8**, 81–104.

Bramley P. A. (1971) Treatment of cysts of the jaws. *Proceedings of the Royal Society of Medicine* **64**, 547–550.

Bramley P. A. (1974) The odontogenic keratocyst – an approach to treatment. *International Journal of Oral Surgery* **3**, 337–341.

Brandao G. S., Ebling H. and Faria e Souza I. (1974) Bilateral nasolabial cyst. *Oral Surgery, Oral Medicine, Oral Pathology* **37**, 480–484.

Brannon R. B. (1976) The odontogenic keratocyst. A clinicopathologic study of 312 cases. Part 1. Clinical features. *Oral Surgery, Oral Medicine, Oral Pathology* **42**, 54–72.

Brannon R. B. (1977) The odontogenic keratocyst. A clinicopathologic study of 312 cases. Part II. Histological features. *Oral Surgery, Oral Medicine, Oral Pathology* **43**, 233–255.

Braun J. P. (1975) Et tilfaelde af en traumatisk knoglecyste. *Tandlaegebladet* **79**, 647–651.

Brons R. and Jongebreur J. W. (1967) Cystis nasoalveolaris. *Nederlandse Tijdschrif van Tandheelkunde* **74**, 537–548.

Brosch F. (1957) Zysten des Kiefer-Gesichtsbereiches. In *Zahn-Mund-Kieferheilk*, Bd. 3/I (eds K. W. Häupl, W. Meyer and K. Schuchardt), p. 446. München, Berlin, Urban und Schwarzenberg.

Brown L. H., Berkman S., Cohen D., Kaplan A. L. and Rosenberg M. (1982) A radiological study of the frequency and distribution of impacted teeth. *Journal of the Dental Association of South Africa* **37**, 627–630.

Brown P. (1990) 'Unnecessary X-rays blamed for cancer deaths.' *New Scientist* **127**, No. 1733, 27. Comment on the report *Patient Dose Reduction in Diagnostic Radiology*, National Radiological Protection Board, 1990, HMSO.

Browne R. M. (1969) The pathogenesis of the odontogenic keratocyst. *Fourth Proceedings of the International Academy of Oral Pathology*, p. 28.

Browne R. M. (1970) The odontogenic keratocyst – clinical aspects. *British Dental Journal* **128**, 225–231.

Browne R. M. (1971a) The odontogenic keratocyst–histological features and their correlation with clinical behaviour. *British Dental Journal* **131**, 249–259.

Browne R. M. (1971b) The origin of cholesterol in odontogenic cysts in man. *Archives of Oral Biology* **16**, 107–113.

Browne R. M. (1972) Metaplasia and degeneration in odontogenic cysts in man. *Journal of Oral Pathology* **1**, 145–158.

Browne R. M. (1975) The pathogenesis of odontogenic cysts: a review. *Journal of Oral Pathology* **4**, 31–46.

Browne R. M. (1976) Some observations on the fluids of odontogenic cysts. *Journal of Oral Pathology* **5**, 74–87.

Browne R. M. and Gough N. G. (1972) Malignant change in the epithelium lining odontogenic cysts. *Cancer* **29**, 1199–1207.

Browne R. M. and Matthews J. B. (1985) Intra-epithelial hyaline bodies in odontogenic cysts: an immunoperoxidase study. *Journal of Oral Pathology* **14**, 422–428.

Browne R. M. and Miller W. A. (1969) Rupture strength of capsules of odontogenic cysts in man. *Archives of Oral Biology* **14**, 1351–1354.

Browne R. M., Rowles S. L. and Smith A. J. (1984) Mineralised deposits in odontogenic cysts. *IRCS Medical Science* **12**, 642–643.

Brüggemann A. (1920) Zysten als Folge von Entwicklungsstörungen im Naseneingang. *Archives of Laryngology and Rhinology* **33**, 101–105. Cited by Allard (1982).

Buchner A. (1973) Granular cell odontogenic cyst. *Oral Surgery, Oral Medicine, Oral Pathology* **36**, 707–712.

Buchner A. (1991) The central (intraosseous) calcifying odontogenic cyst: an analysis of 215 cases *Journal of Oral and Maxillofacial Surgery* **49**, 330–339.

Buchner A., Carpenter W. M., Merrell P. W. and Leider A. S. (1991) Anterior lingual mandibular salivary gland defect. Evaluation of twenty-four cases. *Oral Surgery, Oral Medicine, Oral Pathology* **71**, 131–136.

Buchner A. and David R. (1978) Lipopigment in odontogenic cysts. *Journal of Oral Pathology* **7**, 311–317.

Buchner A. and Hansen L. S. (1979) The histomorphologic spectrum of the gingival cyst in the adult. *Oral Surgery, Oral Medicine, Oral Pathology* **48**, 532–539.

Buchner A. and Hansen L. S. (1980) Lymphoepithelial cysts of the oral cavity. A clinicopathologic study of 38 cases. *Oral Surgery, Oral Medicine, Oral Pathology* **50**, 441–449.

Buchner, A., Merrell P. W., Hansen L. S. and Leider A. S. (1991) Peripheral (extraosseous) calcifying odontogenic cyst. A review of forty-five cases. *Oral Surgery, Oral Medicine, Oral Pathology* **72**, 65–70.

Buchner A. and Ramon Y. (1974) Median mandibular cyst – a rare lesion of debatable origin. *Oral Surgery, Oral Medicine, Oral Pathology* **37**, 431–437.

Burdi A. R. (1968) Distribution of midpalatine cysts – re-evaluation of human palatal closure mechanisms. *Journal of Oral Surgery* **26**, 41–45.

Burke G. W., Feagans W. M., Elzay R. P. and Schwartz L. D. (1966) Some aspects of the origin and fate of midpalatal cysts in human fetuses. *Journal of Dental Research* **45**, 159–164.

Butz S. (1975) Personal communication.

Cahill D. R. and Marks S. C. (1980) Tooth eruption: evidence for the central role of the dental follicle. *Journal of Oral Pathology* **9**, 189–200.

Calonius P. E. B., Hakala P. and Rapola J. (1974) Congenital cervical cysts and fistulas. *Proceedings of the Finnish Dental Society* **70**, 209–216.

Camarda A. J., Pham J. and Forest D. (1989) Mandibular infected buccal cyst: report of two cases. *Journal of Maxillofacial Surgery* **47**, 528–534.

Camilleri A. C. and Lloyd R. E. (1990) Lymphoepithelial cyst of the parotid gland. *British Journal of Oral and Maxillofacial Surgery* **28**, 329–332.

Campbell R. L. and Burkes E. J. (1975) Nasolabial cyst: report of a case. *Journal of the American Dental Association* **91**, 1210–1213.

Cantatore G. (1957) Alcuni considerazioni sin tumori cistici ectodermici odontogenic dei mascellari e sullo loro classificazione con particulare riferimento alle cisti gubernaculari. *Minerva Stomatologica* **7**, 738–741.

Carpenter R. J. (1982) Thymic cyst of the neck with prolongation of the thymus gland. *Otolaryngology Head and Neck Surgery* **90**, 494–496.

Casamassimo P. S. and Lilly G. E. (1980) Mucosal cysts of the maxillary sinus: a clinical and radiographic study. *Oral Surgery, Oral Medicine, Oral Pathology* **50**, 282–286.

Cataldo E. and Mosadomi A. (1970) Mucoceles of the oral mucous membrane. *Archives of Otolaryngology* **91**, 360–365.

Cernéa P., Kuffer R., Baumont M., Brocheriou C. and Guilbert F. (1969) Naevomatose basocellulaire. *Revue de Stomatologie et de Chirurgie Maxillo-Faciale* **70**, 181–226.

Chamda R. A. and Shear M. (1980) Dimensions of incisive fossae on dry skulls and radiographs. *International Journal of Oral Surgery* **9**, 452–457.

Chaudhry A. P., Reynolds D. H., La Chapelle C. F. and Vickers R. A. (1960) A clinical and experimental study of mucocele (retention cyst). *Journal of Dental Research* **39**, 1253–1262.

Chomette G., Mosadomi A., Auriol M. and Vaillant J. M.(1985) Histoenzymological features of epithelial cells in lesions of oral mucosa, in cysts and ameloblastomas of jaws. *International Journal of Oral Surgery* **14**, 61–72.

Christ T. F. (1970) The globulomaxillary cyst – an embryologic misconception. *Oral Surgery, Oral Medicine, Oral Pathology* **30**, 515–526.

Clausen F. P. and Dabelsteen E. (1969) Increase in sensitivity of the rhodamine B method for keratinization by the use of fluorescent light. *Acta Pathologica et Microbiologica Scandinavica (A)* **77**, 169–171.

Clough J. R. and Price C. H. G. (1968) Aneurysmal bone cysts. *Journal of Bone and Joint Surgery (Br.)* **50**, 110–127.

Cohen D. A., Neville B. W., Damm D. D. and White D. K. (1984) The lateral periodontal cyst. *Journal of Periodontology* **55**, 230–234.

Cohen L. (1965) Mucoceles of the oral cavity. *Oral Surgery, Oral Medicine, Oral Pathology* **19**, 365–372.

Cohen M. A. (1979) Pathways of inflammatory cellular exudate through radicular cyst epithelium: a light and scanning electron microscope study. *Journal of Oral Pathology* **8**, 369–378.

Cohen M. A. and Hertzanu Y. (1985) Huge growth potential of the nasolabial cyst. *Oral Surgery, Oral Medicine, Oral Pathology* **59**, 441–445.

Cohen M. A. and Mendelsohn D. B. (1990) CT and MR imaging of myxofibroma of the jaws. *Journal of Computer Assisted Tomography* **14**, 281–285.

Cohen M. A. and Shear M. (1980) Histological comparison of parakeratinized and orthokeratinized primordial cysts (keratocysts). *Journal of the Dental Association of South Africa* **35**, 161–165.

Colmenero C., Patron M. and Colmenero B. (1990) Odontogenic ghost cell tumours. *Journal of Cranio-Maxillo-Facial Surgery* **18**, 215–218.

Constantinides C. G., Davies M. R. Q. and Cywes S. (1982) Intralingual cysts of foregut origin. *South African Journal of Surgery* **20**, 227–232.

Contos J. G., Corcoran J. F., LaTurno S. A., Chiego D. J. and Regezi J. A. (1987) Langerhans cells in apical periodontal cysts: an immunohistochemical study. *Journal of Endodontics* **13**, 52–55.

Correll R. W., Jensen J. L. and Rhyne R. R. (1980) Lingual cortical mandibular defects: a radiographic incidence study. *Oral Surgery, Oral Medicine, Oral Pathology* **50**, 287–291.

Courage G. R., North A. F. and Hansen L. S. (1974) Median palatine cysts. Review of the literature and report of case. *Oral Surgery, Oral Medicine, Oral Pathology* **37**, 745–753.

Cox M., Eveson J. and Scully C. (1991) Human papillomavirus type 16 DNA in an odontogenic keratocyst. *Journal of Oral Pathology and Medicine* **20**, 143–145.

Craig G. T. (1976) The paradental cyst. A specific inflammatory odontogenic cyst. *British Dental Journal* **141**, 9–14.

Craig G. T., Holland C. S. and Hindle M. O. (1980) Dermoid cyst of the mandible. *British Journal of Oral Surgery* **18**, 230–237.

Crawford W. H., Korchin L. and Greskovich F. J. (1968) Nasolabial cyst: report of two cases. *Journal of Oral Surgery* **26**, 582–588.

Dabelsteen E. and Fulling H. J. (1971) A preliminary study of blood group substances A and B in oral epithelium exhibiting atypia. *Scandinavian Journal of Dental Research* **79**, 387–393.

Dascoulis G. (1960) Personal communication.

Daugherty J. W. and Eversole L. R. (1971) Aneurysmal bone cyst of the mandible. Report of a case. *Journal of Oral Surgery* **29**, 737–741.

David V. C. and O'Connell J. E. (1986) Nasolabial cyst. *Clinical Otolaryngology* **11**, 5–8.

Dayan D., Buchner A., Gorsky M. and Harel-Raviv M. (1988) The peripheral odontogenic keratocyst. *International Journal of Oral and Maxillofacial Surgery* **17**, 81–83.

DeGould M. D. and Goldberg J. S. (1991) Recurrence of an odontogenic keratocyst in a bone graft. Report of a case. *International Journal of Oral and Maxillofacial Surgery* **20**, 9–11.

Dent R. J. and Wertheimer F. W. (1967) Hyaline bodies in odontogenic cysts- a histochemical study for hemoglobin. *Journal of Dental Research* **46**, 629.

De Visscher J. G. A. M., van der Wal K. G. H. and Vogel P. L. (1989) The plunging ranula. Pathogenesis, diagnosis and management. *Journal of Cranio-Maxillo-Facial Surgery* **17**, 182–185.

Dewey K. W. (1918) Cysts of the dental system. *Dental Cosmos* **60**, 555–570.

Difiore P. M. and Hartwell G. R. (1987) Median mandibular lateral periodontal cyst. *Oral Surgery, Oral Medicine, Oral Pathology* **63**, 545–550.

Djamshidi M. (1976) The odontogenic cysts: incidence of the primordial cyst. *BSc Dent. Dissertation,* University of Adelaide.

Dominguez F.V. and Keszler A. (1988) Comparative study of keratocysts, associated and non-associated with nevoid basal cell carcinoma syndrome. *Journal of Oral Pathology* **17**, 39–42.

Donatsky O., Hjørting-Hansen E., Philipsen H. P. and Fejerskov J. (1976) Clinical, radiologic and histopathologic aspects of 13 cases of nevoid basal cell carcinoma syndrome. *International Journal of Oral Surgery* **5**, 19–28.

Donath K. (1985) Odontogene und nicht-odontogene Kieferzysten. *Deutsche Zahnärztliche Zeitschrift* **40**, 502–509.

Donoff R. B., Harper E. and Guralnick W. C. (1972) Collagenolytic activity in keratocysts. *Journal of Oral Surgery* **30**, 879–884.

Douglas C. W. I. and Craig G. T. (1986) Recognition of protein apparently specific to odontogenic keratocyst fluids. *Journal of Clinical Pathology* **39**, 1108–1115.

Douglas C. W. I. and Craig G. T. (1987) Evidence for the presence of lactoferrin in odontogenic keratocyst fluids. *Journal of Clinical Pathology* **40**, 914–921.

Douglas C. W. I. and Craig G. T. (1989) Quantitation of lactoferrin in odontogenic cyst fluids. *Journal of Clinical Pathology* **42**, 180–183.

Earl P. D. and Ward-Booth R. P. (1985) A case of branchial (lympho-epithelial) cyst, illustrating the value of ultrasound in diagnosis of cervical swellings. *British Journal of Oral and Maxillofacial Surgery* **23**, 292–297.

Ebling H., Barbachan J. J. O., Quadros O. and Figueiro H. S. (1971) Cisto ceratinizado. *Arch. Cent. Estud. Fac. Odontol. U.M.G.* **8**, 107–113.

El-Bardaie A., Nikai H. and Takata T. (1989) Pigmented nasopalatine duct cyst. Report of 2 cases. *International Journal of Oral and Maxillofacial Surgery* **18**, 138–139.

El-Deeb M., Sedano H. O. and Waite D. E. (1980) Aneurysmal bone cyst of the jaws. Report of a case associated with fibrous dysplasia and review of the literature. *International Journal of Oral Surgery* **9**, 301–311.

Eliasson S., Isacsson G. and Köndell P. A. (1989) Lateral periodontal cysts. Clinical, radiographical and histopathological findings. *International Journal of Oral and Maxillofacial Surgery* **18**, 191–193.

El-Labban N. G. (1979) Electron microscopic investigation of hyaline bodies in odontogenic cysts. *Journal of Oral Pathology* **8**, 81–93.

El-Labban N. G. and Aghabeigi B. (1990) A comparative stereologic and ultrastructural study of blood vessels in odontogenic keratocysts and dentigerous cysts. *Journal of Oral Pathology and Medicine* **19**, 442–446.

Elliott J. N. and Oertel Y. C. (1990) Lymphoepithelial cysts of the salivary glands. Histologic and cytologic features. *American Journal of Clinical Pathology* **93**, 39–43.

Emerson T. G., Whitlock R. I. H. and Jones J. H. (1972) Involvement of soft tissue by odontogenic keratocysts (primordial cysts). *British Journal of Oral Surgery* **9**, 181–185.

Eppley B. L., Bell M. J. and Sclaroff A. (1985) Simultaneous occurrence of dermoid and heterotopic intestinal cysts in the floor of the mouth of a newborn. *Journal of Oral and Maxillofacial Surgery* **43**, 880–883.

Ettinger R. L. and Manderson R. O. (1973) Implantation keratinizing epidermoid cysts. *Oral Surgery, Oral Medicine, Oral Pathology* **36**, 225–230.

Eversole L. R. (1987) Oral sialocysts. *Archives of Otolaryngology Head and Neck Surgery* **113**, 51–56.

Eversole L. R., Sabes W. R. and Rovin S. (1975) Aggressive growth and neoplastic potential of odontogenic cysts. *Cancer* **35**, 270–282.

Ewing J. (1940) *Neoplastic Diseases: A Treatise on Tumours*, 4th edn, Philadelphia, Saunders, p. 323.

Fanibunda K. B. (1970) Bilateral nasolabial cysts: a case report. *Dental Practitioner and Dental Record* **20**, 249–250.

Fantasia J. E. (1979) Lateral periodontal cyst. An analysis of 46 cases. *Oral Surgery, Oral Medicine, Oral Pathology* **48**, 237–243.

Fauchard P. (1746) *The Surgeon Dentist or Treatise on the Teeth* (Tr. Lindsay L. (1946), London, Butterworth, p. 93).

FDI Newsletter (1983) One in every two persons in the middle ages stricken with oral disease. **No. 129**, 9.

Fejerskov O. and Krogh J. (1972) The calcifying ghost cell odontogenic tumor – or the calcifying odontogenic cyst. *Journal of Oral Pathology* **1**, 273–287.

Fell H. (1957) The effect of excess vitamin A on cultures of embryonic chicken skin explanted at different stages of differentiation. *Proceedings of the Royal Society, London (Biol.)* **146**, 242–256.

Ferenczy K. (1958) The relationship of globulomaxillary cysts to the fusion of embryonal processes and to cleft palates. *Oral Surgery, Oral Medicine, Oral Pathology* **11**, 1388–1393.

Ficarra G., Chou L. and Panzoni E. (1990) Glandular odontogenic cyst (sialo-odontogenic cyst). *International Journal of Oral and Maxillofacial Surgery* **19**, 331–333.

Fickling B. W. (1965) Cysts of the jaw – a long term survey of types and treatment. *Proceedings of the Royal Society of Medicine* **58**, 847–854.

Fink H. A. (1963) Retention cyst of the tongue. *Oral Surgery, Oral Medicine, Oral Pathology* **16**, 1290–1293.

Fisher A. D. (1976) Bone cavities in fibro-osseous lesions. *British Journal of Oral Surgery* **14**, 120–127.

Fløe Møller J. and Philipsen H. P. (1958) Et tilfaelde af nasoalveolaer cyste (Klestadt's cyste). A case of nasoalveolar cyst (Klestadt's cyst). *Tandlaegebladet* **62**, 659–668.

Fordyce G. L. (1956) The probable nature of so-called latent haemorrhagic cysts of the mandible. *British Dental Journal* **101**, 40–42.

Forssell K. (1980) The primordial cyst. A clinical and radiographic study. *Proceedings of the Finnish Dental Society* **76**, 129–174.

Forssell K. and Sainio P. (1979) Clinicopathological study of keratinized cysts of the jaws. *Proceedings of the Finnish Dental Society* **75**, 36–45.

Forssell K., Forssell H. and Kahnberg K.-E. (1988) Recurrence of keratocysts. A long-term follow-up study. *International Journal of Maxillofacial and Oral Surgery* **17**, 25–28.

Forssell K., Sorvari T. E. and Oksala E. (1974) An analysis of the recurrence of odontogenic keratocysts. *Proceedings of the Finnish Dental Society* **70**, 135–140.

Fowler C. B. and Brannon R. B. (1989) The paradental cyst: a clinicopathologic study of six new cases and review of the literature. *Journal of Oral and Maxillofacial Surgery* **47**, 243–248.

Freedman P. D., Lumerman H. and Gee J. K. (1975) Calcifying odontogenic cyst. *Oral Surgery, Oral Medicine, Oral Pathology* **40**, 93–106.

Frithiof L. and Hägglund G. (1966) Ultrastructure of the capsular epithelium of radicular cysts. *Acta Odontologica Scandinavica* **24**, 23–34.

Fromm A. (1967) Epstein's pearls, Bohn's nodules and inclusion cysts of the oral cavity. *Journal of Dentistry for Children* **34**, 275–287.

Fujiwara K. and Watanabe T. (1988) Mucus-producing cells and ciliated epithelial cells in mandibular radicular cyst: an electron microscopic study. *Journal of Oral and Maxillofacial Surgery* **46**, 149–151.

Gait C. (1976) Solitary bone cyst of the mandible – report of a case. *British Journal of Oral Surgery* **13**, 250–253.

Galloway R. H., Gross P. D., Thompson S. H. and Patterson A. L. (1989) Pathogenesis and treatment of ranula. Report of three cases. *Journal of Oral and Maxillofacial Surgery* **47**, 299–302.

Gao Z., Mackenzie I. C., Rittman B. R., Korszun A-K., Williams D. M. and Cruchley A. T. (1988a) Immunocytochemical examination of immune cells in periapical granulomata and odontogenic cysts. *Journal of Oral Pathology* **17**, 84–90.

Gao Z., Mackenzie I. C., Williams D. M., Cruchley A. T., Leigh I. and Lane E. B. (1988b) Patterns of keratin-expression in rests of Malassez and periapical lesions. *Journal of Oral Pathology* **17**, 178–185.

Gardner A. F. (1969) The odontogenic cyst as a potential carcinoma: a clinicopathologic appraisal. *Journal of the American Dental Association* **78**, 740–755.

Gardner A. F., Gallagher C. A. and Glaser R. I. (1963) The life history of the oral mucocele. *Northwest Dentistry* **42**, 103–107.

Gardner D. G. (1981) Plexiform unicystic ameloblastoma: a diagnostic problem in dentigerous cysts. *Cancer* **47**, 1358–1363.

Gardner D. G. (1984) Pseudocysts and retention cysts of the maxillary sinus. *Oral Surgery, Oral Medicine, Oral Pathology* **58**, 561–567.

Gardner D. G. (1988) An evaluation of reported cases of median mandibular cysts.*Oral Surgery, Oral Medicine, Oral Pathology* **65**, 208–213.

Gardner D. G. and Corio R. L. (1983) The relationship of plexiform unicystic ameloblastoma to conventional ameloblastoma. *Oral Surgery, Oral Medicine, Oral Pathology* **56**, 54–60.

Gardner D. G. and Corio R.L. (1984) Plexiform unicystic ameloblastoma: a variant of ameloblastoma with a low-recurrence rate after enucleation. *Cancer* **53**, 1730–1735.

Gardner D. G. and Gullane P. J. (1986) Mucoceles of the maxillary sinus. *Oral Surgery, Oral Medicine, Oral Pathology* **62**, 538–543.

Gardner D. G. and O'Neill P. A. (1988) Inability to distinguish ameloblastomas from odontogenic cysts based on expression of blood cell carbohydrates. *Oral Surgery, Oral Medicine, Oral Pathology* **66**, 480–482.

Gardner D.G., Kessler H. P., Morency R. and Schaffner D.L. (1988) The glandular odontogenic cyst: an apparent entity. *Journal of Oral Pathology* **17**, 359–366.

Gardner D. G., Sapp J. P. and Wysocki G. P. (1978) Odontogenic and 'fissural' cysts of the jaws. *Pathology Annual* **13**, 177–200. New York, Appleton-Century-Crofts.

Garlick J. A., Calderon S., Metzker A., Rotem A. and Abramovici A. (1989) Simultaneous occurrence of a congenital lateral upper lip sinus and congenital gingival cyst: a case report and discussion of pathogenesis. *Oral Medicine, Oral Surgery, Oral Pathology* **68**, 317–323.

Gebhardt P. and Lenz W. (1985) Zur Frage der Induktion follikulärer Zysten im Wechselgebiss durch Wurzelbehandlung von Milchzähnen. *Deutsche Zahnärztliche Zeitschrift* **40**, 541–543.

George D. I., Gould A. R. and Behr M. M. (1984) Intraneural epithelial islands associated with a periapical cyst. *Oral Surgery, Oral Medicine, Oral Pathology* **57**, 58–62.

Geschickter C. F. and Copeland M. H. (1949) *Tumors of Bone*, 3rd edn, Philadelphia, Lippincott, p. 316.

Gillette R. and Weinmann J. P. (1958) Extrafollicular stages in dentigerous cyst development. *Oral Surgery, Oral Medicine, Oral Pathology* **11**, 638–645.

Gingell J. C., Levy B. M., Beckerman T. and Tilghman D. M. (1984) Aneurysmal bone cyst. *Journal of Oral and Maxillofacial Surgery* **42**, 527–534.

Giunta J. and Cataldo E. (1973) Lymphoepithelial cysts of the oral mucosa. *Oral Surgery, Oral Medicine, Oral Pathology* **35**, 77–84.

Gold L. and Christ T. (1970) Granular cell odontogenic cyst. *Oral Surgery, Oral Medicine, Oral Pathology* **29**, 437–442.

Gold L. and Sliwkowski A. S. (1973) Lateral periodontal cyst a clinical and histological study. In: Kay L. W. (ed.) *Oral Surgery IV* (Transactions of the Fourth International Conference on Oral Surgery). Copenhagen: Munksgaard, pp. 85–89.

Gorlin R. J. (1957) Potentialities of oral epithelium manifest by mandibular dentigerous cysts. *Oral Surgery, Oral Medicine, Oral Pathology* **10**, 271–284.

Gorlin R. J. and Goltz R. W. (1960) Multiple nevoid basal cell epithelioma, jaw cysts and bifid rib: a syndrome. *New England Journal of Medicine* **262**, 908–912.

Gorlin R. J. and Jirasek J. E. (1970) Oral cysts containing gastric or intestinal mucosa – unusual embryologic accident or heterotopia. *Journal of Oral Surgery* **28**, 9–11.

Gorlin R.J., Yunis J.J. and Tuna W. (1963) Multiple nevoid basal cell carcinoma, odontogenic keratocysts and skeletal anomalies syndrome. *Acta Dermatologica Venereologica (Stockholm)*, **43**, 39–55.

Gorlin R. J., Pindborg J. J., Clausen F. P. and Vickers R. A. (1962) The calcifying odontogenic cyst – a possible analogue of the cutaneous calcifying epithelioma of Malherbe. *Oral Surgery, Oral Medicine, Oral Pathology* **15**, 1235–1243.

Gorlin R. J., Pindborg J. J., Redman R. S., Williamson J. J. and Hansen L. S. (1964) The calcifying odontogenic cyst. A new entity and possible analogue of the cutaneous calcifying epithelioma of Malherbe. *Cancer* **17**, 723–729.

Gothberg K. A. T., Little J. W., King O. R. and Bean L. R. (1976) A clinical study of cysts arising from mucosa of the maxillary sinus. *Oral Surgery, Oral Medicine, Oral Pathology* **41**, 52–58.

Gowgiel J. M. (1979) Simple bone cyst of the mandible. *Oral Surgery, Oral Medicine, Oral Pathology* **47**, 319–322.

Grand N. G. and Marwah A. S. (1964) Pigmented gingival cyst. *Oral Surgery, Oral Medicine, Oral Pathology* **17**, 635–639.

Greer R. O. and Johnson M. (1988) Botryoid odontogenic cyst: clinicopathologic analysis of ten cases with three recurrences. *Journal of Oral and Maxillofacial Surgery* **46**, 574–579.

Gregory G. T. and Shafer W. G. (1958) Surgical ciliated cysts of the maxilla. *J. Oral Surgery, Oral Medicine, Oral Pathology* **16**, 251–253.

Grodjest J. E., Dolinsky H. B., Schneider L. C., Dolinsky E. H. and Doyle J. L. (1987) Odontogenic ghost cell carcinoma. *Oral Surgery, Oral Medicine, Oral Pathology* **63**, 576–581.

Grundy G. E., Adkins K. F. and Savage N. W. (1984) Cysts associated with deciduous molars following pulp therapy. *Australian Dental Journal* **29**, 249–256.

Grupe H. E., jun., Ten Cate A. R. and Zander H. A. (1967) A histochemical and radiobiological study of in vitro and in vivo human epithelial cell rest proliferation. *Archives of Oral Biology* **12**, 1321–1329.

Gruskin S. E. and Dahlin O. C. (1968) Aneurysmal bone cysts of the jaws. *Journal of Oral Surgery* **26**, 523–528.

Gutmann J., Cifuentes C., Gandulfo P. and Guesalaga F. (1978) Intradermal naevus associated with epidermoid cyst in the mucous membrane of the cheek. *Oral Surgery, Oral Medicine, Oral Pathology* **45**, 76–82.

Hall A. M. (1976) The solitary bone cyst. *Oral Surgery, Oral Medicine, Oral Pathology* **42**, 164–168.

Hamilton W. J. and Mossman H. W. (1972) *Human Embryology*, 4th ed. Cambridge, Heffer, p. 302.

Hansen J. (1967) Keratocysts in the jaws. In: Husted E. and Hjørting-Hansen E. (ed.) *Oral Surgery II* (Transactions of the Second International Conference on Oral Surgery). Copenhagen, Munksgaard, pp. 128–134.

Hansen L. S. and Allard R. H. B. (1984) Encysted parasitic larvae in the mouth. *Journal of the American Dental Association* **108**, 632–636.

Hansen J. and Kobayasi T. (1970a) Ultrastructural studies of odontogenic cysts I. Nonkeratinizing cysts. *Acta Morphologica Neerlando-Scandinavica (Lisse)* **8**, 29–42.

Hansen J. and Kobayasi T. (1970b) Ultrastructural studies of odontogenic cysts–II. Keratinizing cysts. *Acta Morphologica Neerlando-Scandinavica (Lisse)* **8**, 43–62.

Hansen L. S., Sapone J. and Sproat R. C. (1974) Traumatic bone cysts of jaws. *Oral Surgery, Oral Medicine, Oral Pathology* **37**, 899–910.

Harada Y., Ueda N., Tashiro T., Sugimoto Y. and Imai M. (1968) Nasoalveolar cyst; report of 3 cases. *Hiroshima Journal of Medical Science* **17**, 15–26.

Harnische H. (1961) *Die Durchfruchstorungen der Weisheitszahne*. Volk und Gesundheit, Berlin.

Harris M. (1978) Odontogenic cyst growth and prostaglandin-induced bone resorption. *Annals of the Royal College of Surgeons of England* **60**, 85–91.

Harris M. and Goldhaber P. (1973) The production of a bone resorbing factor by dental cysts in vitro. *British Journal of Oral Surgery* **10**, 334–338.

Harris M., Jenkins M. V., Bennett A. and Wills M. R. (1973) Prostaglandin production and bone resorption by dental cysts. *Nature* **245**, 213–215.

Harris M. and Toller P. (1975) The pathogenesis of dental cysts. *British Medical Bulletin* **31**, 159–163.

Harrison J. D. (1975) Salivary mucoceles. *Oral Surgery, Oral Medicine, Oral Pathology* **39**, 268–278.

Harrison J. D. and Garrett J. R. (1972) Mucocele formation in cats by glandular duct ligation. *Archives of Oral Biology* **17**, 1403–1414.

Harrison J. D. and Garrett J. R. (1975a) Experimental salivary mucoceles in cat. A histochemical study. *Journal of Oral Pathology* **4**, 297–306.

Harrison J. D. and Garrett J. R. (1975b) An ultrastructural and histochemical study of a naturally occurring salivary mucocele in a cat. *Journal of Comparative Pathology* **85**, 411–416.

Harrison J. D., Sowray J. H. and Smith N. J. D. (1976) Recurrent ranula. *British Dental Journal* **140**, 180–182.

Harvey S. H. (1855) Tumours caused by carious tooth. *American Journal of Dental Surgery* **2**, 589–590.

Hauer A. (1926) Ein Cholesteatom im linken Unterkiefer unter einem retinierten Weisheitszahn. *Zeitschrift fur Stomatologie* **24**, 40–59.

Heath C. (1880) Thirty-five years history of a maxillary tumour. *British Journal of Dental Science* **23**, 502–505.

Heath C. (1887) Cystic diseases of the jaws. *British Journal of Dentistry* **8**, 422–434, 615–626.

Hebda P. A., Alstadt S. P., Hileman W. T. and Eaglstein W. H. (1986) Support and stimulation of epidermal cell outgrowth from porcine skin explants platelet factors. *British Journal of Dermatology* **115**, 529–541. Cited by El-Labban and Aghabeigi (1990).

Hedin M., Klämfeldt A. and Persson G. (1978) Surgical treatment of nasopalatine ducts cysts. A follow-up study. *International Journal of Oral Surgery* **7**, 427–433.

Heikinheimo K., Happonen R.-P., Forssell K., Kuusilehto A. and Virtanen I. (1989) A botryoid odontogenic cyst with multiple recurrences. *International Journal of Oral and Maxillofacial Surgery* **18**, 10–13.

Herbener G. H., Gould A. R., Neal D. C. and Farman A. G. (1991) An electron and optical microscopic study of juxtaposed odontogenic keratocyst and carcinoma. *Oral Surgery, Oral Medicine, Oral Pathology* **71**, 322–328.

Hertzanu Y., Cohen M. and Mendelsohn D. B. (1985) Nasopalatine duct cyst. *Clinical Radiology* **36**, 153–158.

High A. S. and Hirschmann P. N. (1986) Age changes in residual radicular cysts. *Journal of Oral Pathology* **15**, 524–528.

High A. S. and Hirschmann P. N. (1988) Symptomatic residual radicular cysts. *Journal of Oral Pathology* **17**, 70–72.

High A. S., Quirke P., and Hume W. J. (1987) DNA-ploidy studies in a keratocyst undergoing subsequent malignant transformation. *Journal of Oral Pathology* **16**, 135–138.

Higuchi Y., Nakamura N. and Tashiro H. (1988) Clinicopathologic study of cemento-osseous dysplasia producing cysts of the mandible. Report of four cases. *Oral Surgery, Oral Medicine, Oral Pathology* **65**, 339–342.

Hirota J., Maeda Y., Ueta E. and Osaki T. (1989) Immunohistochemical and histologic study of cervical lymphoepithelial cysts. *Journal of Oral Pathology and Medicine* **18**, 202–205.

Hirshberg A., Dayan D. and Horowitz I. (1987) Dentinogenic ghost cell tumor. *International Journal of Oral and Maxillofacial Surgery* **16**, 620–625.

Hjørting-Hansen E., Andreasen J. O. and Robinson L. H. (1969) A study of odontogenic cysts with special reference to location of keratocysts. *British Journal of Oral Surgery* **7**, 15–23.

Hodgkinson D. J., Woods J. E., Dahlin D. C. and Tolman D. E. (1978) Keratocysts of the jaw. Clinicopathologic study of 79 patients. *Cancer* **41**, 803–813.

Hodson J. J. (1962) Epithelial residues of the jaw with special reference to the edentulous jaw. *Journal of Anatomy* **96**, 16–24.

Hoffmeister B. and Härle F. (1985) Zysten im Kiefer-Gesichtbereich–eine katamnestische Studie an 3353 Zysten. *Deutsche Zahnärztliche Zeitschrift* **40**, 610–614.

Hoggins, G. S. and Hutton J. B. (1974) Congenital sublingual cystic swellings due to imperforate salivary ducts. *Oral Surgery, Oral Medicine, Oral Pathology* **37**, 370–373.

Holliday R. A., Cohen W. A., Schinella R. A., Rothstein S. G., Persky M. S., Jacobs J. M. and Som P. M.(1988) Benign lymphoepithelial parotid cysts and hyperplastic cervical lymphadenopathy in AIDS-risk patients: a new CT appearance. *Radiology* **168**, 439–441.

Holtgrave E. and Spiessl B. (1975) Die osteoplastiche Behandlung grosser Kieferzysten. *Schweizerische Monatsschrift fur Zahnheilkunde* **85**, 585–597.

Hong S. P., Ellis G. L. and Hartman, K. S. (1991) Calcifying odontogenic cyst. A review of ninety-two cases with reevaluation of their nature as cysts or neoplasms, the nature of ghost cells, and subclassification. *Oral Surgery, Oral Medicine, Oral Pathology* **72**, 56–64.

Hong S. S., Ogawa Y., Yagi T., Wasaka K., Sakurai M., Sano M. and Harada T. (1990) Benign lymphoepithelial lesion with large cysts:case report. *Journal of Oral Pathology and Medicine* **19**, 266–270.

Hormia M., Ylipaavalniemi P., Nagle R. B. and Virtanen I. (1987) Expression of cytokeratins in odontogenic jaw cyst: monoclonal antibodies reveal distinct variation between different cyst types. *Journal of Oral Pathology* **16**, 338–346.

Hosseini M. (1978–79) Two atypical solitary bone cysts. *British Journal of Oral Surgery* **16**, 262–269.

Howe G. L. (1965) 'Haemorrhagic cysts' of the mandible. *British Journal of Oral Surgery* **3**, 55–75, 77–91.

Howell C. J. T. (1985) The sublingual dermoid cyst. Report of five cases and review of the literature. *Oral Surgery, Oral Medicine, Oral Pathology* **59**, 578–580.

Howell R. E., Handlers J. P., Aberle A. M., Abrams A. M. and Melrose R. J. (1988) CEA immunoreactivity in odontogenic tumors and keratocysts. *Oral Surgery, Oral Medicine, Oral Pathology* **66**, 576–580.

Howie A. J. and Crocker J. (1981) The lining of branchial cysts studied by electron microscopy and enzyme histochemistry. *Journal of Pathology* **135**, 189–197.

Huebner G. R. and Turlington E. G. (1971) So-called traumatic (haemorrhagic) bone cysts of the jaws. *Oral Surgery, Oral Medicine, Oral Pathology* **31**, 354–365.

Hunter J. (1780) Quoted from Palmer J. F. (ed.) (1835) *The Works of John Hunter F.R.S. with Notes*. London, Longman, vol. 1, p. 70.

Hurlen B. and Olsen I. (1985) Scanning electron microscopic observations on the inner surface of jaw cysts. *International Journal of Oral Surgery* **14**, 526–532.

Iatrou I. A., Legakis N., Ioannidou E. and Patrikiou A. (1988) Anaerobic bacteria in jaw cysts. *British Journal of Oral and Maxillofacial Surgery* **26**, 62–69.

Issa M. A. and Davies J. D. (1971) Dermoid cyst of the jaw. *British Dental Journal* **131**, 543–546.

Jaffe H. L. (1950) Aneurysmal bone cyst. *Bulletin of the Hospital for Joint Diseases* **11**, 3–13.

Jaffe H. L. (1953) Giant cell reparative granuloma, traumatic bone cyst and fibrous (fibro-osseous) dysplasia of the jawbones. *Oral Surgery, Oral Medicine, Oral Pathology* **6**, 159–175.

Jaffe H. L. and Lichtenstein L. (1942) Solitary unicameral bone cyst with emphasis on the roentgen picture, the pathologic appearance, and the pathogenesis. *Archives of Surgery* **44**, 1004–1025.

Jensen J. L. and Erickson J. O. (1974) Hyaline bodies in odontogenic cysts: electron microscopic observations. *Journal of Oral Pathology* **3**, 1–6.

Jensen J. L., Wuerker R. B., Correll R. W. and Erickson J. O. (1979) Epithelial islands associated with mandibular nerves. *Oral Surgery, Oral Medicine, Oral Pathology* **48**, 226–230.

Johannessen A. C. (1986) Esterase-positive inflammatory cells in human periapical lesions. *Journal of Endodontics* **12**, 284–288.

Johannessen A. C., Nilsen R. and Skaug N. (1983) Deposits of immunoglobulins and complement factor C3 in human dental periapical inflammatory lesions. *Scandinavian Journal of Dental Research* **91**, 191–199.

Kaneshiro S., Nakajima T., Yoshikawa Y., Iwasaki H. and Tokiwa N. (1981) The postoperative maxillary cyst: report of 71 cases. *Journal of Oral Surgery* **39**, 191–198.

Karmody C. S. and Gallagher J. C.(1972) Nasoalveolar cysts. *Annals of Otology, Rhinology and Laryngology* **81**, 278–283.

Kaugars C. C., Kaugars G. E. and DeBiasi G. F. (1989) Extraosseous calcifying odontogenic cyst: report of case and review of literature. *Journal of the American Dental Association* **119**, 715–718.

Kaugars G. E. (1986) Botryoid odontogenic cyst. *Oral Surgery, Oral Medicine, Oral Pathology* **62**, 555–559.

Kaugars G. E. and Cale A. E. (1987) Traumatic bone cyst. *Oral Surgery, Oral Medicine, Oral Pathology* **63**, 318–324.

Kaugars G. E., Miller M. E. and Abbey L. M. (1989) Odontomas. *Oral Surgery, Oral Medicine, Oral Pathology* **67**, 172–176.

Kay L. W. and Kramer I. R. H. (1962) Squamous cell carcinoma arising in a dental cyst. *Oral Surgery, Oral Medicine, Oral Pathology* **15**, 970–979.

Keene H. J. (1990) Solitary lesion of the mandible resembling a 'Stafne cyst' in human archaeologic material from Mokapu, Hawaii. *Journal of Oral Pathology and Medicine* **19**, 195–196.

Killey H. C. and Kay L. W. (1973) Benign mucosal cysts. In: Kay L. W. (ed.) *Oral Surgery IV* (Transactions of the Fourth International Conference on Oral Surgery). Copenhagen, Munksgaard, pp. 169–174.

Killey H. C., Kay L. W. and Seward G. R. (1977) *Benign Cystic Lesions of the Jaws, their Diagnosis and Treatment*. 3rd edn, Edinburgh and London, Churchill Livingstone.

King E. S. J. (1949) The lateral lymphoepithelial cyst of the neck. *Australian and New Zealand Journal of Surgery* **29**, 109–121.

Kitamura H. (1976) Origin of nonodontogenic cysts: an embryonic consideration of fissural cysts. *Bulletin of the Kanagawa Dental College* **4**, 1–18.

Klammt J. (1972) Die Keratozysten der Kiefer. *Dtsch. Stomat.* **22**, 501–509.

Knapp M. J. (1970a) Oral tonsils: location, distribution, and histology. *Oral Surgery, Oral Medicine, Oral Pathology* **29**, 155–161.

Knapp M. J. (1970b) Pathology of oral tonsils. *Oral Surgery, Oral Medicine, Oral Pathology* **29**, 295–304.

Kniha H. and Gokel M. (1985) Radikuläre Zyste im klinische Bild der medianen Unterkieferläsionen. *Deutsche Zahnärztliche Zeitschrift* **40**, 555–557.

Köndell P-A. and Wiberg J. (1988) Odontogenic keratocysts. A follow-up study of 29 cases. *Swedish Dental Journal* **12**, 57–62.

Kontiainen S., Ranta H. and Lautenschlager I. (1986) Cells infiltrating human periapical inflammatory lesions. *Journal of Oral Pathology* **15**, 544–546.

Koskimies A. I., Ylipaavalniemi P. and Tuompo H. (1975) Polyacrylamide gel electrophoresis of proteins in fluids from jaw cysts. *Proceedings of the Finnish Dental Society* **71**, 6–9.

Kostečka F. (1929) Ein Cholesteatom im Unterkiefer. *Zeitschrift fur Stomatologie (Wien)* **27**, 1102–1108.

Kramer I. R. H. (1963) Ameloblastoma: a clinicopathological appraisal. *British Journal of Oral Surgery* **1**, 13–28.

Kramer I. R. H. (1970) Letter to the editor on the odontogenic keratocyst. *British Dental Journal* **128**, 370.

Kramer I. R. H. (1974) Changing views on oral disease. *Proceedings of the Royal Society of Medicine* **67**, 271–276.

Kramer I. R. H., Pindborg J.J. and Shear M. (1992) *Histological Typing of Odontogenic Tumours.* Berlin, Springer Verlag.

Kramer I. R. H. and Toller P. A. (1973) The use of exfoliative cytology and protein estimations in preoperative diagnosis of odontogenic keratocysts. *International Journal of Oral Surgery* **2**, 143-151.

Kuntz A. A. and Reichart P. A. (1986) Adenomatoid odontogenic tumor mimicking a globulo-maxillary cyst. *International Journal of Oral and Maxillofacial Surgery* **15**, 632–636.

Kuriloff D. B. (1987) The nasolabial cyst – nasal hamartoma. *Otolaryngology Head and Neck Surgery* **96**, 268–272.

Kuusela P., Hormia M., Tuompo H. and Ylipaavalniemi P. (1982) Demonstration and partial characterization of a novel soluble antigen present in keratocysts. *Oncodevelopmental Biology and Medicine* **3**, 283–290.

Kuusela P., Ylipaavalniemi P. and Thesleff I. (1986) The relationship between the keratocyst antigen (KCA) and keratin. *Journal of Oral Pathology* **15**, 287–291.

Kwapis B. W. and Whitten J. B. (1971) Mucosal cysts of the maxillary sinus. *Journal of Oral Surgery* **29**, 561–566.

Lello G. E. and Makek M. (1985) Stafne's mandibular lingual cortical defect. *Journal of Maxillo-facial Surgery* **13**, 172–176.

Levy W. M., Miller A. S., Bonakdarpour A. and Aegerter E. (1975) Aneurysmal bone cyst secondary to other osseous lesions. Report of 57 cases. *American Journal of Clinical Pathology* **63**, 1–8.

Ligthelm A. J. (1989) *Die Ontwikkeling en Evaluering van 'n Experimentele Sistmodel as Biotoetssisteem in Proefdiere.* PhD Thesis, University of Stellenbosch.

Little J. W. and Jakobsen J. (1973) Origin of the globulomaxillary cyst. *Journal of Oral Surgery* **31**, 188–195.

Livingston A. (1927) Observations on the development of the dental cyst. *Dental Record* **47**, 531–538.

Lucas R. B. (1954) Neoplasia in odontogenic cysts. *Oral Surgery, Oral Medicine, Oral Pathology* **7**, 1227–1235.

Lucas R. B. (1972) *Pathology of Tumours of the Oral Tissues*, 2nd edn, Edinburgh and London, Churchill Livingstone.

Lucchesi F. J. and Topazian D. S. (1961) Multilocular median developmental cysts of the mandible. *Journal of Oral Surgery* **19**, 330–338.

Lufkin A. W. (1938) *History of Dentistry*. London, Kimpton, p. 60.

Lund V. J. (1985) Odontogenic keratocyst of the maxilla: a case report. *British Journal of Oral and Maxillofacial Surgery* **23**, 210–215.

Lustmann J., Benoliel R. and Zeltser R. (1989) Squamous cell carcinoma arising in a thyroglossal duct cyst in the tongue. *Journal of Oral and Maxillofacial Surgery* **47**, 81–85.

Lustmann J. and Bodner L. (1988) Dentigerous cysts associated with supernumerary teeth. *International Journal of Oral and Maxillofacial Surgery* **17**, 100–102.

Lustmann J. and Copelyn M. (1981) Oral cysticercosis. Review of the literature and report of 2 cases. *International Journal of Oral Surgery* **10**, 371–375.

Lustmann J. and Shear M. (1985) Radicular cysts arising from deciduous teeth. Review of the literature and report of 23 cases. *International Journal of Oral Surgery* **14**, 153–161.

Lutz J., Cimasoni G. and Held A. J. (1965) Histochemical observations on the epithelial lining of radicular cysts. *Acta Odontologica Scandinavica* **9**, 90–95.

Lysell L. and Molin L. (1972) Tomography in diagnosis of incisive canal cysts. *Swedish Dental Journal* **65**, 321–326.

McClatchey K. D., Appelblatt N. H., Zarbo R. J. and Merrel D. M. (1984) Plunging ranula. *Oral Surgery, Oral Medicine, Oral Pathology* **57**, 408–412.

McIvor J. (1972) The radiological features of odontogenic keratocysts. *British Journal of Oral Surgery* **10**, 110–125.

MacKenzie G. D., Oatis G. W., Mullen M. P. and Grisius R. J. (1985) Computed tomography in the diagnosis of an odontogenic keratocyst. *Oral Surgery, Oral Medicine and Oral Pathology* **59**, 302–305.

MacLeod R. I., Fanibunda K. B. and Soames J. V. (1985) A pigmented odontogenic keratocyst. *British Journal of Oral and Maxillofacial Surgery* **23**, 216–219.

MacLeod R. I. and Soames J. V. (1988) Squamous cell carcinoma arising in an odontogenic keratocyst. *British Journal of Oral and Maxillofacial Surgery* **26**, 52–57.

Machado de Sousa S. O., Campos A. C., Satiago J. L., Jaeger R. G. and Cavalcanti de Araújo V. (1990) Botryoid odontogenic cyst: report of a case with clinical and histogenetic considerations. *British Journal of Oral and Maxillofacial Surgery* **28**, 275–276.

Machtens E., Hjørting-Hansen E., Schmallenbach H. J. and Werz L. (1972) Keratozyste-Ameloblastom, ein klinisch diagnostiches Problem. *Deutsche Zeitschrift fur Mund-, Kiefer-, und Geschichts-Chirurgie (München)* **58**, 157–165.

Maeda Y., Osaki T., Yoneda K. and Hirota J. (1987) Clinico-pathologic studies on postoperative maxillary cysts. *International Journal of Oral and Maxillofacial Surgery* **16**, 682–687.

Magnusson B. C. (1978) Odontogenic keratocysts: a clinical and histological study with special reference to enzyme histochemistry. *Journal of Oral Pathology* **7**, 8–18.

Main D. M. G. (1970a) Epithelial jaw cysts: a clinicopathological reappraisal. *British Journal of Oral Surgery* **8**, 114–125.

Main D. M. G. (1970b) The enlargement of epithelial jaw cysts. *Odontologisk Revy* **21**, 29–49.

Main D. M. G. (1985) Epithelial jaw cysts: 10 years of the WHO classification. *Journal of Oral Pathology* **14**, 1–7.

Markus A. F. (1978–79) Bilateral haemorrhagic bone cysts of the mandible: a case report. *British Journal of Oral Surgery* **16**, 270–273.

Matejka M., Porteder H., Kleinert W., Ulrich W., Watzek G. and Sinzinger H. (1985a) Evidence that PGI_2-generation in human dental cysts is stimulated by leukotrienes C_4 and D_4. *Journal of Maxillofacial Surgery* **13**, 93–96.

Matejka M., Porteder H., Ulrich W., Watzek G. and Sinzinger H. (1985b) Prostaglandin synthesis in dental cysts. *British Journal of Oral and Maxillofacial Surgery* **23**, 190–194.

Matejka M., Ulrich W., Porteder H., Sinzinger H. and Peskar B. A. (1986) Immunohistochemical detection of 6-oxo-$PGF_{1\alpha}$ and PGE_2 in radicular cysts. *Journal of Maxillofacial Surgery* **14**, 108–112.

Mathiesen A. (1973) Preservation and demonstration of mast cells in human apical granulomas and radicular cysts. *Scandinavian Journal of Dental Research* **81**, 218–229.

Matthews J. B. and Browne R. M. (1987) An immunocytochemical study of the inflammatory cell infiltrate and epithelial expression of HLA-DR in odontogenic cysts. *Journal of Oral Pathology* **16**, 112–117.

Matthews J. B., Mason G. I. and Browne R. M. (1988) Epithelial cell markers and proliferating cells in odontogenic jaw cysts. *Journal of Pathology* **156**, 283–290.

Mayer R., Libotte M. and Ruppol P. (1967) La lacune essentielle de la mandibule. *Acta Stomatologica Belgica* **64**, 33–52.

Meerkotter V. (1969) The ameloblastoma in the Witwatersrand area. *Fourth Proceedings of the International Academy of Oral Pathology*, p. 144.

Meerkotter V. A. and Shear M. (1964) Multiple primordial cysts associated with bifid rib and ocular defects. *Oral Surgery, Oral Medicine, Oral Pathology* **18**, 498–503.

Meghji S., Harvey W. and Harris M. (1989) Interleukin 1-like activity in cystic lesions of the jaw. *British Journal of Oral and Maxillofacial Surgery* **27**, 1–11.

Meurman J. H. and Ylipaavalniemi P. (1982) Scanning electron microscopy of the cavity surface in odontogenic jaw cysts. *Proceedings of the Finnish Dental Society* **78**, 194–200.

Meyer A. W. (1931) Median anterior maxillary cysts. *Journal of the American Dental Association* **18**, 1851–1857.

Meyer I. (1955) Dermoid cysts (dermoids) of the floor of the mouth. *Oral Surgery, Oral Medicine, Oral Pathology* **8**, 1149–1164.

Meyer I. (1957) Developmental median cyst of the mandible. *Oral Surgery, Oral Medicine, Oral Pathology* **10**, 75–80.

Mikulicz J. (1876) Beitrag zur Genese der Dermoide am Kopfe. *Wiener Medizinische Wochenschrift* **26**, 953–956, 983–986, 1004–1008. Cited by Forssell (1980).

Miller R. I. and Houston G. D. (1989) Ectopic apocrine cyst in the facial area. *Journal of Oral and Maxillofacial Surgery* **47**, 401–402.

Mitchell D. A. and Ward-Booth R. P. (1984) Atypical presentation of a solitary bone cyst. *International Journal of Oral Surgery* **13**, 256–259.

Monteleone L. and McLellan M. S. (1964) Epstein's pearls (Bohn's nodules) of the palate. *Journal of Oral Surgery* **22**, 301–304.

Moon (1877–78) Radicular odontome. *Odontological Society Transactions 2nd series* **10**, 30–31.

Moreillon M. C. and Schroeder H. E. (1982) Numerical frequency of epithelial abnormalities, particularly microkeratocysts, in the developing human oral mucosa. *Oral Surgery, Oral Medicine, Oral Pathology* **53**, 44–55.

Morgan P. R. and Heyden G. (1975) Enzyme histochemical studies on the formation of hyalin bodies in the epithelium of odontogenic cysts. *Journal of Oral Pathology* **4**, 120–127.

Morgan P. R. and Johnson N.W. (1974) Histological, histochemical and ultrastructural studies on the nature of hyalin bodies in odontogenic cysts. *Journal of Oral Pathology* **3**, 127–147.

Morgan P., Seddon S. and Lane B. (1988) Keratin expression in odontogenic cysts and tumours. *Abstract No. 8 of the 4th Conference of the International Association of Oral Pathologists.*

Morse D. R., Patnik J. W. and Schacterle G. R. (1973) Electrophoretic differentiation of radicular cysts and granulomas. *Oral Surgery, Oral Medicine, Oral Pathology* **35**, 249–264.

Morse D. R., Schacterle G. R. and Wolfson E. M. (1976) A rapid chairside differentiation of radicular cysts and granulomas. *Journal of Endodontics* **2**, 17–20.

Morse D. R., Wolfson E. and Schacterle G. R. (1975) Nonsurgical repair of electrophoretically diagnosed radicular cysts. *Journal of Endodontics* **1**, 158–163.

Mortensen H., Winther J. E. and Birn H. (1970) Periapical granulomas and cysts. An investigation of 1600 cases. *Scandinavian Journal of Dental Research* **78**, 241–250.

Moskow B. S. (1966) The pathogenesis of the gingival cyst. *Periodontics* **4**, 23–28.

Moskow B. S. and Bloom A. (1983) Embryogenesis of the gingival cyst. *Journal of Clinical Periodontology* **10**, 119–130.

Moskow B. S., Siegel K., Zegarelli E. V., Kutscher A. H. and Rothenberg F. (1970) Gingival and lateral periodontal cysts. *Journal of Periodontology* **41**, 249–260.

Moskow B. S. and Weinstein M. M. (1975) Further observations on the gingival cyst. Three case reports. *Journal of Periodontology* **46**, 178–182.

Mourshed F. (1964a) A roentgenographic study of dentigerous cysts. I. Incidence in a population sample. *Oral Surgery, Oral Medicine, Oral Pathology* **18**, 47–53.

Mourshed F. (1964b) A roentgenographic study of dentigerous cysts. II. Role of roentgenograms in detecting dentigerous cyst in the early stages. *Oral Surgery, Oral Medicine, Oral Pathology* **18**, 54–61.

Mourshed F. (1964c) A roentgenographic study of dentigerous cysts. III. Analysis of 180 cases. *Oral Surgery, Oral Medicine, Oral Pathology* **18**, 466–473.

Myall R. W. T., Eastep P. B. and Silver J. G. (1974) Mucous retention cysts of the maxillary antrum. *Journal of the American Dental Association* **89**, 1338–1342.

Nagao Y., Nakajima T., Fukushima M. and Ishiki T. (1983) Calcifying odontogenic cyst: a survey of 23 cases in the Japanese literature. *Journal of Maxillofacial Surgery* **11**, 174–179.

Nanavati S. D. and Gandhi P. R. (1979) Median mandibular cyst. *Journal of Oral Surgery* **37**, 422–425.

Nandakumar H. and Shankaramba K. B. (1989) Hydatid cyst of the mandible: a case report. *Journal of Oral and Maxillofacial Surgery* **47**, 759–761.

Natkin E., Oswald R. J. and Carnes L. I. (1984) The relationship of lesion size to diagnosis, incidence, and treatment of periapical cysts and granulomas. *Oral Surgery, Oral Medicine, Oral Pathology* **57**, 82–94.

Neiburger E. J. (1977) A mandibular cystlike lesion in a prehistoric American Indian. *Oral Surgery, Oral Medicine, Oral Pathology* **43**, 528–529.

Nicolai P., Luzzago F., Maroldi R., Falchetti M. and Antonelli A. R. (1989) Nasopharyngeal cysts. *Archives of Otolaryngology Head and Neck Surgery* **115**, 860–864.

Niemeyer K., Schlien H–P., Habel G. and Mentler C. (1985) Behandlungsergebnisse und Langzeitbeobachtungen bei 62 Patienten mit Keratozysten, *Deutsche Zahnärztliche Zeitschrift*, **40**, 637–640.

Nilsen R., Johannessen A. C., Skaug N. and Matre R. (1984) In-situ characterization of mononuclear cells in human dental periapical inflammatory lesions using monoclonal antibodies. *Oral Surgery, Oral Medicine, Oral Pathology* **58**, 160–165.

Nortjé C. J. and Farman A. G. (1978) Nasopalatine duct cyst. *International Journal of Oral Surgery* **7**, 65–72.

Nortjé C. J. and Wood R. E. (1988) The radiologic features of the nasopalatine duct cyst. An analysis of 46 cases. *Dentomaxillofacial Radiology* **17**, 129–132.

Nxumalo T. N. and Shear M. (1990) Gingival cyst of adults: histogenesis and histopathology. *Abstr. 19, Proceedings of the 24th Annual Meeting of the South African Division of the International Association for Dental Research* p. 60.

Nxumalo T. N. and Shear M. (1992) The gingival cyst of adults. *Journal of Oral Pathology and Medicine*. In press.

Oehlers F. A. C. (1970) Periapical lesions and residual dental cysts. *British Journal of Oral Surgery* **8**, 103–113.

Ohishi M., Ishii T., Shinohara M. and Horinouchi Y. (1985) Dermoid cyst of the floor of the mouth: lateral teratoid cyst with sinus tract in an infant. *Oral Surgery, Oral Medicine, Oral Pathology* **60**, 191–194.

Oikarinen V. J. and Julku M. (1974) An orthopantomographic study of developmental mandibular bone defects (Stafne's idiopathic bone cavities). *International Journal of Oral Surgery* **3**, 71–76.

Oikarinen V. J., Wolf J. and Julku M. (1975) A stereosialographic study of mandibular bone defects (Stafne's idiopathic bone cavities). *International Journal of Oral Surgery* **4**, 51–54.

Olech E. (1957) Median mandibular cysts. *Oral Surgery, Oral Medicine, Oral Pathology* **10**, 69–74.

Olech E., Sicher H. and Weinmann J. P. (1951) Traumatic mandibular bone cysts. *Oral Surgery, Oral Medicine, Oral Pathology* **4**, 1160–1172.

Olsen D. B., Mostofi R. S. and Lagrotteria L. B. (1988) Steatocystoma simplex in the oral cavity: a previously undescribed condition. *Oral Surgery, Oral Medicine, Oral Pathology* **66**, 605–607.

Ostrofsky M. K. (1980) Epithelial residues in the retromolar regions and their possible relationship to the formation of the primordial cyst (odontogenic keratocyst). *MDent. Dissertation,* University of the Witwatersrand, Johannesburg.

Ostrofsky M. K. and Baker M. A. A. (1975) Oral cysticercosis. *Journal of the Dental Association of South Africa* **30**, 535–537.

Packota G. V., Hall J. M., Lanigan D. T. and Cohen M. A. (1990) Paradental cysts on mandibular first molars in children: report of five cases. *Dentomaxillofacial Radiology* **19**, 126–132.

Padayachee A. and Van Wyk C. W. (1987) Two cystic lesions with features of both the botryoid odontogenic cyst and the central mucoepidermoid tumour: sialo-odontogenic cyst? *Journal of Oral Pathology* **16**, 499–504.

Panders A. K. and Hadders H. N. (1969) Solitary keratocysts of the jaws. *Journal of Oral Surgery* **26**, 931–938.

Papanayotou P. H. and Kayavis J. G. (1977) Epidermoid implantation cyst of the lower lip: report of case. *Journal of Oral Surgery* **35**, 585–586.

Partridge M. and Towers J. F. (1987) The primordial cyst (odontogenic keratocyst): its tumour-like characteristics and behaviour. *British Journal of Oral and Maxillofacial Surgery* **25**, 271–279.

Partsch C. (1892) Uber Kieferzysten. *Deutsche Monatsschrift fur Zahnheilkunde* **10**, 19; 271–304.

Partsch C. (1910) Zur Behandlung der Kieferzysten. *Deutsche Monatsschrift fur Zahnheilkunde* **28**, 252–259.

Patron M., Colmenero C. and Larrauri J. (1991) Glandular odontogenic cyst: clinicopathological analysis of three cases. *Oral Surgery, Oral Medicine, Oral Pathology* **72**, 71–74.

Patten B. M. (1961) The normal development of the facial region. In: *Congenital Anomalies of the Face and Associated Structures*, (ed. S. Prizansky), Springfield, Thomas. pp. 11–45. (Quoted by Little and Jakobsen, 1973.)

Payne T. F. (1972) An analysis of the clinical and histopathologic parameters of the odontogenic keratocyst. *Oral Surgery, Oral Medicine, Oral Pathology* **33**, 538–546.

Pearcey R. G. (1985) Squamous cell carcinoma arising in dental cysts. *Clinical Radiology* **36**, 387–388.

Pedley N. (1886) Cyst of the upper jaw. *British Dental Association Journal* **7**, 289.

Perl P., Perl T. and Goldberg B. (1972) Hydatid cyst in the tongue. *Oral Surgery, Oral Medicine, Oral Pathology* **33**, 579–581.

Perrini N. and Fonzi L. (1985) Mast cells in human periapical lesions: ultrastructural aspects and their possible physiopathological implications. *Journal of Endodontics* **11**, 197–202.

Persson G. (1973) Remarkable recurrence of a keratocyst in a bone graft. *International Journal of Oral Surgery* **2**, 69–76.

Persson G. (1985) An atypical solitary bone cyst. *Journal of Oral and Maxillofacial Surgery* **43**, 905–907.

Phelan J. A., Kritchman D., Fusco-Ramer M., Freedman P. D. and Lumerman H. (1988) Recurrent botryoid odontogenic cyst (lateral periodontal cyst). *Oral Surgery, Oral Medicine, Oral Pathology* **66**, 345–348.

Philippou S., Rühl G. H. and Mandelartz E. (1990) Scanning electron microscopic studies and x-ray microanalysis of hyaline bodies in odontogenic cysts. *Journal of Oral Pathology and Medicine* **19**, 447–452.

Philipsen H. P. (1956) Om keratocyster (kolesteatom) i kaeberne. *Tandlaegebladet* **60**, 963–981.

Philipsen H. P., Fejerskov O., Donatsky O. and Hjørting-Hansen E. (1976) Ultrastructure of epithelial lining of keratocysts in nevoid basal cell carcinoma syndrome. *International Journal of Oral Surgery* **5**, 71–81.

Pindborg J. J. and Hansen J. (1963) Studies on odontogenic cyst epithelium. 2. Clinical and roentgenologic aspects of odontogenic keratocysts. *Acta Pathologica et Micobiologica Scandinavica (A)* **58**, 283–294.

Pindborg J. J. and Hjørting-Hansen E. (1974) *Atlas of Diseases of the Jaws*, 1st edn, Copenhagen, Munksgaard.

Pindborg J. J., Philipsen H. P. and Henriksen J. (1962) Studies on odontogenic cyst epithelium – keratinization in odontogenic cysts. In: *Fundamentals of Keratinization*, p.151, Washington DC, American Association for the Advancement of Science.

Poker I. D. and Hopper C. (1990) Salivary extravasation cyst of the tongue. *British Journal of Oral and Maxillofacial Surgery* **28**, 176–177.

Pollard Z. F., Harley R. D. and Calhoun J. (1976) Dermoid cysts in children. *Pediatrics* **57**, 379–382.

Poyton H. G. and Morgan G. A. (1965) The simple bone cyst. *Oral Surgery, Oral Medicine, Oral Pathology* **20**, 188–197.

Praetorius F. (1975) Calcifying odontogenic cyst: range, variations and neoplastic potential. Paper delivered at a Symposium on Maxillofacial Bone Pathology, Brussels, 30–31 March 1974, organized by Committee on Maxillofacial Bone Pathology. *International Journal of Oral Surgery* **4**, 89 (Abstr.).

Praetorius F. and Hammarström L. (1974) A new concept of the pathogenesis of oral mucous cysts based upon a study of 200 cysts. Personal communication.

Praetorius F., Hjørting-Hansen E., Gorlin R. J. and Vickers R. A. (1981) Calcifying odontogenic cyst. Range, variations and neoplastic potential. *Acta Odontologica Scandinavica* **39**, 227–240.

Pullon, P. A., Shafer W. G., Elzay R. P., Kerr D. A. and Corio R. L. (1975) Squamous odontogenic tumor. *Oral Surgery, Oral Medicine, Oral Pathology* **40**, 616–630.

Pulver W. H., Taubman M. A. and Smith D. H. (1978) Immune components in human dental periapical lesions. *Archives of Oral Biology* **23**, 435–443.

Quinn J. H. (1960) Congenital epidermoid cyst of anterior half of tongue. *Oral Surgery, Oral Medicine, Oral Pathology* **13**, 1283–1287.

Rachanis C. C., Altini M. and Shear M. (1979) A clinicopathological comparison of primordial cyst (keratocysts) in two different age groups. *Journal of Dental Research* **58D**, 2324 (Abstr.).

Rachanis C. C. and Shear M. (1978) Age standardized incidence rates of primordial cyst (keratocyst) on the Witwatersrand. *Community Dentistry and Oral Epidemiology* **6**, 296–299.

Radden B. G. and Reade P. C. (1973) Odontogenic cysts. A review and clinicopathological study of 368 odontogenic cysts. *Australian Dental Journal* **18**, 218–225.

Ramanathan J. and Philipsen H. P. (1981) *In vivo* behaviour of intraosseously implanted oral epithelium in rats. *International Journal of Oral Surgery* **10**, 180–188.

Rasmusson L. G., Magnusson B. C. and Borrman H. (1991) The lateral periodontal cyst. A histopathological and radiographic study of 32 cases. *British Journal of Oral and Maxillofacial Surgery* **29**, 54–57.

Redman R. S. (1974) Nasopalatine duct cyst with pigmented lining suggestive of olfactory epithelium. *Oral Surgery, Oral Medicine, Oral Pathology* **37**, 421–428.

Reeve C. M. and Levy B. P. (1968) Gingival cysts: a review of the literature and a report of four cases. *Periodontics* **6**, 115–117.

Reff-Eberwein G., Donath K. and Schmitz R. (1985) Die odontogene Keratozyste (OKC). *Deutsche Zahnärztliche Zeitschrift* **40**, 514–520.

Rhodus N. L. (1990) The prevalence and clinical significance of maxillary sinus mucous retention cysts in a general clinic population. *Ear, Nose and Throat Journal* **69**, 82–90.

Rickles N. H. and Little J. W. (1967) The histogenesis of the branchial cyst. *American Journal of Pathology* **40**, 533–547.

Ritchey B. and Orban B. (1953) Cysts of the gingivae. *Oral Surgery, Oral Medicine, Oral Pathology* **6**, 765–771.

Rittersma J. (1972) *Het Basocellulaire Nevus Syndroom*. Groningen, NV Boekdrukkerij Dÿstra Niemeyer.

Riviere G. R. and Sabet T. Y. (1973) Experimental follicular cysts in mice – a histologic study. *Oral Surgery, Oral Medicine, Oral Pathology* **36**, 205–213.

Robinson H. B. G. (1945) Classification of cysts of the jaws. *American Journal of Orthodontics and Oral Surgery* **31**, 370–375.

Robinson L. and Hjørting-Hansen E. (1964) Pathologic changes associated with mucous retention cysts of minor salivary glands. *Oral Surgery, Oral Medicine, Oral Pathology* **18**, 191–205.

Robinson L. and Martinez M. G. (1977) Unicystic ameloblastoma. A prognostically distinct entity. *Cancer* **40**, 2278–2285.

Robinson P. D. (1985) Aneurysmal bone cyst. *British Journal of Oral and Maxillofacial Surgery* **23**, 220–226.

Rodu B., Tate A. L. and Martinez M. G. (1987) The implications of inflammation in odontogenic keratocysts. *Journal of Oral Pathology* **16**, 518–521.

Roediger W. E. W., Lloyd P. and Lawson H. H. (1973) Mucous extravasation theory as a cause of plunging ranulas. *British Journal of Surgery* **60**, 720–722.

Roed-Petersen B. (1969) Nasolabial cysts. *British Journal of Oral Surgery* **7**, 84–95.

Roggan R. and Donath K. (1985) Klinik und Pathomorphologie odontogener follikulärer Zysten -- Nachuntersuchung von 239 Fällen. *Deutsche Zahnärztliche Zeitschrift* **40**, 536–540.

Roper-Hall H. T. (1938) Cysts of developmental origin in the premaxillary region, with special reference to their diagnosis. *British Dental Journal* **65**, 405–436.

Rosai J. (1981) Ackerman's *Surgical Pathology*, 6th edn, St Louis, Mosby, p. 103.

Rosencrans M. and Barak J. (1969) Parasitic infection of the mouth. A case report of *Cysticercus cellulosae*. *New York State Dental Journal* **35**, 271–273.

Rubin M. M. and Murphy F. J. (1989) Simple bone cyst of the mandibular condyle. *Journal of Oral and Maxillofacial Surgery* **47**, 1096–1098.

Rud J. and Pindborg J. J. (1969) Odontogenic keratocysts: a follow-up study of 21 cases. *Journal of Oral Surgery* **27**, 323–330.

Rudick A. (1981) The distribution of jaw cysts accessioned in the Department of Oral Pathology, University of the Witwatersrand, 1974–1978. *MSc (Dent.) Dissertation,* University of the Witwatersrand, Johannesburg.

Ruffer M. A. (1921) *Studies in the Palaeopathology of Egypt*, (ed. R. L. Moodie) Chicago, University of Chicago Press.

Rühl G. H., Philippou S. and Mandelartz E. (1989) Zur Histogenese von hyalinen Bodies in odontogenen Zysten. *Deutsche Zeitschrift fur Mund, Kiefer, Gesichts Chururgie* **13**, 145–154

Ruiter D. J., van Rijssel Th. G. and van der Velde E. A. (1977) Aneurysmal bone cysts. A clinicopathological study of 105 cases. *Cancer* **39**, 2231–2239.

Rushton M. A. (1955) Hyaline bodies in the epithelium of dental cysts. *Proceedings of the Royal Society of Medicine* **48**, 407–409.

Sadeghi E. M. and Bell W. A. (1980) Developmental cyst of floor of mouth: soft tissue variety of median mandibular cyst. *Journal of Oral Surgery* **38**, 841–843.

Sadeghi E. M., Weldon L. L., Kwon P. H. and Sampson E. (1991) Mucoepidermoid odontogenic cyst. *International Journal of Oral and Maxillofacial Surgery* **20**, 142–143.

Saku T., Shibata Y., Koyama Z., Cheng J., Okabe H. and Yeh Y. (1991) Lectin histochemistry of cystic jaw lesions: an aid for differential diagnosis between cystic ameloblastoma and odontogenic cysts. *Journal of Oral Pathology and Medicine* **20**, 108–113.

Sakuma T. (1973) An immunological study of radicular cysts. *Journal of the Tokyo Dental College Society* **19**, 312–322.

Salama N. and Hilmy A. (1951) Ancient Egyptian skull and a mandible showing cysts. *British Dental Journal* **90**, 17–18.

Santora E., Ballantyne A. J. and Hinds E. C. (1970) Nasoalveolar cyst: report of case *Journal of Oral Surgery* **28**, 117–120.

Sapp J. P. and Gardner D. G. (1977) An ultrastructural study of the calcifications in calcifying odontogenic cysts and odontomas. *Oral Surgery, Oral Medicine, Oral Pathology* **44**, 754–766.

Saunders I. D. F. (1972) Bohn's nodules – a case report. *British Dental Journal* **132**, 457–458.

Schajowicz F. (1981) *Tumors and Tumor-like Lesions of Bone and Joints*, New York, Springer Verlag, p. 439.

Scharffetter K., Balz-Herrmann C., Lagrange W., Koberg W. and Mittermayer Ch. (1989) Proliferation kinetics-study of the growth of keratocysts. *Journal of Cranio-Maxillo-Facial Surgery* **17**, 226–233.

Schiødt M. and Friis-Hasché E. (1972) Fire tilfaede af oral lymfoepiteliale cyster. *Tandlaegebladet* **76**, 1075–1081.

Scholfield J. J. (1971) Unusual recurrence of an odontogenic keratocyst. *British Dental Journal* **130**, 487–489.

Schroeder H. E. (1976) Gingival tissue. In: *Scientific Foundations of Dentistry*, 1st ed., (ed. B. Cohen and I. R. H. Kramer) Ch. 36. London, Heinemann.

Schwenzer N., Ehrenfeld M. and Roos R. (1985) Über die sogenannte solitäre Knochenzyste. *Deutsche Zahnärztliche Zeitschrift* **40**, 573–575.

Scott J. and Wood G. D. (1989) Aggressive calcifying odontogenic cyst--a possible variant of ameloblastoma. *British Journal of Oral and Maxillofacial Surgery* **27**, 53–59.

Sedano H. O. and Gorlin R. J. (1968) Hyaline bodies of Rushton; some histochemical considerations concerning their etiology. *Oral Surgery, Oral Medicine, Oral Pathology* **26**, 198–201.

Seifert G., Thomsen S. T. and Donath K. (1981) Bilateral dysgenetic polycystic parotid glands: morphological analysis and differential diagnosis of a rare disease of salivary glands. *Virchows Archives A* **390**, 273–288.

Seward G. R. (1962a) Nasolabial cysts and their radiology. *Dental Practitioner* **12**, 154–161.

Seward G. R. (1962b) Surgical significance of odontogenic epithelium. *Paper presented to the 82nd Annual Conference of the British Dental Association, Nottingham.*

Seward G. R. (1964) *Radiology in General Dental Practice*. London: British Dental Association.

Seward G. R. (1965) Dermoid cysts of the floor of the mouth. *British Journal of Oral Surgery* **3**, 36–47.

Seward M. H. (1973) Eruption cyst: an analysis of its clinical features. *Journal of Oral Surgery* **31**, 31–35.

Seward M. H. and Seward G. R. (1968) Observations on Snawdon's technique for the treatment of cysts in the maxilla. *British Journal of Oral Surgery* **6**, 149–159.

Sewerin I. and Praetorius F. (1974) Keratin-filled pseudocysts of ducts of sebaceous glands of the vermilion border of the lip. *Journal of Oral Pathology* **3**, 279–283.

Shafer W. G., Hine M. K. and Levy B. M. (1983) *A Textbook of Oral Pathology*, 4th edn, Philadelphia and London, Saunders.

Shamaskin R. G., Svirsky J. A. and Kaugars G. E. (1989) Intraosseous and extraosseous calcifying odontogenic cyst. *Journal of Oral and Maxillofacial Surgery* **47**, 562–565.

Shaw W., Smith M. and Hill F. (1980) Inflammatory follicular cysts. *Journal of Dentistry for Children* **47**, 97–101.

Shear M. (1960a) Primordial cysts. *Journal of the Dental Association of South Africa* **15**, 211–217.

Shear M. (1960b) Secretory epithelium in the lining of dental cysts. *Journal of the Dental Association of South Africa* **15**, 117–122.

Shear M. (1961a) Clinical statistics of dental cysts. *Journal of the Dental Association of South Africa* **16**, 360–364.

Shear M. (1961b) The hyaline and granular bodies in dental cysts. *British Dental Journal* **110**, 301–307.

Shear M. (1963a) The histogenesis of the dental cyst. *Dental Practitioner* **13**, 238–243.

Shear M. (1963b) Cholesterol in dental cysts. *Oral Surgery, Oral Medicine, Oral Pathology* **16**, 1465–1473.

Shear M. (1963c) The microscopic features of the fibrous walls of dental cysts. *Diastema* **1**, 9–13.

Shear M. (1964) Inflammation in dental cysts. *Oral Surgery, Oral Medicine, Oral Pathology* **17**, 750–767.

Shear M. and Altini M. (1976) The possible inductive role of ectomesenchyme in the pathogenesis of some odontogenic lesions. *Journal of the Dental Association of South Africa.* **31**, 649–654.

Shear M. and Pindborg J. J. (1975) Microscopic features of the lateral periodontal cyst. *Scandinavian Journal of Dental Research* **83**, 103–110.

Shear M. and Singh S. (1978) Age-standardized incidence rates of ameloblastoma and dentigerous cyst on the Witwatersrand, South Africa. *Community Dentistry and Oral Epidemiology* **6**, 195–199.

Shteyer A., Lustmann J. and Lewis-Epstein J. (1978) The mural ameloblastoma: a review of the literature. *Journal of Oral Surgery* **36**, 866–872.

Shugar J. M. A., Som P. M., Ryan J. R., Jacobson A. L., Bernard P. J. and Dickman S. H. (1988) Multicentric parotid cysts and cervical adenopathy in AIDS patients. A newly recognized entity: CT and MR manifestations. *Laryngoscope* **98**, 772–775.

Shuler C. F. and Shriver B. J. (1987) Identification of intermediate filament keratin proteins in parakeratinized odontogenic keratocysts. *Oral Surgery, Oral Medicine, Oral Pathology* **64**, 439–444.

Siar C. H. and Ng K. H. (1988) Orthokeratinized odontogenic keratocysts in Malaysians. *British Journal of Oral and Maxillofacial Surgery* **26**, 215–220.

Sicher H. (1962) Anatomy and oral pathology. *Oral Surgery, Oral Medicine, Oral Pathology* **15**, 1264–1269.

Simon J. H. S. (1980) Incidence of periapical cysts in relation to the root canal. *Journal of Endodontics* **6**, 845–848.

Simon J. H. S. and Jensen J. L. (1985) Squamous odontogenic tumor-like proliferations in periapical cysts. *Journal of Endodontics* **11**, 446–448.

Skaug N. (1973) Proteins in fluid from nonkeratinizing jaw cysts. 2. Concentrations of total protein, some protein fractions and nitrogen. *Journal of Oral Pathology* **2**, 280–291.

Skaug N. (1974) Proteins in fluid from nonkeratinizing jaw cysts. 4. Concentrations of immunoglobulins (IgG, IgA and IgM) and some non-immunoglobulin proteins – relevance to concepts of cyst wall permeability and clearance of cystic proteins. *Journal of Oral Pathology* **3**, 47–61.

Skaug N. (1976a) Intracystic fluid pressure in nonkeratinizing jaw cysts. *International Journal of Oral Surgery* **5**, 59–65.

Skaug N. (1976b) Lipoproteins in fluid from nonkeratinizing jaw cysts. *Scandinavian Journal of Dental Research* **84**, 98–105.

Skaug N. (1977) Soluble proteins in fluid from nonkeratinizing jaw cysts in man. *International Journal of Oral Surgery* **6**, 107–121.

Skaug N. and Hofstad T. (1972) Demonstration of glycosaminoglycans in fluid from jaw cysts. *Acta Pathologica et Microbiologica Scandinavica Section A* **80**, 285–286.

Skaug N. and Hofstad T. (1973) Proteins in fluid from non-keratinizing jaw cysts. 1. Separation patterns on cellulose acetate membranes and percentage distribution of the electrophoretic fractions. *Journal of Oral Pathology* **2**, 112–125.

Skaug N., Johannessen A.C., Matre R. and Nilsen R. (1984a) *In-situ* characterization of cell infiltrates in human dental periapical granulomas 2. Demonstration of receptors for the complement components of C3b and C3d. *Journal of Oral Pathology* **13**, 111–119.

Skaug N., Johannessen A. C., Nilsen R. and Matre R. (1984b) *In-situ* characterization of cell infiltrates in human dental periapical granulomas. 3. Demonstration of T lymphocytes. *Journal of Oral Pathology* **13**, 120–127.

Smith G., Matthews J. B. , Smith A. J. and Browne R. M. (1987) Immunoglobulin-producing cells in human odontogenic cysts. *Journal of Oral Pathology* **16**, 45–48.

Smith G., Smith A. J. and Basu M. K. (1989) Mast cells in human odontogenic cysts. *Journal of Oral Pathology and Medicine* **18**, 274–278.

Smith G., Smith A. G., Basu M. K. and Rippen J. W. (1988) The analysis of fluid aspirate glycosaminoglycans in diagnosis of the postoperative maxillary cyst (surgical ciliated cyst). *Oral Surgery, Oral Medicine, Oral Pathology* **65**, 222–224.

Smith G., Smith A. J. and Browne R. M. (1983) Protein differences in odontogenic cyst fluids. *IRCS Medical Science* **11**, 117.

Smith G., Smith A. J. and Browne R. M. (1984) Glycosaminoglycans in fluid aspirates from odontogenic cysts. *Journal of Oral Pathology* **13**, 614–621.

Smith G., Smith A. J. and Browne R. M. (1986) Analysis of odontogenic cyst fluid aspirates. *IRCS Medical Science* **14**, 304.

Smith G., Smith A. J. and Browne R. M. (1988a) Histochemical studies on glycosaminoglycans of odontogenic cysts. *Journal of Oral Pathology* **17**, 55–59.

Smith G., Smith A. J. and Browne R. M. (1988b) Quantification and analysis of the glycosaminoglycans in human odontogenic cyst linings. *Archives of Oral Biology* **33**, 623–626.

Smith I. and Shear M. (1978) Radiological features of mandibular primordial cysts (keratocysts). *Journal of Maxillofacial Surgery* **6**, 147–154.

Sorsa T., Ylipaavalniemi P., Suomalainen K., Vauhkonen M. and Lindy S. (1988) Type-specific degradation of interstitial collagens by human keratocyst capsule collagenase. *Medical Science Research* **16**, 1189–1190.

Soskolne W. A., Bab J. and Sochat S. (1976) Production of keratinizing cysts within mandibles of rats with autogenous gingival epithelial grafts. *Journal of Oral Pathology* **5**, 122–128.

Soskolne W. A. and Shear M. (1967) Observations on the pathogenesis of primordial cysts. *British Dental Journal* **123**, 321–326.

Soskolne W. A. and Shteyer A. (1977) Median mandibular cyst. *Oral Surgery, Oral Medicine, Oral Pathology* **44**, 84–88.

Southam J. C. (1974) Retention mucoceles of the oral mucosa. *Journal of Oral Pathology* **3**, 197–202.

Spence C. B. (1853–54) Diseases of the surrounding tissues originating in carious teeth. *American Journal of Dental Surgery* 2nd series, 278–282.

Spitzer W. J. and Steinhäuser E. W. (1985) Röntgenbefunde bei odontogenen Keratozysten. *Deutsche Zahnärztliche Zeitschrift* **40**, 602–605.

Spouge J. D. (1966) Sebaceous metaplasia in the oral cavity occurring in association with dentigerous cyst epithelium. *Oral Surgery, Oral Medicine, Oral Pathology* **21**, 492–498.

Stafne E. C. (1942) Bone cavities situated near the angle of the mandible. *Journal of the American Dental Association* **29**, 1969–1972.

Stafne E. C. (1969) *Oral Roentgenographic Diagnosis*, 3rd edn, Philadelphia and London, Saunders, p. 159.

Stam F. C., van der Waal I. and van der Kwast W. A. M. (1979) Pigment in the lining of nasopalatine duct cysts: report of two cases. *Journal of Oral Pathology* **8**, 170–175.

Standish S. M. and Shafer W. G. (1957) Serial histologic effects of rat submaxillary and sublingual gland duct and blood vessel ligation. *Journal of Dental Research* **36**, 866–879.

Standish S. M. and Shafer W. G. (1958) The lateral periodontal cyst. *Journal of Periodontology* **29**, 27–33.

Standish S. M. and Shafer W. G. (1959) The mucous retention phenomenon. *Journal of Oral Surgery* **17**, 15–22.

Stanley H. R., Krogh H. and Pannuk E. (1965) Age changes in the epithelial components of follicles (dental sacs) associated with impacted third molars. *Oral Surgery, Oral Medicine, Oral Pathology* **19**, 128–139.

Steidler N. E., Cook R. M. and Reade P. C. (1979–80) Aneurysmal bone cyst of the jaws. *British Journal of Oral Surgery* **16**, 254–261.

Stenman G., Magnusson B., Lennartsson B. and Juberg-Ode M. (1986) *In-vitro* growth characteristics of human odontogenic keratocysts and dentigerous cysts. *Journal of Oral Pathology* **15**, 143–145.
Stern M. H., Dreizen S., Mackler B. F. and Levy B. M. (1981) Antibody-producing cells in human periapical granulomas and cysts. *Journal of Endodontics* **7**, 447–452.
Stern M. H., Dreizen S., Mackler B. F. and Levy B. M. (1982) Isolation and characterization of inflammatory cells from the human periapical granuloma. *Journal of Dental Research* **61**, 1408–1412.
Stockdale C. R. and Chandler N. P. (1988) The nature of the periapical lesion – a review of 1108 cases. *Journal of Dentistry* **16**, 123–129.
Stoelinga P. J. W. (1971a) Over kaak-kysten. *MD Thesis,* University of Nijmegen. Nijmegen, Centrale Drukkerij N.V.
Stoelinga P. J. W. (1971b) Laterale ontwikkelings-(fissurale) kysten in de bovenkaak. *Nederlandse Tijdschrif van Tandheelkunde* **78**, 258–264.
Stoelinga P. J. W. (1973) Recurrences and multiplicity of cysts. In: Kay L. W. (ed.) *Oral Surgery IV* (Transactions of the Fourth International Conference on Oral Surgery). Copenhagen, Munksgaard, pp. 77–80.
Stoelinga P. J. W. (1976) Studies on the dental lamina as related to its role in the etiology of cysts and tumors. *Journal of Oral Pathology* **5**, 65–73.
Stoelinga P. J. W. and Bronkhorst F. B. (1988) The incidence, multiple presentation and recurrence of aggressive cysts of the jaws. *Journal of Cranio-Maxillo-Facial Surgery* **16**, 184–195.
Stoelinga P. J. W., Cohen M. M. and Morgan A. F. (1975) The origin of keratocysts in the basal cell nevus syndrome. *Journal of Oral Surgery* **33**, 659–663.
Stoelinga P. J. W. and Peters J. H. (1973) A note on the origin of keratocysts of the jaws. *International Journal of Oral Surgery* **2**, 37–44.
Stoneman D. W. and Worth H. M. (1983) The mandibular infected buccal cyst – molar area.*Dental Radiography and Photography* **56**, 1–14.
Stout F. W., Lunin M. and Calonius P. E. B. (1968) A study of epithelial remnants in the maxilla. *Abstracts of the 46th General Meeting of the International Association for Dental Research*. Abstracts 419, 420, 421, pp. 142–143.
Struthers P. J. (1980) Aneurysmal bone cyst of the jaws. *M Dent Dissertation,* University of the Witwatersrand, Johannesburg.
Struthers P. J. and Shear M. (1976) Root resorption produced by the enlargement of ameloblastomas and cysts of the jaws. *International Journal of Oral Surgery* **5**, 128–132.
Struthers P. J. and Shear M. (1984a) Aneurysmal bone cyst of the jaws. (I) Clinicopathological features. *International Journal of Oral Surgery* **13**, 85–89.
Struthers P. J. and Shear M. (1984b) Aneurysmal bone cyst of the jaws. (II) Pathogenesis. *International Journal of Oral Surgery* **13**, 92–100.
Sugar A. W., Walker D. M. and Bounds G. A. (1990) Surgical ciliated (postoperative maxillary) cysts following mid-face osteotomies. *British Journal of Oral and Maxillofacial Surgery* **28**, 264–267.
Sugimura M., Kashibayashi Y., Tsubakimoto M., Ban I. and Kawakatsu K. (1976) Fibrinolytic activity in cystic lesions of jaw bones. *International Journal of Oral Surgery* **5**, 166–171.
Summers L. (1972) Cavitation of apical cysts. *Journal of Dental Research* **51**, 12–47.
Summers L. (1974) The incidence of epithelium in periapical granulomas and the mechanism of cavitation in apical dental cysts in man. *Archives of Oral Biology* **19**, 1177–1180.
Summers L. and Papadimitriou J. (1975) The nature of epithelial proliferation in apical granulomas. *Journal of Oral Pathology* **4**, 324–329.
Suzuki M. (1975) A study of biological chemistry on the nature of jaw cysts (I). *Journal of Maxillofacial Surgery* **3**, 100–118.
Suzuki M. (1984) A biochemical study of the nature of jaw cysts (II). *Journal of Maxillofacial Surgery* **12**, 213–224.
Suzuki M. (1988) A biochemical study on the nature of jaw cysts (III). Instrumental analysis of the viscous component of fluids in ciliated cysts of the maxilla. *Journal of Cranio-Maxillo-Facial Surgery* **16**, 85–88.
Swanson K. S., Kaugars G. E. and Gunsolley J. C. (1991) Nasopalatine duct cyst: an analysis of 334 cases. *Journal of Oral and Maxillofacial Surgery* **49**, 268–271.

Swartz J. D., Abaza N. A., Hendler B. H., Tidwell O. and Popky G. L. (1985) High resolution computed tomography: Part 4, Evaluation of odontogenic lesions. *Head and Neck Surgery* **7**, 409–417.

Takeda Y. (1985) Hyaline bodies and secondary dental cuticle in dentigerous cyst. *Journal of Oral Pathology* **14**, 268–269.

Takeda Y. (1991) Duct-like structures in odontogenic epithelium of compound odontoma. *Journal of Oral Pathology and Medicine* **20**, 184–186.

Takeda Y., Kikuchi H. and Suzuki A. (1985) Hyaline bodies in ameloblastoma: histological and ultrastructural observations. *Journal of Oral Pathology* **14**, 639–643.

Takeda Y., Suzuki A. and Yamamoto H. (1990) Histopathologic study of epithelial components in the connective tissue wall of unilocular type of calcifying odontogenic cyst. *Journal of Oral Pathology and Medicine* **19**, 108–113.

Tal H., Altini M. and Lemmer J. (1984) Multiple mucous retention cysts of the oral mucosa. *Oral Surgery, Oral Medicine, Oral Pathology* **58**, 692–695.

Tanimoto K., Fujita M., Wada T. and Yamasaki A. (1983) Radiographic appearance of cystic lesion in the median mandibular region. *Japanese Society of Dental Radiology* **22**, 241–250.

Tanimoto K., Tomita S., Aoyama M., Furuki Y., Fujita M. and Wada T. (1988) Radiographic characteristics of the calcifying odontogenic cyst. *International Journal of Oral and Maxillofacial Surgery* **17**, 29–32.

Telfer M. R., Jones G. M., Pell G. M. and Eveson J. W. (1990) Primary bone cyst of the mandibular condyle. *British Journal of Oral and Maxillofacial Surgery* **28**, 340–343.

Ten Cate A. R. (1972) The epithelial cell rests of Malassez and the genesis of the dental cyst. *Oral Surgery, Oral Medicine, Oral Pathology* **34**, 950–964.

Thoma K. (1937) Facial cleft or fissural cyst. *International Journal of Orthodontics* **23**, 83–89.

Tillman B. P., Dahlin D. C., Lipscomb P. R. and Stewart J. R. (1968) Aneurysmal bone cyst: an analysis of ninety-five cases. *Mayo Clinic Proceedings* **43**, 478–495.

Timosca G. and Gavrilită L. (1974) Cysticercosis of the maxillofacial region. *Oral Surgery, Oral Medicine, Oral Pathology* **37**, 390–400.

Toida M., Tsai C-S., Okumura Y., Tatematsu N. and Oka N. (1990) Distribution of Factor XIIIa-containing cells and collagenous components in radicular cysts: histochemic and immunohistochemic studies. *Journal of Oral Pathology and Medicine* **19**, 155–159.

Toljanic J. A., Lechewski E., Huvos A. G., Strong E. W. and Schweiger J. W. (1987) Aneurysmal bone cysts of the jaws: a case study and review of the literature. *Oral Surgery, Oral Medicine, Oral Pathology* **64**, 72–77.

Toller P. A. (1948) Experimental investigations into factors concerning the growth of cysts of the jaws. *Proceedings of the Royal Society of Medicine* **41**, 681–688.

Toller P. A. (1964) Radioactive isotope and other investigations in a case of haemorrhagic cyst of the mandible. *British Journal of Oral Surgery* **2**, 86–93.

Toller P. A. (1966a) Epithelial discontinuities in cysts of the jaws. *British Dental Journal*, **120**, 74–78.

Toller P. A. (1966b) Permeability of cyst walls in vivo: investigations with radioactive tracers. *Proceedings of the Royal Society of Medicine* **59**, 724–729.

Toller P. A. (1967) Origin and growth of cysts of the jaws. *Annals of the Royal College of Surgeons of England* **40**, 306–336.

Toller P. A. (1970a) Protein substances in odontogenic cyst fluids. *British Dental Journal* **128**, 317–322.

Toller P. A. (1970b) The osmolality of fluids from cysts of the jaws. *British Dental Journal* **129**, 275–278.

Toller P. A. (1971) Autoradiography of explants from odontogenic cysts. *British Dental Journal* **131**, 57–61.

Toller P. A. and Holborrow E. J. (1969) Immunoglobulins and immunoglobulin containing cells in cysts of the jaws. *Lancet* **ii**, 178.

Tolman D. E. and Stafne E. C. (1967) Developmental bone defects of the mandible. *Oral Surgery, Oral Medicine, Oral Pathology* **24**, 488–490.

Torabinejad M. (1983) The role of immunological reactions in apical cyst formation and the fate of epithelial cells after root canal therapy: a theory. *International Journal of Oral Surgery* **12**, 14–22.

Torabinejad M. and Kettering J. D. (1985) Identification and relative concentration of B and T lymphocytes in human chronic periapical lesions. *Journal of Endodontics* **11**, 122–125.

Torabinejad M., Kettering J. D. and Bakland L. K. (1981) Localization of IgE immunoglobulin in human dental periapical lesions by the peroxidase antiperoxidase method. *Archives of Oral Biology* **26**, 677–681.

Toto P. D., Wortel J. P. and Joseph G. (1982) Lymphoepithelial cysts and associated immunoglobulins. *Oral Surgery, Oral Medicine, Oral Pathology* **54**, 59–65.

Traeger K. A. (1961) Cyst of the gingiva (mucocele): report of a case. *Oral Surgery, Oral Medicine, Oral Pathology* **14**, 243–245.

Trask G. M., Sheller B. L. and Morton T. H.(1985) Mandibular buccal infected cyst in a six-year-old girl: report of a case. *Journal of Dentistry for Children* **52**, 377–379.

Trott J. R., Chebib F. and Galindo Y. (1973) Factors related to cholesterol formation in cysts and granulomas. *Journal of the Canadian Dental Association* **39**, 550–555.

Trott J. R. and Esty C. (1972) An analysis of 105 dental cysts. *Journal of the Canadian Dental Association* **38**, 75–78.

Trueta J. (1968) *Studies of the Development and Decay of the Human Frame*, 1st edn, pp.78–79. London, Heinemann. Cited by Hosseini (1978–79).

Turner J. G. (1898) Dental cysts. *Journal of the British Dental Association* **19**, 711–734.

Uitto V-J. and Ylipaavalniemi P. (1977) Alterations in collagenolytic activity caused by jaw cyst fluids. *Proceedings of the Finnish Dental Society* **73**, 197–202.

Ulmansky M., Azaz B. and Sela J. (1969) Calcifying odontogenic cyst. *Journal of Oral Surgery* **27**, 415–419.

Unal T., Gomel M. and Gunel O. (1987) Squamous odontogenic tumor-like islands in a radicular cyst: report of a case. *Journal of Oral and Maxillofacial Surgery* **45**, 346–349.

Valderhaug J. (1972) A histologic study of experimentally induced radicular cysts. *International Journal of Oral Surgery* **1**, 137–147.

Valderhaug J. (1974) A histologic study of experimentally induced periapical inflammation in primary teeth in monkeys. *International Journal of Oral Surgery* **3**, 111–113.

Van Bruggen A. P., Shear M., du Preez I. J., van Wyk D. P., Beyers D. and Leeferink G. A. (1985) Nasolabial cysts. A report of 10 cases and a review of the literature. *Journal of the Dental Association of South Africa* **40**, 15–19.

Van der Wal N., Wiener J.D., Allard R. H. B., Henzen-Logmans S. C. and van der Waal I. (1987) Thyroglossal cysts in patients over 30 years of age. *International Journal of Oral and Maxillofacial Surgery* **16**, 416–419.

Van der Waal I., Rauhamaa R., van der Kwast W. A. M. and Snow G. B. (1985) Squamous cell carcinoma arising in the lining of odontogenic cysts. Report of 5 cases. *International Journal of Oral Surgery* **14**, 146–152.

Vedtofte P. and Dabelsteen E. (1975) Blood group antigens A and B in ameloblastomas, odontogenic keratocysts and nonkeratinizing cysts. *Scandinavian Journal of Dental Research* **83**, 96–102.

Vedtofte P. and Holmstrup P. (1989) Inflammatory paradental cysts in the globulomaxillary region. *Journal of Oral Pathology and Medicine* **18**, 125–127.

Vedtofte P., Pindborg J. J. and Hakomori S. I. (1985) Relation of blood group carbohydrates to differentiation patterns of normal and pathological odontogenic epithelium. *Acta Pathologica Microbiologica et Immunologica Scandinavica Section A* **93**, 25–34.

Vedtofte P., Holmstrup P. and Dabelsteen E. (1982) Human odontogenic keratocyst transplants in nude mice. *Scandinavian Journal of Dental Research* **90**, 306–314.

Vedtofte P. and Praetorius F. (1979) Recurrence of the odontogenic keratocyst in relation to clinical and histological features. A 20-year follow-up study of 72 patients. *International Journal of Oral Surgery* **8**, 412–420.

Vedtofte P. and Praetorius F. (1989) The inflammatory paradental cyst. *Oral Surgery, Oral Medicine, Oral Pathology* **68**, 182–188.

Vickers R. A. and Gorlin R. J. (1970) Ameloblastoma: delineation of early histopathologic features of neoplasia. *Cancer* **26**, 699–710.

Vickers R. A. and von der Muhll O. H (1966) An investigation concerning inducibility of lymphoepithelial cysts in hamsters by autogenous epithelial transplantation. *Journal of Dental Research* **45**, 1029–1032.

Voorsmit R. A. C. A. (1984) The incredible keratocyst. *MD Dissertation,* University of Nijmegen. Naarden, Los Printers.

Voorsmit R. A. C. A. (1986) The art of treating keratocysts: fixation before enucleation. *Abstract, 8th Congress of the European Association for Maxillofacial Surgery,* Madrid, p. 68.

Voorsmit R. A. C. A., Stoelinga P. J. W. and van Haelst U. J. G. M. (1981) The management of keratocysts. *Journal of Maxillofacial Surgery* **9**, 228–236.

Waldron C. A. (1969) Some observations on the jaw cysts in the basal cell nevoid carcinoma syndrome. *Fourth Proceedings of the International Academy of Oral Pathology*, p. 220.

Waldron C. A. and Koh M. L. (1990) Central mucoepidermoid carcinoma of the jaws: report of four cases with analysis of the literature and discussion of the relationship to mucoepidermoid, sialodontogenic, and glandular odontogenic cysts. *Journal of Oral and Maxillofacial Surgery* **48**, 871–877.

Wampler H. W., Krolls S. O. and Johnson R. P. (1978) Thyroglossal-tract cyst. *Oral Surgery, Oral Medicine, Oral Pathology* **45**, 32–38.

Ward T. G. and Cohen B. (1963) Squamous carcinoma in a mandibular cyst. *British Journal of Oral Surgery* **1**, 8–12.

Warwick R. and Williams P. L. (eds.) (1973) *Gray's Anatomy*, 35th edn, London, Longman, p. 116.

Wassmund M. (1935) The fusion of the flap and cyst wall. In *Lehrbuch der Praktische Chirurgie des Munde und der Kiefer, Volume 1*, Leipzig, Von Herran Meusser, p. 93.

Weathers D. R. and Waldron C. A. (1973) Unusual multilocular cysts of the jaws (botryoid odontogenic cysts). *Oral Surgery, Oral Medicine, Oral Pathology* **36**, 235–241.

Webb D. J. and Brockbank J. (1984) Treatment of the odontogenic keratocyst by combined enucleation and cryosurgery. *International Journal of Oral Surgery* **13**, 506–510.

Weidner N., Geisinger K. R., Sterling R. T., Miller T. and Yen T. S. B.(1986) Benign lymphoepithelial cysts of the parotid gland. A histologic, cytologic and ultrastructural study. *American Journal of Clinical Pathology* **85**, 395–401.

Wertheimer F. W. (1966) A histologic comparison of apical cuticles, secondary cuticles and hyaline bodies. *Journal of Periodontology* **37**, 91–94.

Wertheimer F. W., Fullmer H. M. and Hansen L. S. (1962) A histochemical study of hyaline bodies in odontogenic cysts and a comparison to the human secondary dental cuticle. *Oral Surgery, Oral Medicine, Oral Pathology* **15**, 1466.

Wesley R. K., Scannell T. and Nathan L. E. (1984) Nasolabial cyst: presentation of a case with a review of the literature. *Journal of Oral and Maxillofacial Surgery* **42**, 188–192.

White D. K., Lucas R. M. and Miller A. S. (1975) Median mandibular cyst: review of the literature and report of two cases. *Journal of Oral Surgery* **33**, 372–375.

Wilk A. E., Milobsky S., Reynolds D., Princiotto J. and Zapolski E. J. (1983) The demonstration of $alpha_1$ antitrypsin in periapical lesions. *Oral Surgery, Oral Medicine, Oral Pathology* **55**, 86–90.

Wilson D. F. and Ross A. S. (1978) Ultrastructure of odontogenic keratocysts. *Oral Surgery, Oral Medicine, Oral Pathology* **45**, 887–893.

Wolf J. and Hietanen J. (1990) The mandibular infected buccal cyst (paradental cyst). A radiographic and histological study. *British Journal of Oral and Maxillofacial Surgery* **28**, 322–325.

Woo S.-B., Eisenbud L., Kleiman M. and Assael N. (1987) Odontogenic keratocysts in the anterior maxilla: report of two cases, one simulating a nasopalatine cyst. *Oral Surgery, Oral Medicine and Oral Pathology* **64**, 463–465.

Wood R. E., Nortjé C. J., Padayachee A. and Grotepass F. (1988) Radicular cysts of primary teeth mimicking premolar dentigerous cysts: report of three cases. *Journal of Dentistry for Children* **55**, 288–290.

Woolgar J. A., Rippin J. W. and Browne R. M. (1987a) A comparative histological study of odontogenic keratocysts in basal cell naevus syndrome and control patients. *Journal of Oral Pathology* **16**, 75–80.

Woolgar J. A., Rippin J. W. and Browne R. M. (1987b) The odontogenic keratocyst and its occurrence in the nevoid basal cell carcinoma syndrome. *Oral Surgery, Oral Medicine, Oral Pathology* **64**, 727–730.

Woolgar J. A., Rippen J. W. and Browne R. M. (1987c) A comparative study of the clinical and histological features of recurrent and non-recurrent odontogenic keratocysts. *Journal of Oral Pathology* **16**, 124–128.

Wright B. A., Wysocki G. P. and Larder T. C. (1983) Odontogenic keratocysts presenting as periapical disease. *Oral Surgery, Oral Medicine, Oral Pathology* **56**, 425–429.

Wright J. M. (1979a) The A and B blood group substances on odontogenic epithelium. *Journal of Dental Research* **58**, 624–628.

Wright J. M. (1979b) Squamous odontogenic tumorlike proliferations in odontogenic cysts. *Oral Surgery, Oral Medicine, Oral Pathology* **47**, 354–358.

Wright J. M. (1981) The odontogenic keratocyst: orthokeratinized variant. *Oral Surgery, Oral Medicine, Oral Pathology* **51**, 609-618.

Wysocki G. P. (1981) The differential diagnosis of globulomaxillary radiolucencies. *Oral Surgery, Oral Medicine, Oral Pathology* **51**, 281–286.

Wysocki G. P., Brannon R. B., Gardner D. G. and Sapp P. (1980) Histogenesis of the lateral periodontal cyst and the gingival cyst of the adult. *Oral Surgery, Oral Medicine, Oral Pathology* **50**, 327–334.

Wysocki G. P. and Sapp J. P. (1975) Scanning and transmission electron microscopy of odontogenic keratocysts. *Oral Surgery, Oral Medicine, Oral Pathology* **40**, 494–501.

Yamada K., Tatemoto Y., Okada Y. and Mori M. (1989) Immunostaining of involucrin in odontogenic epithelial tumors and cysts. *Oral Surgery, Oral Medicine, Oral Pathology* **67**, 564–568.

Yamamoto H. and Takagi M. (1986) Clinicopathologic study of the postoperative maxillary cyst. *Oral Surgery, Oral Medicine, Oral Pathology* **62**, 544–548.

Yamasoba T.,Tayama N., Syoji M. and Fukuta M. (1990) Clinicostatistical study of lower lip mucoceles. *Head and Neck* **12**, 316–320.

Yanagisiwa S. (1980) Pathologic study of periapical lesions 1. Periapical granulomas: clinical, histopathologic and immunohistopathologic studies. *Journal of Oral Pathology* **9**, 288–300.

Yeschua R., Bab I. A., Wexler M. R. and Neuman Z. (1977) Dermoid cyst of the floor of the mouth in an infant. *Journal of Maxillofacial Surgery* **5**, 211–213.

Ylipaavalniemi P. (1977) Cyst fluid concentrations of immunoglobulins α_2-macroglobulin and α_1-antitrypsin. *Proceedings of the Finnish Dental Society* **73**, 185–188.

Ylipaavalniemi P. and Tuompo H. (1977) Effect of proteolytic digestion on jaw cyst fluids. *Proceedings of the Finnish Dental Society* **73**, 179–184.

Ylipaavalniemi P., Tuompo H. and Calonius P. E. B. (1976) Proteins and inflammation in jaw cysts. *Proceedings of the Finnish Dental Society* **72**, 191–195.

Ylipaavalniemi P., Tuompo H. and Koskimies A. I. (1976) Immunoelectrophoresis of proteins in fluids from jaw cysts. *Proceedings of the Finnish Dental Society* **72**, 7–10.

Yoshikawa Y., Nakajima T., Kaneshiro S. and Sakaguchi M. (1982) Effective treatment of the postoperative maxillary cyst by marsupialization. *Journal of Oral and Maxillofacial Surgery* **40**, 487–491.

Yoshimura Y., Takada K., Takeda M., Mimura T. and Mori M. (1970) Congenital dermoid cysts of the sublingual region. Report of a case. *Journal of Oral Surgery* **28**, 366–370.

Zachariades N., Papanikolaou S. and Koundouris I. (1982) Median mandibular cyst. *International Journal of Oral Surgery* **11**, 201–204.

Zachariades N., Papanikolaou S. and Triantafyllou D. (1985) Odontogenic keratocysts: review of the literature and report of 16 cases. *Journal of Oral and Maxillofacial Surgery* **43**, 177–182.

Zegarelli D. J. and Zegarelli E. V. (1973) Radiolucent lesions in the globulomaxillary region. *Journal of Oral Surgery* **31**, 767–771.

Index

AIDS:
  lympho-epithelial cyst of parotid gland in, 203
Adenomatoid odontogenic tumour, 89, 127
Alcianophilia, 18
Allergy:
  mucosal cyst of maxillary sinus and, 189
Ameloblastic fibroma:
  in calcifying odontogenic cyst, 106
Ameloblastic fibro-odontome
  in calcifying odontogenic cyst, 106
Ameloblastoma, 245
  cytokeratin in, 91
  in calcifying odontogenic cyst, 106
  involving unerupted teeth, 92
  plexiform unicystic, 90, 93, 95
  possible origin from dentigerous cyst, 92
  recurrence of, 246
  unicystic, 90, 93–8
    age distribution, 95
    histological classification, 95–7
    sex distribution, 95
    site distribution, 95
    treatment, 98
  unilocular, 75
  Vickers–Gorlin criteria, 95
  with ghost cells, 110
Ameloblastomatoid features in keratocysts, 38
Ameloblasts:
  gingival cysts from, 60
Aneurysmal bone cyst, 179–86
  clinical features, 179
  frequency of, 179
  histology, 184
  malignant form of, 183
  pathogenesis of, 181
  pathology, 184
  pre-existing lesions, 182, 186
  radiology, 180
  recurrence, 186
  site of, 180
  treatment, 186
Anterior median lingual cyst, 208
Antikeratin monoclonal antibodies, 40, 42, 91, 92
Apical granulomas, 140
  biochemical studies of, 141
  immunological studies of, 143
Autoradiography:
  studies in cysts, 17

Bay cyst, 159
Blood group antigens:
  dentigerous cysts and, 91
  in keratocysts, 36
Blood vessels in median palatine cysts, 124
Bohn's nodules, 46
Bone:
  contour defects of, 250
  perforation of, 11
Bone cyst:
  aneurysmal, 179–86
    clinical features, 179
    frequency of, 179
    histology, 184
    malignant form of, 183
    pathogenesis, 181
    pathology, 184
    pre-existing lesions, 182, 186
    radiology, 180
    recurrence, 186
    site of, 180
    treatment, 186
  haemorrhagic, *see under Bone cyst, solitary*
  solitary, 127, 171–6
    age distribution, 171
    clinical features, 171
    clinical presentation, 173
    frequency of, 171
    haematoma and, 174, 175
    multiple, 173
    pathogenesis, 173–5
    radiology, 173
    sex distribution, 172
    site of, 172
    spontaneous regression, 175
    trauma and, 173, 174
    treatment of, 250
  traumatic, *see under Bone cyst, solitary*

Bone grafting, 250
Bone resorption:
  prostaglandins in, 84, 150
Botryoid odontogenic cyst, 69–71
  frequency, 70
  recurrence, 70
  treatment, 71
Branchial cleft cysts, 201–5
  treatment, 253
  see also Lympho-epithelial cysts
Breathing:
  problems from cysts, 131, 198
Buccal cysts:
  mandibular infected, 167–70
Buccal vestibule:
  lympho-epithelial cyst of, 204

Calcification:
  in cysticercosis, 225
  in radicular cysts, 160
Calcifying odontogenic cyst, 102–10, 129
  age distribution, 103
  classification of, 106
  clinical features, 102
  clinical presentation, 104
  epithelial lining, 106–9
  extraosseus, 104
  frequency of, 102
  melanin deposits in, 109
  pathogenesis and pathology, 105
  radiology, 105
  satellites of, 109
  site of, 104
  treatment, 110
  ultrastructure of, 109
  unilocular and multicystic, 107
Caldwell–Luc operation:
  postoperative maxillary cyst following, 193, 195
Carcinoembryonic antigen:
  in odontogenic cysts, 40, 41, 92
Celcus, 1
Ceroid:
  in radicular cysts, 159
Children:
  cystic hygroma in, 210
  eruption cysts in, 99
  mucoceles in, 99
    gingival cysts in, 46–50
  oral alimentary tract cysts in, 210
  radicular cysts in, 87, 137, 139
Cholesteatoma, 4
Cholesterol clefts in keratocysts, 38
Cholesterol crystals in radicular cysts, 157, 158
Chondroitin-4-sulphate in cyst fluid, 18, 88, 195
Classification of cysts, xi
Collagen:
  in keratocysts, 19
  in radicular cysts, 159
Collagenase, in keratocyst, 19
Collateral cyst:
  inflammatory, 63, 136, 162
  variety of keratocyst, 25
Congenital intralingual cyst, 208, 210
Congenital sublingual cysts, 221
Cortical plate:
  perforation of, 105
CT scanning, 26
Cyst fluids:
  constituents of, 18
  glycosaminoglycans in, 18, 19, 88, 89, 151
  keratinized squames in, 42
  lactoferrin in, 44
  osmolality of, 17
  prostaglandins in, 84
  protein in, 18, 42, 43, 88, 148, 149, 195
Cysticercosis, 224–6
Cystic hygroma, 210
Cysticercus cellulosae, 224
Cysts:
  classification of, xi
  definition of, xi
  distribution of, 6
  frequency of, 6
  regression without treatment, 227
  treatment, 227–256
  see also under bone cysts and specific names
Cytokeratins:
  in dentigerous cysts, 91, 92
  in keratocysts, 40
  in lateral periodontal cyst, 63, 64
  in Malassez rests, 145
Cytology, in diagrams of keratocysts, 42

Deciduous teeth:
  radicular cysts associated with, 87, 137, 139
Dental lamina:
  development of keratocysts from, 73, 247
  disintegration of, 47, 48
  epithelial remnants, 47, 56
  formation of, 67
  gingival cysts originating from, 54, 55, 56
  keratin formation in, 47
  lateral periodontal cysts originating from, 63, 64
  proliferation of, 49
    in keratocysts, 38
Dentigerous cysts, 5, 75–98, 128
  age incidence, 77
  anatomical distribution, 79, 80
  animal experiments on, 86
  around unerupted teeth, 88
  as potential ameloblastoma, 92
  blood vessels in, 31
  carcinomatous changes in, 161
  central, 80, 81, 82
  circumferential, 80, 82
  clinical features, 76
  clinical presentation, 80
  cytokeratins in, 91, 92
  deciduous teeth and, 87
  definition of, 75
  diagnosis, 23, 75
  enucleation, 238
  epithelial lining, 90, 91

Dentigerous cysts (*continued*)
 extrafollicular origin, 85, 86
 frequency of, 76
 fluids in, 148
 growth of, 80
 glycosaminoglycans in, 88
 immunoglobulins in, 88
 impacted teeth and, 85
 inflammation in, 91
 inflammatory origin, 87, 88
 interleukin 1 in, 84
 intrafollicular origin, 85
 keratin in, 41, 90, 161
 lateral type, 80, 81, 82
 mast cells in, 39
 origin of, 86, 87, 88, 92
 pathogenesis, 84
 pathology, 89
 prostaglandins in, 84, 89
 protein in fluid, 88
 racial frequency, 79, 85
 radiology, 80
 regression of, 228
 root resorption in, 82, 83
 sex distribution, 78, 85
 site of, 79, 80
 teeth involved in, 77
 treatment, 243, 246
Dentinogenic ghost cell ameloblastoma, 107
Dentinogenic ghost cell tumour, 107
DNA in keratocysts, 35
Dermoid cysts, 196–201
 clinical presentation, 198
 frequency of, 196
 pathogenesis, 198
 site of, 197
 treatment, 251, 252, 253
Developmental cysts of soft tissues, 196–211, *see also specific cysts and sites*
Developmental defects of mandible, 177, 178
Discharge:
 from keratocysts, 10
 from lympho-epithelial cysts, 204
 from maxillary cysts, 193
 from nasopalatine duct cysts, 114

Echinococcus spp, 223
Enamel:
 hypoplasia in dentigerous cysts, 86
 projections and paradental cysts, 165, 167
Enucleation of cysts, 227
 drainage, 243
 incision for, 235, 241
 primary closure, 234, 239, 240
 recurrence after, 247
 removal of lining, 236, 237, 242, 244
 through palate, 238
 with packing, 234
Epidermal cyst, of the skin, 201
Epidermoid cysts, 196–201
 implantation keratinizing, 198
 frequency of, 196
 keratin-filled, 198
 pathogenesis, 198
 pathology, 198
 site of, 197
Epithelial membrane antigen:
 in odontogenic cysts, 40, 41, 92
Epithelial plaques in cysts, 57, 64, 65, 66, 67
Epstein's pearls, 46
Eruption cyst, 99–101
 clinical features, 99
 epithelial lining, 100
 pathology, 100
 treatment, 101
Experimental production of cysts:
 dentigerous, 86
 keratocyst, 30, 31
 lympho-epithelial, 204
 radicular, 151

Face:
 dermoid cysts of, 197
 keratinous cysts of, 201
Facial processes, 127
Factor XIIIa in radicular cysts, 159
Fauchard, P, 2
Fibrinolysis in cyst growth, 150
Fibromas:
 bone cysts and, 182, 186
Fibrosarcomas:
 bone cysts and, 182, 183
Fibrous dysplasia, 186
Flatworms, 223
Follicular ameloblastoma, 68
Follicular cyst, *see Dentigerous cyst*
Follicular keratocyst, 23
Foramen caecum:
 cyst of, 207
Foregut:
 intralingual cyst of, 208
Frequency of various jaw cysts, 6

Gastric epithelium:
 oral cysts with, 209
Ghost cells in calcifying odontogenic cyst, 107, 108
Giant cell granuloma:
 aneurysmal bone cyst and, 182, 186
 mistaken for globulomaxillary cyst, 129
Giant cell tumours:
 aneurysmal bone cyst and, 181
Gingiva:
 cytokeratins in, 91
 epithelial nests in, 54
 trichinosis, 226

Gingival cysts, 46–50
  of adults, 51–60
    age frequency of, 53
    bone erosion and, 51
    clinical features, 52
    clinical presentation, 54
    epidermoid and keratocyst varieties, 57
    epithelial plaques in, 57
    from ameloblasts, 60
    histology, 57
    incidence of, 53
    lined with epithelium, 55
    multicystic form, 56
    pathogenesis, 54
    radiology, 54
    relation to lateral periodontal cyst, 57, 58, 60
    sex frequency of, 53
    site of, 54
    treatment, 60
  of infants, 46–50
    age distribution, 46
    clinical features, 46
    frequency of, 46
    pathology and treatment, 50
Glandular odontogenic cyst, 71–4
  histology, 72
  radiology, 72
  treatment, 74
Globulomaxillary cyst, 126
  critical studies of, 127
  embryological aspects of, 127
  keratocysts and, 10, 26
Glycosaminoglycans in cyst fluids, 18, 19, 88, 89, 151
Goblet cells:
  in dermoid cysts, 199
  in glandular odontogenic cysts, 73, 74
  in nasolabial cysts, 134, 135
  in nasopalatine duct cysts, 120
Gorlin cyst, *see Calcifying odontogenic cyst*
Gorlin–Goltz syndrome, 11

Haemorrhagic bone cyst, 171, *see also Solitary bone cyst*
Haemosiderin in radicular cysts, 157
Heparin in cyst fluid, 18, 88, 195
Historical background, 1
Hunter, John, 3
Human immunodeficiency virus, 203
Hyaline bodies:
  in dentigerous cysts, 90
  in keratocytes, 38
  in radicular cysts, 154, 155, 156
  origin of, 155, 156, 157
  ultrastructure of, 156
Hyaline cartilage in cyst walls, 123
Hyaluronic acid in cyst fluid, 18, 19, 88, 195
Hydatid cysts, 223–4
Hydatid sand, 224
Hyoid bone:
  cysts near, 207

Immune mechanisms in radicular cysts, 139, 143–5, 148, 149
Immunoglobulins:
  in antral cysts, 190
  in cyst fluids, 88
  in keratocysts, 44
  in mucosal cysts of the antrum, 190
  in radicular cysts, 143–5, 148, 149
Incisive canal cyst, *see Nasopalatine duct cyst*
Incisive fossae, 115
Infection:
  in nasopalatine duct cyst, 115
  maxillary antral cyst and, 190
  in radicular cyst, 139
Inflammation:
  antral cysts and, 190, 191
  in cyst formation, 162
  in eruption cyst, 100, 101
  in keratocyst, 37
  in radicular cyst, 139, 140, 160
Inflammatory collateral cyst, 63, 136, 162
Interleukin 1 in cysts, 84
Intralingual cyst of foregut origin, 208

Keratin:
  and carcinomatous change, 33
  in cell rests of Malassez, 145
  in dentigerous cysts, 90, 91
  in dermoid and epidermoid cysts, 198
Keratin-containing microcysts, 49
Keratinization, 4
Keratinous cysts, of the skin, 201
Keratocyst:
  aetiology of, 28
    mesenchymal capsule in, 31
  age distribution of, 4, 6, 8, 14, 15
  age-specific morbidity rates, 7, 8
  ameloblastomatous change in, 38
  and so-called fissural cysts, 126, 128
  arising from basal cell proliferation, 14
  arising from dental lamina, 13
  blood group antigens in, 36
  blood vessels in, 31
  bony expansion, 10
  budding of basal layer, 38
  CT scanning, 26
  carbohydrate constituents of, 36
  carcinoembryonic antigen (CEA) in, 40, 41
  carcinomatous potential, 13, 16, 33
  cholesterol clefts in, 38
  clinical features, 6
  clinical presentation, 10
  collateral, 25
  crystalline deposits in, 45
  cytokeratins in, 40
  definitions, 5
  deflecting roots, 26
  development from dental lamina, 247
  devitalizing lining cells with Carnoy's fluid, 247
  DNA in, 35

Keratocyst (*continued*)
diagnosis, 42, 43, 44
differential diagnosis, 4
enlargement of, 16
cyst fluid and, 17
enucleation of, 248
envelopmental, 25, 75, 81, 86, 245
treatment, 248, 249
epithelial cells, 40
epithelial dysplasia in, 33
epithelial lining:
growth potential, 13
histology, 41
infolding of, 37
proliferation, 17
sources of, 27
experimental investigation, 31
epithelial membrane antigens (EMA) in, 40, 41
extraneous, 25
family history and, 28
fibrous capsule, 37
fluids:
constituents of, 18
lactoferrin in, 44
osmolality, 17
protein in, 42, 43
follicular, 86
growth of, 31
growth rate, 16, 17
histochemistry of cell membrane carbohydrates, 36
histology of, 30, 32
human papilloma virus and, 35
hyaline bodies in, 38
immunoglobulins in, 44
incidence of, 6, 7, 8
incomplete eradication, 13
infected, 10
inflammatory exudate, 18
inflammatory processes in, 37
keratinized layer in, 30
keratocyst antigen (KCA), 43
lining of, 247
marsupialization, 248
mast cells in, 39
melanin pigmentation in, 38
mitotic activity in, 17
mucous metaplasia in, 38
multilocular, 21, 246, 248
multiple, 11, 13, 16
definition, 15
recurrences and, 14
orthokeratinization, 13, 36
pathogenesis, 27
pathology, 32
peripheral, 10
prognosis:
size and, 13
proliferating dental lamina in, 38
racial distribution, 9
radiology, 19

Keratocyst (*continued*)
rat liver antigen (RLA) in, 40, 41
recurrences, 11, 13
incidence of, 12
multiple cysts and, 14
radiology, 26
rate of, 16
treatment affecting, 11, 13
relation to naevoid basal cell carcinoma syndrome, 9, 15
multiple cysts in, 11, 16
recurrences and, 13
satellite cysts in, 15
replacement, 25, 28
satellite cysts in, 15, 28, 38
sex distribution of, 9, 14, 15
simulating nasopalatine cyst, 118
site of, 5, 10, 15
size of, 10
prognosis and, 13
recurrence and, 12
terminology, 4
treatment:
affecting recurrences, 11, 13
enucleation, 16
excision of epithelium, 30
ultrastructural studies, 39
varieties of, 25
Keratocyst antigen, 43

Lactoferrin, 44
Latent bone cyst, 177
Lateral dentigerous cyst:
regression of, 228
Lateral periodontal cyst, 60–9, 126, 128, 129
age distribution of, 61
botryoid type, 68
clinical features, 60
clinical presentation, 62
cytokeratin composition, 63
encapsulated multilocular, 71
epithelial lining, 65, 68
epithelial plaques in, 57, 66
frequency, 60
growth potential, 64
histochemistry, 68
histology, 65
lateral radicular cyst and, 63
multicystic form, 56, 68
pathogenesis, 63
radiology, 62
relation to gingival cyst, 51, 56, 60
sex distribution of, 61
site of, 61
thickening of epithelium in, 66
treatment, 68
unicystic type, 68
Lateral sublingual dermoid cysts, 253
Leucine aminopeptidase, in keratocyst wall, 19
Lingual mandibular bone defect, 177–8

Lip:
  cysticercosis of, 225
  mucoceles on, 214
  paraesthesia from bone cyst, 173
Lipofuscin in nasopalatine duct cysts, 123
Lymphocytes in radicular cysts, 143, 144, 145, 159
Lympho-epithelial cysts, 201–5
  intraoral, 204
  of parotid gland, 202
    AIDS-related, 203
  treatment, 253

Malassez, cell rests of, 63, 65, 142, 160
  keratin in, 145
  paradental cyst from, 167
  proliferation, 163
Malherbe, calcifying epithelioma of, 102, 106, 108
Mandibular condyle:
  bone cyst in, 173
  epidermoid cyst of, 198
Mandibular infected buccal cyst, 136, 166, 167–70
  diagnosis, 169
  treatment, 170
Marsupialization of cysts, 228–34
  advantages of, 228
  difficulties of, 229
  incisions, 229, 230
  recurrence after, 247
  suturing, 231
  weakness of operation, 229, 232
Mast cells:
  in keratocysts, 39
  in radicular cysts, 160
Maxillary antrum:
  benign mucosal cyst of, 187–91
    age and sex distribution, 188
    allergy and, 189
    clinical features, 187
    clinical presentation, 189
    immunoglobulins in, 190
    incidence of, 187
    inflammatory origin, 190, 191
    pathogenesis, 190
    pathology, 190
    radiology, 189
    site of, 188
    treatment, 191
  cyst of floor, 188
  cysts associated with, 187–95
  lymphangiectatic cysts, 187
  mesothelial cysts, 187
  mucocele, 187
  postoperative cyst, 192–5
  retention cyst, 187, 191
Median alveolar cyst, 124, 125
Median mandibular cyst, 125–6
Median palatal raphe, 127
Median palatine cyst, 111, 124
  diagnosis, 116
Melanin-containing cells, 68
Melanin deposits in cysts, 38, 109, 123
Midline sublingual dermoid cyst, 197, 251
Midpalatal raphe cysts:
  of infants, 46–50
    clinical features, 46
    origin of, 49
    pathogenesis, 47, 124
    pathology and treatment, 50
Mouth:
  floor of:
    dermoid cysts of, 196, 197
    epidermoid cyst of, 196, 197
    lympho-epithelial cyst of, 204, 206
    ranula, 221, 256
  lympho-epithelial cysts of, 204, 205, 206
Mucoceles, 212–21
  age distribution of, 212
  clinical features, 212
  clinical presentation, 214
  definitions, 212
  epithelial lining, 216
  frequency, 212
  histology, 217
  pathogenesis, 214
  pathology, 217
  racial distribution, 213
  sex distribution, 213
  site of, 214
  traumatic origin, 214, 216
  treatment, 221
Mucoepidermoid odontogenic cyst, 71–4, *see also Glandular odontogenic cyst*
Mucopapillary cysts, 219
Mucosal cyst of maxillary antrum, 187, *see also Maxillary antrum, benign mucosal cyst*
Mucous extravasation cysts, 212, 217
  treatment of, 255
Mucous gland cysts, 46
Mucous retention cysts, 212, 215, 217, 219
Myxoma, 127, 129

Naevoid basal cell carcinoma syndrome:
  blood group antigens in keratocysts, 36
  description of, 11
  relation to keratocysts, 9, 14–16
    aetiology of, 28
    epithelial islands in, 15
    multiple cysts, 11, 16
    orthokeratization in, 36
    recurrences in, 13
    satellite cysts in, 15
Nasoalveolar cyst, *see Nasolabial cyst*
Nasolabial cyst, 130–5
  age distribution, 130
  clinical features, 130
  epithelial lining, 134
  frequency of, 130
  histology, 134
  origin of, 133
  pathogenesis, 133

Nasolabial cyst (*continued*)
sex distribution, 130, 134
treatment, 250
Nasopalatine duct:
as organ of smell, 119
fetal, 119
Nasopalatine duct cyst, 111–23, 124
aetiology, 119
age distribution, 112
CT scan of, 118
clinical features, 111
clinical presentation, 113
diagnosis, 121
epithelial cell nests in, 123
epithelium, 120, 121
extension of, 124
frequency of, 111
growth of, 120
histology of, 120
hyaline cartilage in walls, 123
inflammatory origin, 119, 123
melanin and lipofuscin in, 123
nerves and blood vessels in, 121, 122, 123
pathogenesis, 118
racial distribution, 112
radiology, 115
sex distribution, 112
treatment, 123, 248
Nasopharyngeal cysts, 211
Neck:
branchial cysts of, 205
dermoid cysts of, 197, 198
keratinous cysts, 201
lympho-epithelial cysts, 201

Odontogenic ghost cell ameloblastoma, 107
Odontogenic ghost cell carcinoma, 107
Odontogenic keratocyst, *see Keratocyst*
Odontomes, 105, 106, 110
Oral alimentary tract cyst, 199, 209–10
Oral tonsils, 204
Osteoclast activating factor, 84
Osteosarcoma, 181, 182

Paget's disease of bone, 182
Pain:
causes:
bone cyst, 173
branchial cyst, 201
calcifying odontogenic cyst, 104
cyst of maxillary antrum, 189
dentigerous cyst, 80
keratocysts, 10
lateral periodontal cyst, 62
mandibular infected buccal cyst, 169
nasolabial cyst, 131
palatine duct cyst, 114
postoperative cyst of maxilla, 193
radicular cyst, 139, 140
Palate:
lympho-epithelial cyst of, 204
Palatine papilla:
cysts of, 111, 115, 121
Palatine pillar:
lympho-epithelial cyst of, 204
Paradental cyst, 136, 162–7, 170
age distribution, 166
clinical features, 166
epithelial lining, 165
frequency of, 166
inflammatory origin, 165
pathogenesis, 167
pathology and histology, 167
radiology, 164, 166
sex distribution, 166
site of, 166
treatment of, 167
Parasitic cysts, 223–6
Parotid gland,
calcifying odontogenic cyst in, 104
dysgenetic disease, 221
lympho-epithelial cyst, 202
AIDS-related, 203
polycystic (dysgenetic) disease, 221
Periapical granuloma, 129, 139
fluids in, 162
formation of, 143
treatment, 162
Pericoronitis:
in paradental cyst, 163, 164
Peripheral granuloma, 145
Peripheral odontogenic keratocyst, 10
Pigmented cells in radicular cysts, 159
Pilar cyst, of the skin, 201
Plasma lipids in radicular cysts, 157
Plasma proteins in radicular cysts, 149
Postoperative maxillary cyst, 192–5
age distribution, 192
clinical presentation, 193
frequency, 192
radiological features, 193
sex distribution, 193
site of, 193
Pre-maxillary-maxillary cysts, 126
Primordial cysts, *see Odontogenic keratocysts*
Prostaglandins:
in cyst growth and bone resorption, 84, 89, 150
Protein in cyst fluid, 18, 42, 43, 88, 148, 149, 195
Proteoglycans in cyst fluid, 18
Pulp infection:
periodontal cyst and, 63

Radicular cysts, 5, 87, 126, 128, 129, 136–62
age distribution, 136, 140
anatomical distribution of, 138
calcification in, 160
carcinomatous change in, 161
cholesterol crystals in, 157, 158
ciliated cells in, 152, 154

Radicular cysts (*continued*)
clinical features, 136
clinical presentation, 139
cyst-prone individuals, 139
cytokeratins in, 41
in deciduous teeth, 139
diagnosis, 139, 141
endodontic therapy, 162
enlargement of, 148
enucleation, 238
epithelial lining, 152, 153
carcinomatous change in, 161
formation of, 145
Langerhans cells in, 144
proliferation of, 144, 145, 151
experimental, 148, 151
factor XIIIa in, 159
frequency, 136
giant cells in, 157, 158
haemosiderin in, 157
hyaline bodies in, 154, 155, 156
immune mechanisms in, 139, 143–9
in ancient Egypt, 1
infected fluids in, 160
infection in, 139
inflammation in, 139, 140, 160
initiation of, 147
interleukin 1 in, 84
involucrin in, 159
keratinized linings, 152
keratin metaplasia and malignant change, 161
light and dark cells in, 160
lymphocytes in, 159
malignant change in, 161
marsupialized, 234
mast cells in, 39, 160
microcysts in, 147
mimicing dentigerous cysts, 82
mucous cells in, 152, 153, 154
mural nodules, 159
non-surgical treatment of, 161
pathogenesis, 142
pathology, 151
permeability of walls, 149
phases of initiation, 142
pigmented cells, 159
plasma lipids in, 157
plasma proteins in, 149
pressures within, 150
prostaglandins in, 84, 150
proteins in fluids, 148, 149
racial distribution, 138
radiology, 140
regression of, 227
residual, 140
diagnosis, 141
epithelial proliferation in, 151
marsupialization, 234
proteins in, 148
role of lymphocytes, 143
root canal fluids from, 141

Radicular cysts (*continued*)
satellite microcysts in, 160
secretory characteristics in, 152, 153
sex distribution, 138, 140
site of, 138
treatment of, 161, 227
vascular walls of, 160
Ranula, 220, 221
superficial or plunging, 221
treatment, 256
Rathke's pouch:
cysts from, 211
Reactive oncocytoid cysts, 219
Regression of cysts, 227
Residual cysts, *see under Radicular cycts*
Roundworms, 223, 226
Rushton's hyaline bodies, 154, 155, 156

Salivary glands:
cysts of, 212–22, *see also Ranula, Mucoceles, Mucous extravasation cysts and Mucous retention cysts*
ligation of ducts causing mucoceles, 214, 216
lympho-epithelial cysts of, 203
Scalp:
keratinous cyst of, 201
Sebaceous cyst, 201
Serres, glands of, 47
Sialocyst, 212
Sialo-odontogenic cyst, 71–4
Simple bone cyst, 171, *see also Solitary bone cyst*
Sjögren's syndrome, 203
Skin:
cysts of, 201
Soft tissue cysts:
developmental, 196–211
treatment, 251
see also Specific cysts and sites
Solitary bone cyst, 171
age distribution, 171
clinical presentation, 173
frequency, 171
pathogenesis, 173
pathology, 176
radiological features, 173
sex distribution, 172
site distribution, 172
treatment, 250
Stafne cavity, 177–8
Static bone cavity, 177
Steatocytoma simplex, 199
Submandibular gland:
ranula of, 256
Surgical ciliated cyst of the maxilla, *see Postoperative maxillary cyst*

Taenia spp, 223
Taenia solium, 224
Tapeworms, 223

Teeth:
aplasia of, 28
displacement:
by aneurysmal bone cysts, 180
by calcifying odontogenic cyst, 105
by dentigerous cyst, 83
by keratocysts, 26
by nasopalatine duct cyst, 118
by solitary bone cyst, 175
enamel hypoplasia, 86
eruption:
keratocysts and, 24
imapcted:
dentigerous cysts on, 79, 80
distribution of, 85
unerupted:
ameloblastoma in, 92
dentigerous cysts around, 78, 84
follicle, 81
Teeth roots:
deflected by keratocysts, 26
radicular cysts and, 239
resorption, 82, 83
by bone cyst, 180
by calcifying odontogenic cyst, 105
in palatine duct cyst, 118
in radicular cysts, 142
Teratoid cyst, 199
Thyroglossal duct cyst, 205, 207, 208
malignant change, 207
treatment of, 208
Tongue:
anterior median lingual cyst, 208
cysticercosis of, 225
intralingual cyst of foregut origin, 208
lympho-epithelial cysts of, 204
mucoceles in, 213
oral alimentary tract cyst, 209, 210
Tonsils, oral, 204
Tornwaldt's bursa, 211
Trauma:
bone cysts and, 171, 173, 174
causing mucoceles, 214, 216
Trichilemmal keratinous cyst, 201
Trichinella spiralis, 226
Trichinosis, 226

Vickers–Gorlin criteria, for ameloblastoma, 97
Vomer-nasal organ of Jacobson, 119, 123

Water-clear cells, 57, 64, 65, 66, 67
Wisdom teeth:
dentigerous cyst and, 77, 78